PEDIATRICS, CHILD AND ADOLESCENT HEALTH

PAIN MANAGEMENT YEARBOOK 2013

PEDIATRICS, CHILD AND ADOLESCENT HEALTH

JOAV MERRICK – SERIES EDITOR –
NATIONAL INSTITUTE OF CHILD HEALTH AND HUMAN DEVELOPMENT, MINISTRY OF SOCIAL AFFAIRS, JERUSALEM

Positive Youth Development: Theory, Research and Application
Daniel TL Shek, Rachel CF Sun and Joav Merrick (Editors)
2012. ISBN: 978-1-62081-305-8 (Hardcover)

Tropical Pediatrics: A Public Health Concern of International Proportions
Richard R Roach, Donald E Greydanus, Dilip R Patel, Douglas N Homnick and Joav Merrick (Editors)
2012-September.
ISBN: 978-1-61942-831-7 (Hardcover)

Positive Youth Development: A New School Curriculum to Tackle Adolescent Developmental Issues
Hing Keung Ma, Daniel TL Shek and Joav Merrick (Editors)
2012- October. ISBN: 978-1-62081-384-3 (Hardcover)

Understanding Autism Spectrum Disorder: Current Research Aspects
Ditza A Zachor and Joav Merrick (Editors)
2012- November.
ISBN: 978-1-62081-353-9 (Hardcover)

Transition from Pediatric to Adult Medical Care
David Wood, John G. Reiss, Maria E. Ferris, Linda R. Edwards and Joav Merrick (Editors)
2012- November.
ISBN: 978-1-62081-409-3 (Hardcover)

Child and Adolescent Health Yearbook 2012
Joav Merrick (Editor)
2012- November.
ISBN: 978-1-61942-788-4 (Hardcover)

Child Health and Human Development Yearbook 2011
Joav Merrick (Editor)
2012- December.
ISBN: 978-1-61942-969-7 (Hardcover)

Child and Adolescent Health Yearbook 2011
Joav Merrick (Editor)
2013- January.
ISBN: 978-1-61942-782-2 (Hardcover)

Child Health and Human Development Yearbook 2012
Joav Merrick (Editor)
2013- March. ISBN: 978-1-61942-978-9 (Hardcover)

Developmental Issues in Chinese Adolescents
Daniel TL Shek, Rachel CF Sun and Joav Merrick (Editors)
2012-September.
ISBN: 978-1-62081-262-4 (Hardcover)

Guidelines for the Healthy Integration of the Ill Child in the Educational System: Experience from Israel
Yosefa Isenberg (Author)
2013 - 3rd Quarter.
ISBN: 978-1-62808-350-7 (Hardcover)

PEDIATRICS, CHILD AND ADOLESCENT HEALTH

PAIN MANAGEMENT YEARBOOK 2013

JOAV MERRICK
EDITOR

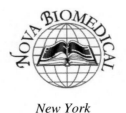

New York

NOTICE TO THE READER

The Publisher has taken reasonable care in the preparation of this book, but makes no expressed or implied warranty of any kind and assumes no responsibility for any errors or omissions. No liability is assumed for incidental or consequential damages in connection with or arising out of information contained in this book. The Publisher shall not be liable for any special, consequential, or exemplary damages resulting, in whole or in part, from the readers' use of, or reliance upon, this material. Any parts of this book based on government reports are so indicated and copyright is claimed for those parts to the extent applicable to compilations of such works.

Independent verification should be sought for any data, advice or recommendations contained in this book. In addition, no responsibility is assumed by the publisher for any injury and/or damage to persons or property arising from any methods, products, instructions, ideas or otherwise contained in this publication.

This publication is designed to provide accurate and authoritative information with regard to the subject matter covered herein. It is sold with the clear understanding that the Publisher is not engaged in rendering legal or any other professional services. If legal or any other expert assistance is required, the services of a competent person should be sought. FROM A DECLARATION OF PARTICIPANTS JOINTLY ADOPTED BY A COMMITTEE OF THE AMERICAN BAR ASSOCIATION AND A COMMITTEE OF PUBLISHERS.

Additional color graphics may be available in the e-book version of this book.

Library of Congress Cataloging-in-Publication Data

ISBN: 978-1-63117-944-0

Published by Nova Science Publishers, Inc. † New York

Contents

Contents

Introduction

Dental pain

Joav Merrick, MD, MMedSc, DMSc[1,2,3,4] *

[1]National Institute of Child Health and Human Development, Jerusalem
[2]Office of the Medical Director, Health Services, Division for Intellectual and
Developmental Disabilities, Ministry of Social Affairs and Social Services, Jerusalem,
[3]Division of Pediatrics, Hadassah Hebrew University Medical Center,
Mt Scopus Campus, Jerusalem, Israel and [4]Kentucky Children's Hospital,
University of Kentucky College of Medicine, Lexington, Kentucky,
United States of America

When a new dentist set up in a small town he quickly acquired a reputation of being the "painless" dentist. But a local kid quickly disputed this. "He's a fake!" he told his friends. "He's not painless at all. When he stuck his finger in my mouth I bit him - he just yelled like anyone else."

A toothache is a pain in or around a tooth that can be caused by tooth decay, an abscessed tooth, tooth fracture, a damaged filling, repetitive motions, such as chewing gum or grinding teeth or infected gums. Tooth pain may be sharp, throbbing or constant and in some people, pain results only when pressure is applied to the tooth. Swelling around the tooth, fever or headache and foul-tasting drainage from the infected tooth are other pain manifestations.

Oral health is very important to our everyday lives without us even being aware of the importance. If everything is functioning in our oral area we can eat, speak, smile, smell, taste, touch, chew and swallow. But many people around the world are not taking care of their teeth and the results are tooth decay and periodontal disease and resulting decrease in quality of life for that person.

* Correspondence: Professor Joav Merrick, MD, MMedSci, DMSc, Medical Director, Health Services, Division for Intellectual and Developmental Disabilities, Ministry of Social Affairs and Social Services, POBox 1260, IL-91012 Jerusalem, Israel. E-mail: jmerrick@zahav.net.il.

Many children and adults are suffering, even though we today have interventions that can prevent oral diseases and reduce dental costs. One example is water fluoridation.

Information from the CDC in Atlanta shows that tooth decay affects more than one-fourth of children in the United States aged 2–5 years and half of those aged 12-15 years. About half of all children and two-thirds of adolescents aged 12-19 years from lower-income families have had decay. Children and adolescents of some racial and ethnic groups and those from lower-income families have more untreated tooth decay, like for example, 40% of Mexican American children aged 6-8 years have untreated decay, compared with 25% of non-Hispanic whites. Among all adolescents aged 12-19 years, 20% currently have untreated decay. Advanced gum disease affects 4-12% of adults in the United States. Half of the cases of severe gum disease in the United States are the result of cigarette smoking. The prevalence of gum disease is three times higher among smokers than among people who have never smoked. One-fourth of adults in the United States aged 65 years or older have lost all of their teeth and more than 7,800 people, mostly older Americans, die from oral and pharyngeal cancers each year.

The CDC has several recommendations for maintaining a good oral health:

1. Drink fluoridated water and use a fluoride toothpaste. Fluoride's protection against tooth decay works at all ages.
2. Take care of your teeth and gums. Thorough tooth brushing and flossing to reduce dental plaque can prevent gingivitis—the mildest form of gum disease.
3. Avoid tobacco. In addition to the general health risks posed by tobacco, smokers have four times the risk of developing gum disease compared to non-smokers. Tobacco use in any form—cigarette, pipes, and smokeless (spit) tobacco—increases the risk for gum disease, oral and throat cancers, and oral fungal infection (candidiasis). Spit tobacco containing sugar increases the risk of tooth decay.
4. Limit alcohol. Heavy use of alcohol is also a risk factor for oral and throat cancers. When used alone, alcohol and tobacco are risk factors for oral cancers, but when used in combination the effects of alcohol and tobacco are even greater.
5. Eat wisely. Adults should avoid snacks full of sugars and starches. Limit the number of snacks eaten throughout the day. The recommended five-a-day helping of fiber-rich fruits and vegetables stimulates salivary flow to aid remineralization of tooth surfaces with early stages of tooth decay.
6. Visit the dentist regularly. Check-ups can detect early signs of oral health problems and can lead to treatments that will prevent further damage, and in some cases, reverse the problem. Professional tooth cleaning (prophylaxis) also is important for preventing oral problems, especially when self-care is difficult.
7. Diabetic patients should work to maintain control of their disease. This will help prevent the complications of diabetes, including an increased risk of gum disease.
8. If medications produce a dry mouth, ask your doctor if there are other drugs that can be substituted. If dry mouth cannot be avoided, drink plenty of water, chew sugarless gum, and avoid tobacco and alcohol.
9. Have an oral health check-up before beginning cancer treatment. Radiation to the head or neck and/or chemotherapy may cause problems for your teeth and gums. Treating existing oral health problems before cancer therapy may help prevent or limit oral complications or tissue damage.

A final word on patients and dental pain:

A man walks into the dentist's office and after the dentist examines him, he says, "that tooth has to come out. I'm going to give you a shot of Novocain and I'll be back in a few minutes."

The man grabs the dentist's arm, "No way. I hate needles I'm not having any shot!"

So the dentist says, "Okay, we'll have to go with the gas."

The man replies, "Absolutely not. It makes me very sick for a couple of days. I'm not having gas."

So the dentist steps out and comes back with a glass of water, "here," he says. "Take this pill."

The man asks "What is it?"

The doc replies, "Viagra."

The man looks surprised, "Will that kill the pain?" he asks.

"No," replies the dentist, "but it will give you something to hang on to while I pull your tooth!"

References

[1]   CDC. Oral health. Preventing cavities, gum disease, tooth loss and oral cancers at a glance 2011.
        URL: http://www.cdc.gov/chronicdisease/resources

SECTION ONE: PAIN AND ONCOLOGY

In: Pain Management Yearbook 2013
Editor: Joav Merrick

ISBN: 978-1-63117-944-0
© 2014 Nova Science Publishers, Inc.

Chapter 1

Pain control after total knee arthroplasty in continuous femoral nerve infusion group versus single shot group

Syed Irfan Qasim Ali, MD and David E Landry, MD*

Department of Anesthesia, Maine General Medical Center,
Waterville, Maine, United States of America

Abstract

Our study looked at post operative opioid use in patients undergoing unilateral knee arthroplasty in a community setting comparing total opioid dose in patients having single shot femoral nerve block (SFNB) to those having continuous femoral nerve block (CFNB) for post-operative pain relief. Methods: A retrospective chart review was conducted to examine post operative opioid use in patients undergoing unilateral knee arthroplasty and having either SFNB or a CFNB in addition to intravenous or oral opioids for post-operative pain control. The records were divided into two groups. Group 1 consisted of 40 patients receiving SFNB. Group 2 consisted of 42 patients receiving CFNB for 48 hours. The primary outcome for the study was total opioid usage during the first 48 hours after surgery in both groups. Results: The difference in opioid use in the first 48 hours in patients receiving a SFNB compared to those receiving a CFNB was less than 6 mg of morphine. This was not a statistically significant difference. Conclusion: In this study patients received either a SFNB or a CFNB using accepted techniques in addition to intravenous and oral opioids. Those patients receiving post operative analgesia with a CFNB following unilateral knee arthroplasty did not require less opioid than patients receiving only a SFNB pre operatively. The use of CFNB in this retrospective chart review did not result in lower opioid use.

* Correspondence: David E Landry, MD, Maine General Medical Center, 149 North Street, Waterville, Maine 04901, US. E-mail: David.landry@mainegeneral.org

Keywords: Pain, opioid, knee arthroplasty, orthopedics

Introduction

Two recent studies suggested that a continuous femoral nerve block (CFNB) provided better pain relief in the first 48 hours post-operatively than a single shot femoral nerve block (SFNB) for patients undergoing unilateral total knee arthroplasty (1). But a more recent meta-analysis (2) suggested that addition of a sciatic nerve block or CFNB to a SSFNB did not reduce morphine consumption or pain scores. Since there is wide institutional variability in local anesthetic choice and concentration, catheter type, and insertion techniques for CFNB not all techniques may yield similar results.

Studies of patients undergoing unilateral total knee arthroplasty which evaluate the quality and outcomes of analgesia provided by either CFNB or SFNB have involved low number of patients in tertiary centers. Only one randomized controlled trial directly compared these two approaches (1). In that study it was demonstrated that patients receiving a CFNB had lower pain scores and lower post operative opioid use than patients receiving a SFNB. A second study Kadic (3) found patients receiving a CFNB also had less pain and lower opioid use in first 48 hours postoperatively. Whether the results of these studies would translate into improved pain control in a less controlled setting is unproven. A retrospective chart review study was designed and conducted of patients undergoing unilateral total knee arthroplasty at one 120 bed community hospital in central Maine

Methods

After local IRB approval of the study, patient records were selected randomly from a list of 425 people who had undergone unilateral total knee arthroplasty between June 2005 and June 2007. Patients were divided into two groups. Group 1 consisted of 40 patients receiving a SFNB. Group 2 consisted of 42 patients receiving a CFNB. The choice of anesthesia for surgery was at the discretion of the anesthesiologist with the preference being spinal anesthesia. The anesthesiology department has five anesthesiologists with an average duration of practice of 18.5 years and significant regional anesthesia experience.

No attempt was made to randomize patient selection by attending anesthesiologist. Records from 110 patients were randomly selected for the study and initially reviewed for inclusion. Potential exclusion criteria included incomplete postoperative opioid data, lack of data to confirm successful catheter placement, inability to obtain stimulation of the mid-portion of the quadriceps with a current of 0.5mA or less, or removal of the femoral nerve catheter prior to 48 hours post operatively. All of the patients were enrolled in the institutional knee arthroplasty pathway and admitted to the same orthopedic floor. All patients had pain assessment every 4 hours using a numeric pain intensity 0-10 scale (0=no pain, 10=worst pain) and were encouraged to request opioid medication if the pain score was greater than or equal to 4/10 and there was no observed somnolence. By protocol morphine 2 mg IV Q 2 hours PRN or hydromorphone 0.5mg Q 2 hours PRN were used initially for pain control. When the patients were able to take fluids, oxycodone 5-10 mg Q 4 hours was utilized. All patients received preoperative education regarding methods of post-operative pain control and the institution's pain scale.

Single shot femoral nerve block

Forty patients received a SFNB by one of three techniques chosen by the attending anesthesiologist. The position and placement of needle tip was confirmed by using either ultrasound alone (n=1), ultrasound combined with femoral nerve stimulation (n=11) or femoral nerve stimulation alone (n=28).

Femoral nerve stimulation was done utilizing a Braun Medical Stimuplex variable output nerve stimulator and a 21 gauge Braun Stimuplex insulated needle. After sterile prep and drape the skin 1cm lateral to the femoral pulsation and slightly below the inguinal skin crease was infiltrated with local anesthetic and the stimulating needle advanced to obtain contraction of the mid portion of the quadriceps with a current of 0.5mA or less.

The average current to obtain a quadriceps muscle twitch was 0.33mA with a range from 0.1mA-0.5mA. Blocks in the combined ultrasound nerve stimulation group were placed as previously described and relied on quadricep stimulation as an end point. All thirty-nine patients had nerve stimulation evidenced by muscle twitch at 0.5mA or less.

The ultrasound only nerve block was performed utilizing a Sonosite Titan ultrasound and a Braun 21 gauge Stimuplex needle using similar insertion technique as previously described. Direct visualization of the needle tip was attempted followed by visualization of local anesthetic flow around the femoral nerve.

Table 1.

Single Shot Femoral Nerve Block Group		
Methods To Insert FN Catheter		
US (Ultra sound) Only	US with Nerve Stimulation	Nerve Stimulation Only
1	11	28
Total = 40		

Table 2.

Single Shot Femoral Nerve Block Group	
Current in mA to obtain a quadriceps muscle twitch	
The range of current in mA (Milli Amps)	0.1mA - 0.5mA
The average current in mA to achieve quadriceps muscle twitch	0.33mA
Number of patients with quadriceps muscle twitch at 0.5mA or less	39
Number of patients with quadriceps muscle twitch at > 0.5mA	None
mA	N=2
0.2 mA	N=4
0.3 mA	N=15
0.35 mA	N=2
0.4 mA	N=12
0.5 mA	N=4

Local anesthetics

Either ropivacaine or bupivacaine, were used in the SFNB group at the discretion of the anesthesiologist. Ropivacaine was used in 28 patients. The average concentration of ropivacaine used in these patients was 0.33% with the range of concentration from 0.2% - 0.5%.

The average volume of ropivacaine used was 30.5cc and the range of volume was from 20-40cc. Bupivacaine was used in 12 patients.

The average concentration used was 0.30%.The range of concentration was 0.25%-0.5%.The average volume of bupivacaine was 30.25cc with the range of volume from 25-40cc.

Table 3.

Anesthetic Agent Used in SFNB Group					
Medicine Used	Number of Patients	Range of Concentration	Average Concentration	Range of Volume	Average Volume
Ropivacaine	28	0.2%-0.5%	0.33%	20-40cc	30.5cc
Bupivacaine	12	0.25%-0.5%	0.30%	25-40cc	30.25cc

Continuous femoral nerve block

Forty two patients received a CFNB by one of three techniques chosen by the attending anesthesiologist including ultrasound only, ultrasound with nerve stimulation, or nerve stimulation only. The position and placement of the catheter was confirmed by using either ultrasound alone (n=2), ultrasound combined with femoral nerve stimulation (n=33) or femoral nerve stimulation alone (n=7)

In all cases a Braun polyamide closed tip epidural catheter was utilized and was advanced 3-5cm beyond the needle tip. Nerve stimulation was done using the previously mentioned technique except that a Braun Medical 18 gauge insulated Touhy needle with integrated wire was utilized. Attempts were made to obtain stimulation of the mid-portion of the quadriceps with a current of 0.5mA or less. The average stimulating current was 0.46mA.The range was from 0.2mA -1mA. Thirty seven patients had nerve stimulation evidenced by quadriceps muscle twitch at 0.5mA or less. Three patients had nerve stimulation at > 0.5mA. These three patients had confirmation of catheter placement with ultrasound as well. These three patients had good evidence of local anesthetic flow around the femoral nerve. Ultrasound guided nerve blocks were performed in the previously mentioned manner except that a Braun Medical 18 gauge insulated Touhy needle was utilized (4-8).

Table 4.

Continuous Femoral Nerve Block Group		
Methods To Insert FN Catheter		
US (Ultra sound) Only	US with Nerve Stimulation	Nerve Stimulation Only
4	31	7
Total = 42		

Table 5.

Continuous Femoral Nerve Block Group	
Current in mA to obtain a quadriceps muscle twitch	
The range of current (note change)	0.2mA - 1mA
The average current to achieve quadriceps muscle twitch (note change)	0.46mA

Number of patients with quadriceps muscle twitch at 0.5mA or less	35
Number of patients with quadriceps muscle twitch at > 0.5mA	3 (All three had confirmation with US as well)
mA	N=1
0.3 mA	N=1
0.4 mA	N=18
0.45 mA	N=1
0.48 mA	N=1
0.5mA	N=13
0.6 mA	N=2
1 mA	N=1

Table 6.

Anesthetic Agent Used in CFNB Group					
Medicine Used	Number of Patients	Range of Concentration	Average Concentration	Range of Volume	Average Volume
Ropivacaine	42	0.2-0.5%	0.37%	20-40cc	29.57cc.

Local anesthetic

All 42 CFNB patients received ropivacaine as local anesthetic agent during catheter placement. The average concentration of ropivacaine used was 0.37%. Range of concentration was 0.2%-0.5%. The initial average volume was 29.57cc, and the range for initial anesthetic volume was 20-40cc. In all 42 patients the CFNB was continued for 48 hours postoperatively and the patients were evaluated daily by member of the anesthesia team for analgesia adequacy and signs of complications and muscle weakness.

Continuous infusion management

Prior to discharge from the recovery room the femoral catheter was connected to an infusion pump. All patients received a continuous infusion of 0.2% ropivacaine starting at 6ml/hr. Through Anesthesia Department protocol the orthopedic floor nursing staff could incrementally increase the infusion up to a maximum of 10ml/hr for patient's complaint of pain greater than or equal to 4 out of 10 on a numeric pain scale.

Measures

The types and quantities of local anesthetics were extracted for each group. Similarly, data for opioid use was also extracted. The period of opioid usage was from the time the patient left the recovery room until 48 hours post surgery. All opioid medications used during this 48 hour period by any route (oral, intramuscular or intravenous) were extracted. All opioids were converted to intravenous morphine equivalent and summed for each patient. These conversions were done using the C-tools 2.0 drug conversion calculator. The conversions were verified and rechecked by hospital pharmacists. Patients' demographics were also recorded.

Analyses

Based on results from the Salinas, et al., a difference of more than 10mg of morphine equivalent over the 48 hour post-operative period would be considered clinically significant. A sample size power calculation was performed assuming 30 versus 40 morphine equivalents, a standard deviation of 15, $p < 0.05$, with a power of 0.80, which resulted in a requirement of 36 or more patients in each group. A t-test was used to calculate the mean difference in morphine equivalent use between groups.

Results

Initially 110 records were selected in the study, but 28 records were excluded. Reasons for exclusion included incomplete postoperative narcotic usage data (n=7), unavailability of data to confirm the successful catheter placement (n=8), inability to obtain stimulation of the mid-portion of the quadriceps with a current of 0.5mA or less (n=5), or because the catheter was removed before 48 hours (n=8). A total of 18 patients were excluded from CFNB group.

A total of 10 patients were excluded from SFNB group. This resulted in two groups, a SFNB group of 40 patients and CFNB group of 42 patients. There were no observed complications from therapy in either group.

Group demographics

The two study groups were very similar. Of the 40 SFNB patients, 27 (67.5%) were females and 13 (32.5%) were males, compared to 42 CFNB patients of which 30 (71%) were females and 12 (29%) were males. The average age of SFNB females was 70.4 years with the age range from 55-84 years. The average age of SFNB males was 71.1 years with the age range from 56-86 years. This compared to the average age of CFNB females of 68.47 years of age with a range of age 49-84 years. The average age of CFNB males was 72.58 years with a range of 61-83 years. For SFNB, 27 (68%) patients received spinal anesthesia and 13 (32%) general anesthesia. In the CNFB group, 25 (60%) patients received spinal anesthesia and 17 (40%) general anesthesia. None of the differences were statistically significant.

Table 7.

Study Demographics							
Group	Patients	SEX M F		Mean Age Yrs M F		Anesthesia Spinal Gen	
SFNB	40	13(32.5%)	27 (67.5%)	71.1	70.4	27 (68%)	13 (32%)
CFNB	42	12 (29%)	30 (71%)	72.5	68.4	25 (60%)	17 (40%)

Table 8.

Opioid Used as Intravenous Morphine Equivalent			
Group	Patients	Mean Opioid /Patient	Total Group Use
SFNB	40	45.99	1839.6
CFNB	42	40.82	1714.50

Opioid usage

Comparing post-operative opioid use in the SFNB group to the CFNB group it was determined that the opioid use between the two groups was similar. Patients in the SFNB group received a mean of 45.99mg of morphine equivalent per patient (sd=21.4).Patients in the CFNB group received a mean of 40.82.mg of morphine equivalent per patient (s.d.23.11).This study noted a 5.17mg morphine equivalent difference in opioid use between the SFNB group and CFNB group. The value was less than the calculated 10mg difference between groups needed to be statistically significant. The result of the group mean difference t-test was t = 1.04, 80 df (degree of freedom), two tailed p= .307 which is not statistically significant.

Discussion

The use of single shot peripheral nerve blocks to provide postoperative pain relief is well recognized (9). It is a relatively recent practice to place peripheral nerve catheters in an attempt to provide better or longer lasting analgesia in the post-operative period (1,3) and it can result in lowered pain scores and reduced opioid use in first 48 hours post operatively. Here in a community hospital in a retrospective study we did not find similar results despite utilizing similar techniques. Since placing peripheral nerve catheters are more time intensive, utilize more equipment and potentially expose the patient to a heightened risk of infection (4) and possibly more falls 10, careful refinement of technique may be needed to see any significant reduction in opioid utilization. Technical limitations of this study include the fact that several different techniques were used to place both the SFNB's and the CFNB's, but this is the nature of private practice. Additionally no comparison of pain scores between groups were undertaken .While both groups of patients had blocks placed by experienced anesthesiologist using accepted techniques there was no assessment of block success such as a decrease in sensory function in the femoral nerve distribution in the early post-operative period. This might have provided valuable information in this study. In this study reduced opioid use may not be an accurate reflection of improved pain levels as ongoing pain scores were not assessed by this study and secondly differences in nursing assessment that the anesthesiologists were not aware of may have impacted opioid use between study groups. If indeed the results of this study are valid it may be more difficult to obtain decreased opioid use and by inference reduced pain scores than one would imply from reading the well done studies by Salinas (1) and Kadic (3).

The continued practice in this community setting is to preferentially place CFNB's with the technique being heartily endorsed by the institution's orthopedic surgeons and patients having second knee arthroplasty who had a CFNB for the first surgery.

Acknowledgment

The authors would like to thank Daniel Meyer MPH for the assistance with statistics. Additionally thanks are extended to Michael Bushey M.D., Chief Dept. of Anesthesia at Maine General Medical Center and Dr James Gagnon at Maine Medical Center for their thoughtful review of the paper. Contributions: Dr David Landry designed the original study and guided in data collection and also did extensive editing of manuscript. Dr Syed Ali did all data collection and tables and wrote the initial manuscript and wrote the drafts again based on suggestions from Dr Landry. Financial Support: None. Conflict of Interest: None. Implications statement: In our retrospective chart review the efficacy of post-operative analgesia provided by continuous femoral nerve block was compared to that provided by a single shot femoral nerve block in patients undergoing unilateral knee arthroplasty. No significant difference in total opioid dose was noted between the two groups during the first 48 hours post- surgery.

References

[1]   Salinas FV, Liu SS, Mulroy MF. The effect of single-injection femoral nerve block versus continuous femoral nerve block after total knee arthroplasty on hospital length of stay and long-term functional recovery within an established clinical pathway. Anesth Analg 2006;102(4):1234-9.

[2]   Paul A. Femoral nerve block improves analgesia outcomes after total arthroplasty. Anesthesiology 2010;113:1014-5.

[3]   Kadic L, Boonstra MC, De Wall Malefijt MC, Lako SJ, Van Egmond J, Driessen JJ. Continuous femoral nerve block after total knee arthroplasty. Acta Anaesthesiol Scand 2009;53(7):914-20.

[4]   Capdevila X, Bringuier S, Borgeat A. Infectious risk of continuous peripheral nerve blocks. Am Soc Anesthesiol 2009;110(1):182-8.

[5]   Beaudoin FL, Nagdev A. Ultrasound guided femoral nerve blocks in elderly patients with hip fractures. Am J Emerg Med 2010;28(1):76-81.

[6]   Osaka Y, Kashiwagi M. Ultrasound guided combined femoral-obturator nerve block for the knee arthroscopic surgery of meniscal lesion. Masui 2010;59(8):1042-4.

[7]   Hotta K, Sata N, Suzuki H. Ultrasound guided combined femoral nerve and lateral femoral cutaneous nerve blocks for femur neck fracture surgery. Masui 2008;57(7):892-4.

[8]   Ito H, Shibata Y. Ultrasound guided femoral nerve block. Masui 2008; 57(5):575-9.

[9]   Szczukowski MJ, Hines JA, Snell JA, Sisca TS. Femoral nerve block for total knee arthroplasty patients: A method to control postoperative pain. J Arthroplasty 2004;19(6):720-5.

[10]   Ilfeld BM, Duke KB, Donohue MC. The association between lower extremity continuous peripheral nerve blocks and patients falls after knee and hip replacement. Anesth Analg 2010;111(6):1552-4.

[11]   Reeves M, Skinner MW. Continuous intraarticular infusion of ropivacaine after unilateral total knee arthroplasty. Anaesth Intensive Care 2009;37(6):918-22.

[12]   Bunburaphong P, Niruthisard S, Werawatganon T, Keeyapaj W, Vimuktanandana A, Toleb K. Postoperative analgesia for total knee replacement: Comparing between pre and post operative "3-in-1" femoral nerve block. J Med Assoc Thai 2006;89(4):462-7.

[13]   Capdevila X, Barthelet Y, Biboulet P, Ryckwaert Y, Rubenovitch J, d'Athis F. Effects of perioperative analgesic technique on the surgical outcome and duration of rehabilitation after major knee surgery. Anesthesiology 1999;91:8-15.

[14]   Singelyn FJ, Deyaert M, Joris D, Pendeville E, Gouverneur JM. Effects of intravenous patient controlled analgesia with morphine, continuous epidural analgesia, and continuous three in one block on post operative pain and knee rehabilitation after total knee arthroplasty. Anesth Analg 1998:87:88-92.

[15]   Seet E, Leong EL, Yeo AS, Fook-Chong S. Effectiveness of 3-in-1 continuous femoral nerve block of differing concentrations compared to patient controlled intravenous morphine for post total knee arthroplasty analgesia and knee rehabilitation. Anesth Intensive Care 2006;34:25-30.

[16]   Chelly JE, Ben-David B. Do continuous femoral nerve blocks affect the hospital length of stay and functional outcome. Anesth Analg 2007;104:996-7.

[17]   Navas AM, Gutierrez TV, Moreno ME. Continuous peripheral nerve blockade in lower extremity surgery. Acta Anaesthesiol Scand 2005; 49:1048-55.

In: Pain Management Yearbook 2013
Editor: Joav Merrick

ISBN: 978-1-63117-944-0
© 2014 Nova Science Publishers, Inc.

Chapter 2

Comparing the non-communicating adult pain checklist (NCAPC) with the pain and discomfort scale (PADS) in evaluating pain in adults with intellectual disability

Meir Lotan, MScPT, PhD, Archi Benishvily, BPT
and Elad Gefen, BPT*
School of Health Sciences, Department of Physical Therapy,
Ariel University Center of Samaria, Ariel and Army Medical Services, Zrifin, Israel

Abstract

Pain is a difficult phenomenon to measure especially in individuals with intellectual and developmental disabilities (IDD), thereby compromising pain management for this population. Despite that fact, measures that evaluate pain in adults with IDD are scarce. Recently two scales have been constructed to evaluate pain behaviors in adults with IDD, the Non-Communicating Adult's Pain Checklist (NCAPC) and the Pain and Discomfort Scale (PADS). Aim: The aim of the present article was to compare the NCAPC and PADS in evaluating procedural pain in adults with IDD, in regards to reliability, sensitivity, clinical usability and internal consistency. Procedure: 52 vignettes were randomly picked out of a pull of videos of 228 individuals recorded during annual flew vaccination. Two observers separately scored pain behaviors using the PADS and the NCAPC. Results: Both scales showed high interrater reliability (PADS $ICC_{1,3} = 0.86$-0.87, NCAPC $ICC_{1,3} = 0.81$-0.84), Sensitivity to pain behaviors in adults with IDD (SRM PADS = 0.52, SRM NCAPC = 0.57), high correlation among the scales ($r1 = 0.9$, $r2 = 0.95$), and high internal consistency (PADS $\alpha = 0.74$-0.78, NCAPC $\alpha = 0.78$-0.85).

* Correspondence: Meir Lotan, BPT, MScPT, PhD, Rehov Rothchild 67, IL-44201 Kfar-Saba, Israel. E-mail: ml_pt_rs@netvision.net.il

Discussion: Most findings are favorable for the NCAPC accept for interrater reliability. These results are probably due to the fact this scale was constructed from this group of client's pain reactions. The fact that both scales show very similar outcomes validate both scales as appropriate for measuring pain in adults with IDD. The fact that two inexperienced observers were able to use both scales and come up with such good psychometric results, support the clinical usability of both scales, hopefully contributing to better pain management in this population.

Keywords: Pain, scale, pain behavior, intellectual and developmental disability

Introduction

The prevalence of pain in the people with intellectual and developmental disability (IDD) is unclear, mainly due to communication problems that makes the recognition of pain difficult (1). People with IDD are vulnerable to the same range of pain-inflicting procedures as the non-IDD adult population, but in addition they are also vulnerable to experiencing pain from falls, leg braces, and ill-fitting wheelchairs (2). A study investigating the frequency, duration, intensity, and location of pain, as well as the interference of pain with activities, in adults with cerebral palsy (CP) and IDD, found that pain was a significant problem for the majority of participants (3). Of the 93 participants (with an average age of 38 years), the majority had quadriplegia (84%) and were non-ambulatory (94%). One or more areas of chronic pain (minimum of three months' duration) were reported by 67% of the participants, and 53% experienced moderate to severe pain on an almost daily basis. Lower-extremity pain (66%) and back pain (63%) were the most common complaints. The duration of pain ranged from a mean of 7.5 years for upper-extremity pain to a mean of 20 years for hip or buttock pain. Likewise, McGrath et al. (4) investigated the pain experience of 64 children with IDD and found that they suffered pain on a regular basis, with 83% suffering constant pain at a level higher than 3 on a 10-point scale.

Thus, the accumulating evidence suggests that individuals with IDD suffer from more pain incidents than the general population and can be considered as a population at risk in regards to pain. However, it is clear that better pain management should start with proper pain evaluation and that it is essential for the clinician to use reliable evaluation tools to initiate the pain assessment and intervention processes.

Assessing pain in individuals with IDD is a challenging task and can become extremely difficult at the levels of severe and profound IDD, when the ability to verbally communicate pain experience is severely compromised (5). Without objective assessment, pain can be misinterpreted or underestimated, which might lead to inadequate management and undermine quality of life (6).

Very few studies on pain in individuals with IDD have been published. Available findings suggest that pain in people with severe intellectual disability is common, yet rarely actively treated (7). Studies in this field also indicate that people with IDD have 2.5 times more health problems than people without IDD (8). Individuals with severe or profound levels of IDD are more likely to have additional disabling conditions or multiple complex medical problems coupled with communication difficulties. Such medical problems, whether directly or indirectly linked to the disability, often necessitate painful procedures, including physical therapy treatments and various medical interventions. Recent data reveals that "sick days" in this population were associated with higher levels of pain and discomfort than "well days" (9) and that people with severe cognitive impairments and low communication abilities are likely to experience the most pain over time (10).

Despite the increased research attention focused on expressive behavior related to pain in individuals with IDD (11-14), research on this topic is still scarce and there are but few pain assessment scales available for use in this specific population.

When reviewing pain assessment scales for individuals with IDD we find that they mostly target the pediatric population. One scale was developed for the general population, but has been used for individuals with IDD in the past. The following scales are ordered chronologically.

1) *The Facial Action Coding System (FACS;* 15): The FACS is a list of facial actions (action units – AUs) based on movements of specific muscles or groups of muscles in the face. FACS was repeatedly found to be highly reliable by Craig and associates (16, 17). This scale has been was found suitable for detecting pain behaviors in individuals with mild to moderate levels of IDD undergoing influenza injection (5).

2) *The Evaluation Scale for Pain in Cerebral Palsy (ESPCP;* (18): The ESPCP consists of 22 items of pain behaviors derived from physicians' reports of cues considered to be indicative of pain during medical examination. The items included various facial expressions: crying, movements and posture (increase in muscular tone and/or involuntary movements, analgesic postures); protective reactions (movement towards painful areas), and social behaviors (e.g., reduced interest in surroundings). Although there appears to be a common set of pain behaviors in people with cerebral palsy and severe intellectual disabilities, the importance of the different items in determining pain is dependent on the individual's level of development.

Using the ESPCP, Collignon et al. (19) developed a 10-item observational scale to evaluate pain and facilitate therapeutic decision-making in children with severe handicaps and adults with cerebral palsy. Collignon and Giusiano (20) then further developed the tool to better fit an adolescent population with IDD. These researchers investigated pain behaviors in 100 individuals, ranging in age from 2 to 33 years (mean 16 years), with multiple physical disabilities and profound IDD and without speech or any means of communication ability through symbols. Pain could only be detected by observing global behavioral changes, rather than by the presence of a single sign. In addition, each combination of disabilities appeared to evoke a specific set of behaviors. For instance, behaviors associated with the voluntary protection of painful areas were more likely to occur in individuals with a lesser degree of motor impairment. This tool was not further investigated for psychometric properties.

3) *The Non-Communicating Children's Pain Checklist (NCCPC;* (21): The collection of pain items for this scale was initiated by McGrath and associates (22). This group of researchers interviewed twenty parents or caregivers of cognitively impaired children, ranging in age from 6 to 29 years, regarding cues they considered to be indicative of pain in their children. The interviews included instances of short, sharp pain, such as needle pain, as well as longer-lasting pain, such as headache or injury. A list of 31 cues was elicited. While specific behaviors often differed from one child to another, classes of behaviors (vocal, eating/sleeping, social/personality, facial expressions, body and limbs activity, and physiological reactions) were common to almost all children.

The NCCPC was developed from this initial study (21). It was comprised of 30 items and was to be tested in a home setting. Parents and caregivers assessed whether the pain cues were 'present' or 'absent' in four situations: acute pain, long-term pain, a non-painful but distressing situation, and a non-painful, calm situation. On the average, more than four times as many pain cues were present in painful situations than in calm (no-pain) situations. The total number of present cues did not differ between painful and distressed states, but scores for the 'eating/sleeping' and 'body/limb' subscales were higher during acute pain than during distress.

A second version of the NCCPC checklist, the NCCPC-PV (PV = Postoperative Version), was evaluated in a postoperative setting (23). In this study, items related to eating and sleeping were omitted and each of the remaining items was scored on a four-point ordinal scale according to frequency of occurrence. Twenty-four children, ranging in age from 3 to 19 years, were each observed by one of their caregivers and one of the researchers for 10 minutes both before and after surgery. When available, nurses also provided their assessments. Each observer completed the NCCPC-PV independently in addition to giving a global rating of the intensity of the child's pain using a Visual Analogue Scale. The NCCPC-PV was found to show very high internal consistency (Cronbach's alpha=0.91) and good interrater reliability (ICC 0.78 to 0.82). A moderate correlation (from 0.39 to 0.53) was observed preoperatively between scores on the NCCPC-PV and global assessments of the child's pain through the VAS. A score of 11 on the NCCPC-PV provided 0.88% sensitivity and 0.81% specificity for classifying children who were rated at a moderate-severe level of pain on a verbal rating scale (VRS).

A third revised version of this scale, the NCCPC-R (R= revised), used ordinal ratings according to frequency of occurrence as above, but this time included the items related to eating and sleeping. This version was evaluated in home settings (24). Using the NCCPC-R, 55 caregivers of 71 children with severe cognitive impairments, ranging in age from 3 to 18 years, conducted observations of their children during a time of pain and a time without pain. The NCCPC-R was found to have high internal consistency (Cronbach's alpha=0.93), as well as a moderate correlation with the pain intensity ratings provided by caregivers (Pearson's r=0.46).

Sensitivity (0.84) and specificity (0.77) for pain were optimized at a cut-off point of 7 out of a possible total score of 90.

4) *The Pain Indicator for Communicatively Impaired Children* (*PICIC*; (25): The PICIC uses six core items to assess the expression of chronic pain in non-communicative children with significant IDD. A significant relationship was demonstrated between five of the six core items and the presence and severity of pain (25). However, further research is needed before the PICIC can be established as a tool holding proper psychometric values.

5) *The Pediatric Pain Profile* (*PPP*; 26): The PPP is a 20-item behavior rating scale designed to assess pain in children with severe neurological and cognitive disability. The validity and reliability of the scale was assessed in 140 children, ranging in age from 1 to 18 years, who were unable to communicate through speech or augmentative communication. Parents used the PPP to retrospectively rate their child's behavior when 'at their best' and when in pain. Children were found to display significantly higher scores when in pain than in a non-pain situation, and their scores increased in line with global evaluations of pain.

In order to assess interrater reliability, two raters concurrently observed and individually rated each child's behavior. Interrater reliability by ICC values was found to range between

0.74 and 0.89. In order to assess the construct validity and responsiveness of the scale, the behavior of 41 children was rated before and four hours after the administration of an analgesic. The PPP scores were found to be significantly higher before than after analgesic administration ($p< 0.001$). As part of this process, the behavior of 30 children was rated before and five days after surgery. Internal consistency ranged from 0.75 to 0.89 (Cronbach's alpha), and sensitivity (1.00) and specificity (0.91) were optimized at a cut-off point of 14 on a 60-point scale. Although there was no significant difference between the mean preoperative and postoperative scores, the highest PPP score occurred in the first 24 hours after surgery in 14 (47%) children. Yet, the authors claim that the PPP should be considered as reliable and valid and suggest that it has potential for both clinical and research purposes.

Despite such claims, it seems that more rigorous psychometric properties need to be established for the PPP and that further research is required in order to evaluate the acceptability, feasibility, and usefulness of the PPP as a tool in clinical settings for children with severe to profound neurological and cognitive disabilities. Further validation as an evaluative tool is also required. Finally, it has yet to be determined whether the PPP is also useful for pain assessment in adults with similar degrees of disability (26).

There are only two scales developed for adults with IDD to date, the PADS and the NCAPC, and both are based on the Non-Communicating children's pain checklist (NCCPC).

1) *The Pain and Discomfort Scale (PADS*; (27): This scale is based on previous research on facial expressions and body movements as indicators of acute pain and discomfort in children (24). The PADS was developed to assess pain in individuals without capacity to convert internal experiences into expressed language. This scale was also designed to aid health care professionals in recognizing, diagnosing, and more effectively treating pain in patients with severe and profound communication difficulties.

Bodfish et al. (27) conducted three validation studies on PADS. In the first study, 22 adults with severe and profound IDD were assessed with the PADS before and during acute medical procedures known to produce pain and discomfort (i.e., a gastronomy-tube insertion or a toenail removal). The total scores increased significantly during the medical procedures ($p<0.01$) as compared to the baseline, and the PADS was interpreted by the authors as being sensitive to pain and discomfort in this population (27). In the second study, the scores in a group of patients with painful chronic medical conditions and physical disabilities were significantly higher ($p<0.01$) than in patients with severe and profound levels of IDD alone (Bodfish et al., 2001). In the last study, eight adults with a profound level of IDD as well as other medical conditions were assessed with the PADS both before and after pain treatment. In all cases, there was a significant reduction in the score from baseline to treatment, which the authors interpreted as indicative of treatment effects and reduced pain (27).

The work of Bodfish et al. (27) was later used to detect pain and discomfort during a dental scaling procedure. Twenty-eight subjects with cognitive and communication deficits were assessed at multiple baselines as well as during and after the procedure. Reliability was found to be between 93.6%–99.7%. The results indicated that scores on the PADS were significantly higher during the procedure than during all other non-pain situations quantified by the PADS. An optimal cut-off point for sensitivity and specificity (28) has not yet been demonstrated for the PADS (29). However, the accumulating evidence suggests that the PADS is a sensitive measure of pain in adults with IDD (27, 29).

2). *The Non-Communicating Adults Pain Checklist (NCAPC;30-32)*- The NCCPC was created for children with IDD (21, 23, 24) Yet, advanced age, previous pain experiences and potentially reduced health state may necessitate specific adaptation of the pediatric scale in adults with the same diagnosis (27). The later assumption was confirmed during our initial investigation (33), as we found behaviors that were present in the NCCPC-R that did not appear in the adult population and pain behaviors that were commonly observed in adults, but not captured by the NCCPC-R. Therefore, an item by item investigation was performed on the 27 items of the NCCPC-R, observing pain behaviors of 228 adults with IDD. A new scale was than constructed, termed the Non-Communicating Adult's Pain Checklist (NCAPC), which evaluates the pain experience of adults with IDD. The scale is divided into six subscales: Vocal expression, emotional reaction, facial expression, body language, protective reactions, and physiological signs, and contains 18 items, each rated on an ordinal 4-point scale (0-3), the total score ranging from 0 (no pain behavior observed) to 54 (maximum expression of pain behaviors). The new NCAPC scale with the same number of sub-categories, yet with fewer items than the NCCPC-R, was found to hold promising psychometric properties such as: high internal consistency (Alpha =0.77), sensitivity of each item to pain behaviors ($p<0.05$) as well as high sensitivity to register pain behaviors of adults at all levels of IDD (SRM=2.05) (31), very high intra- and inter-rater reliability (ICC= 0.94-0.91 correspondingly) (32), as well as sensitivity to distinguish between pain and non-pain situations, and between different pain situations and pain experiences (30).

Present study

The study aimed to compare the sensitivity, reliability and clinical usability of two pain evaluation scales for adults with IDD.

Research population

The present research population included video vignettes of 52 adults at variable genders, age, level of intellectual disability and mobility and functional level (see table 1).

Table 1. Demographic data of participants

Level of IDD	# of participants	Age range	AA (SD)	WC (%)	PA	Gender (Males)
Mild	4	40-72	57 (±11.44.)	0 (0%)	4 (100%)	3 (75%)
Moderate	24	21-70	45(±13.48)	5 (21%)	19 (79%)	15 (62%)
Sever	15	16-64	37 (±12.74)	2 (13%)	13 (87%)	10 (67%)
Profound	9	19-52	37 (±16.76)	5 (55%)	4 (45%)	5 (55%)
All participants	52	19-72	42 (±13.74)	12(23%)	40 (67%)	33 (63%)
	AA= Average age		WC= wheelchair users		PA= pedal ambulation	

These videos were extracts from a group of participants who were part of a larger cohort of 228 individuals living in several residential settings and their videos were used to construct the NCAPC (31, 33). All videos were numbered from 1-228, and the numbers were pulled out of a close container (each number was retrieved to the closed container before the next pull).

Inclusion criteria

1   Adults with IDD
2   Participated in previous research project
3   Had clear pain reaction on videotaping samples
4   Had their number drawn through a random shuffle

Exclusion criteria

Individuals whose numbers were not pulled through the random shuffle

The scales

The PADS and the NCAPC, two scales that were originally built for adults with IDD.
Similarities between the two scales:

1   Designated and created for adults
2   Originated from the NCCPC
3   Contain 18 items
4   Similar sub-sections
5   Hold good psychometric properties (sensitivity, reliability, Validity)

Differences between the two scales:

1   There is less emphasis on protective reactions in the PADS
2   The PADS was evaluated on small number of participants, while the NCAPC was tested and constructed based on observation of pain behaviors of over 200 participants.
3   The PADS was evaluated in a variety of pain situations (procedural, chronic, with and without pain reduction medication), while the NCACP was used in two setting of procedural pain (vaccination and a dental clinic).

Research hypothesis

It is expected that the NCAPC and the PADS will achieve closely related outcomes, it might be possible that the NCAPC will achieve slightly better outcomes in regards to the PADS due to the following fact:

1   The NCACP was constructed on video vignettes of the same pain stimulus (an injection) and based on that same population
2   The PADS was constructed using manual manipulation of adults with IDD, and therefore the participants have less free body movements in comparison to the NCAPC

Research procedure

After the random number pulling two observers watched the different videos describing participants during yearly mandatory (by the ministry of health) flew vaccination.

Each observer independently evaluated pain reaction of participants by the two pain evaluation scales. In each viewing the order of the scales was reversed (if for participant one, observer 1 used the PADS as his first scale, than he used the NCAPC as the first scale for the next viewing). The order of scales will be different for both observers (when observer 1 will start with the NCAPC observer 2 will start for the same viewing with the PADS).

Statistical procedures

The results of the observers will undergo 5 statistical procedures:

1   Interrater reliability - In order to evaluate the stability of scores between different raters (interrater reliability), ICC(1,1) was used. ICC(1,1) is based on one-way analysis of variance, in which all variation between occasions is regarded as measurement error (34). In a slightly different model ICC(3,1), using the "two-way random mixed consistency" model, the effect of any systematic shift in data is not considered part of the error of measurement (34, 35). There is no consensus of how to judge ranges of correlation coefficients, yet Currier (36) have suggested that ICCs in the range of 0.60-0.79 might be considered as moderate reliability, while ICCs in the range of 0.80-0.89 are considered as high reliability.

2   Pearson correlation was used to assess correlation between the scores of the different scales used by a single observer (37).

3   Sensitivity to change of the scales - Sensitivity to change of the total of each scale was examined by calculating the Standardized Response Mean (SRM), dividing the score of each participant by the standard deviation of the total change scores (38). Benchmarks of change have been proposed by Cohen (39), suggesting an effect size of ≥ 0.8 to be large.

4   Internal consistency - internal consistency for the different items on each scale was performed using Cronbach's Alpha. The suggested values for α for this test are in the range of 0.9-0.7 (39).

Results

Interrater reliability

Interrater reliability for both scales was found high:
PADS: (0.86)ICC (1,1) ; (0.87)ICC (3,1).
NCAPC: (0.81)ICC (1,1); (0.84)ICC (3,1). (see graph 1 and 2)

1   *Correlation of the two scales within each observer* - A very high correlation between both scales pain scores was found within each observer, observer 1 (r=0.95) and observer 2 (r=0.90).

2   *Sensitivity of the scales to pain behavior of participants (SRM)* - The NCAPC was found more sensitive than the PADS at all levels of IDD (see table 2).

3   *Internal consistency (Cronbach α)* - High internal consistency was found for all items in both questionnaires:

PADS – An α of   0.7was found for observer 1 without items negatively influencing the α, An α of 0.74 was found for observer 2, with 2 items negatively influencing the α (2, & 12).

NCAPC - An α of 0.85 was found for observer 1 without items negatively influencing the α, and an α of 0.78 was found for observer 2, with 3 items negatively influencing the α (2, 7 & 10).

Table 2. Comparison of sensitivity to pain of both scales

	NCAPC	PADS
Interrater reliability	0.84-0.81	0.87-0.86
Sensitivity (SRM) of all groups	0.57	0.52
Sensitivity for level of profound IDD	0.66	0.59
Sensitivity for level of severe IDD	0.37	0.31
Sensitivity for level of moderate IDD	0.80	0.73
Sensitivity for level of mild IDD	-0.16	-0.16
Internal consistency (Cronbach α)	0.85-0.78	0.78-0.74

Index: The items showing better results is marked with a gray background

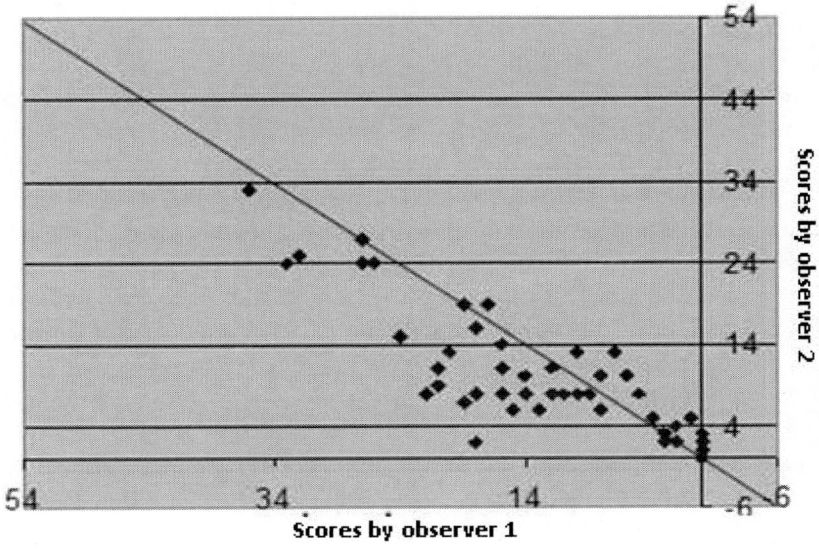

Graph 1. Interrater reliability for the PADS.

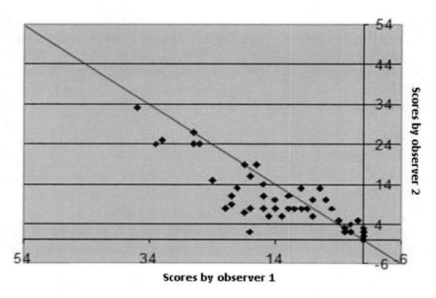

Graph 2. Interrater reliability for the NCAPC.

Conclusion

The aim of the study was to compare two pain scales designed to evaluate pain in adults with IDD in regards to sensitivity, internal consistency, and usability. Present findings confirmed the original findings suggesting that both scales hold high psychometric values, with slightly better values in all measures examined for the NCAPC, apart from interrater reliability which was found slightly improved for the PADS. The results indicated that both scales are efficient in measuring procedural pain within the designated population.

Interrater reliability – Both scales showed high interrater reliability (ICC>0.8). The original interrater reliability for the PADS was reported as 0.63 (29). The findings in the present article suggest higher values. In a research by Lotan et al. (32) interrarter reliability for the NCAPC was found at 0.91-0.92 by therapists and caregivers (Higher than the present findings). The difference in interrarter reliability results might lie in the fact that the observers had no prior familiarity with individuals with IDD and with pain scales. Another possible factor that influenced interrarter reliability was the fact that the observers underwent only a 1 hour tutorial for each scale. It was estimated that in order for a user to achieve proper acquaintance with the NCAPC a 2.5 hour tutorial is warranted (32).

Correlation found between scores within each observer – From the high correlation found in both observers between the scales (Observer 1 – 0.95; Observer 2 – 0.90) we can deduce that both scales are measuring the same phenomenon. Such high correlations received from two scales that were built by two teams using completely different pain stimulus (The PADS- manual manipulation; The NCAPC - an injection) and different participants across the globe support the validity of the two scales for capturing the measured behavior; pain in adults with IDD.

Sensitivity to pain – was examined with SRM. The comparison between the two scales showed a slightly higher sensitivity for the NCAPC, yet the authors believe that the differences found were related to the fact that the NCAPC was designed with the same population and the same pain stimulus. There are no reports regarding the sensitivity of the PADS, yet the present findings are inferior to previously reported sensitivity measured for the NCAPC (31). It seems that those measures could be attributed to the small number of participants in each group (especially within the mild IDD group; N=4) and the large impact of standard deviation on this measure.

Internal consistency – both scales were found to show satisfactory levels of internal consistency (within the range of 0.9-0.7), thereby, suggesting that the items on both scales are generally supportive of the observed phenomenon; pain behavior in adults with IDD.

Observer's comments – The high psychometric values presented by both scales were received with but little use of the items related to physiological response (breathing, change in facial color), and the authors question the need for those items.

The NCAPC was found more sensitive than the PADS despite the fact that the PADS has 5 levels of pain behavior for each item (0=not present, 1=Difficult to detect or only occurs once or twice during assessment, 2= Occurs infrequently and is easy to detect, 3= Occurs frequently and is easy to detect, 4= Occurs almost continuously during assessment and is easy to detect) and the NCAPC has only 4 levels (0=Not at all, 1= Not at all, 2=fairly often, 3=Very often).

Limitations of the study

1   As the observed phenomenon was procedural pain, the outcome of the present investigation can be held relevant only to procedural pain – therefore future investigations should look into other types of pain

2   The present investigation used video vignettes that were part of the construction of the NCAPC. Future investigations should use video observations from non-related populations.

3   The observers in the present investigation had undergone only an hour tutorial on using the scales. It is recommended that lengthier tutorial will be used in the future. Nevertheless, the fact that the observers were able to use the scales without previous acquaintance with the population, and with such short tutorials regarding the pain scales imply that the scales can be easily used.

References

[1]   Reid BC, Chenette R, Macek MD. Prevalence and predictors of untreated caries and oral pain among Special Olympic athletes. Spec Care Dentist 2003;23:139–42.

[2]   Regnard C, Mathews D, Gibson L, Clarke C. Difficulties in identifying distress and its causes in people with severe communication problems. Int J Palliat Nurs 2003;9:173–6.

[3]   Schwartz L, Engel JM, Jensen MP. Pain in persons with cerebral palsy. Arch Phys Med Rehabil 1999;80:1243-6.

[4]   McGrath PJ, Breau LM, Camfield C, Finley GA. Caregivers management of pain in cognitively impaired children with severe speech impairments. Poster presented at the 5th international symposium on pediatric pain. London, England. June 18-21, 2000.

[5]   Lachapelle DL, Hadijistavropoulos R, Craig KD. Pain measurement in persons with intellectual disability. Clin J Pain 1999;15:13-23.

[6]   Malviya S, Voepel-Lewis T, Trait AR, Merkel S, Lauer A, Munro H, Farley F. Pain management in children with and without cognitive impairment following spine fusion surgery. Pediatr Anesthesia 2001;11:453–8.

[7]   Stallard P, Williams L, Lenton S, Velleman R. Pain in cognitively impaired, non-communicating children. Arch Dis Child 2001;85:460–2.

[8]   Van Schrojenstein Lantman-De Valk HMJ, Metsemakers JFM, Haveman MJ, Crebolder HFJM. Health problems in people with intellectual disability in general practice: a comparative study. Fam Pract 2000;17:405–7.

[9]   Carr EG, Jamie Æ, Owen-DeSchryver S. Physical illness, pain, and problem behavior in minimally verbal people with developmental disabilities. J Autism Dev Disord 2007;37:413–24.

[10]   Breau LM, Camfield CS, McGrath PJ, Finley A. The incidence of pain in children with severe cognitive impairments. Arch Pediatr Adolesc Med 2003;157:1219–26.

[11]   Carter B, McArthur E, Cunliffe M. Dealing with uncertainty: parental assessment of pain in their children with profound special needs. J Adv Nurs 2002;38,449–57.

[12]   Donovan JD. Learning disability nurses' experiences of being with clients who may be in pain. J Adv Nurs 2002;38:458–66.

[13]   Oberlander TF, O'Donnell ME. Beliefs about pain among professionals working with children with significant neurological impairment. Dev Med Child Neurol 2001;43:136–40.

[14]   Stallard P, Williams L, Velleman R, Lenton S, McGrath P.J. Brief report: behaviors identified by caregivers to detect pain in noncommunicating children. J Pediatr Psychol 2002;27:209–14.

[15]   Ekman P, Friesen W. Investigators guide to the facial action coding system. Palo Alto, CA: Consulting Psychologist Press, 1978.

[16]   Craig KD, Korol CT, Pillai RR. Challenges of judging pain in vulnerable infants. Clin Perinatol 2002; 29:445–57.

[17]   Craig KD, Prkachin KM, Grunau R. The facial expression of pain. In: Turk D, Melzack R. (Eds). Handbook of pain assessment. New York: Guilford, 1992: 257–76.

[18]   Giusiano B, Jimeno MT, Collignon P, Chau Y. Utilization of neural network in the elaboration of an evaluation scale for pain in cerebral palsy. Methods Inf Med 1995;34:498–502.

[19]   Collignon P, Giusiano B, Boutin AM, Combes JC. Utilisation d'une échelle d'hétéroévaluation de la doleur chez le sujet sévérement polyhandicapé. Douleur et Analgesie 1997;1:27–32. [French]

[20]   Collignon P, Giusiano B. Validation of a pain evaluation scale for patients with severe cerebral palsy. Eur J Pain 2001;5:433–42.

[21]   Breau LM, McGrath PJ, Camfield C, Rosmus C, Finley GA. Preliminary validation of an observational pain checklist for persons with cognitive impairments and inability to communicate verbally. Dev Med Child Neurol 2000;42:609–16.

[22]   McGrath PJ, Rosmus C, Canfield C, Campbell MA, Hennigar A. Behaviours caregivers use to determine pain in nonverbal, cognitively impaired individuals. Dev Med Child Neurol 1998;40:340–3.

[23]   Breau LM, Finley GA, McGrath PJ, Camfield CS. Validation of the Non-communicating Children's Pain Checklist-Postoperative Version. Anesthesiology 2002;96:528–35.

[24]   Breau LM, McGrath PJ, Camfield CS, Finley GA. Psychometric properties of the non-communicating children's pain checklist-revised. Pain 2002;99:349–57.

[25]   Stallard P, Williams L, Velleman R, Lenton S, McGrath PJ, Taylor G. The development and evaluation of the pain indicator for communicatively impaired children (PICIC). Pain 2002;98:145–9.

[26]   Hunt A. Goldman A. Seers K, Crichton N, Mastroyannopoulou K, Moffat V, Oulton K, Brady M. Clinical validation of the Paediatric Pain Profile. Dev Med Child Neurol 2004;46(1):9-18.

[27]   Bodfish JW, Harper VN, Deacon JR, Symons FJ. Identifying and measuring pain in persons with developmental disabilities: a manual for the Pain and Discomfort Scale (PADS). Western Carolina Center Research Reports, 2001.

[28]   Groth-Marnat, G. Handbook of psychological assessment. 3rd edition, Hoboken: NJ, John Wiley, 1997:21–2.

[29]　Phan A, Edwards CL, Robinson EL. The assessment of pain and discomfort in individuals with mental retardation. Res Dev Disabil 2005;26(5):433-9.

[30]　Lotan M, Moe-Nilssen R, Ljunggren AE, Strand LI: Psychometric properties and usability of the Non-Communicating Adult Pain Checklist (NCAPC) a pain scale for adults with Intellectual and Developmental Disabilities in a clinical setting (dental treatments). Res Dev Disabil 2010;31(2):367-75.

[31]　Lotan M, Ljunggren AE, Johnsen TB, Defrin R, Pick CG, Strand LI. A modified version of the Non-Communicating Children Pain Checklist-Revised (NCCPC-R), adapted to adults with intellectual and developmental disabilities. Sensitivity to pain and internal consistency. J Pain 2009;10(4):398-407.

[32]　Lotan M, Moe-Nilssen R, Ljunggren AE, Strand LI. Reliability of the Non-Communicating Adult Pain Checklist (NCAPC), assessed by different groups of health workers. Res Dev Disabil 2009;30(4):735-45.

[33]　Defrin R, Lotan M, Pick CG. The evaluation of acute pain in individuals with cognitive impairment: a differential effect of the level of impairment. Pain 2006;124(3):312-20.

[34]　Shrout PE, Fleiss FL. Intraclass correlations: uses in assessing rater reliability. Psychol Bull 1979;86:420–8.

[35]　Moe-Nilssen, R. Test-retest reliability of trunk accelerometry during standing and walking. Arch Phys Med Rehabil 1998;79,1377-85.

[36]　Currier DP. Elements of research in physical therapy. Baltimore: Williams Wilkins, 1990.

[37]　Nicewander WA. Thirteen ways to look at the correlation coefficient. Am Statistician 1988;42(1):59–66.

[38]　Finch E, Brooks D, Stratford PW, Mayo NE. Physical rehabilitation outcome measures: A guide to enhanced clinical decision making, 2nd ed. Hamilton, BC: Decker, 2002.

[39]　Cohen J. Statistical power analysis for behavioral sciences, 2nd ed. Hillsdale, NJ: Lawrence Erlbaum, 1988.

In: Pain Management Yearbook 2013
Editor: Joav Merrick

Chapter 3

Chasing the ghosts: The impact of diagnostic labeling on self-management and pain-related guilt in chronic low back pain patients

Danijela Serbic, MSc and Tamar Pincus, PhD*

Department of Psychology, Royal Holloway,
University of London, Egham, Surrey, United Kingdom

Abstract

In the majority of chronic low back pain (CLBP) patients a clear diagnosis cannot be established; as a result patients are given labels such as non-specific low back pain. There is some evidence to suggest that lack of a clear diagnosis is associated with negative psychological, clinical and behavioural outcomes. The main aim of this study was to examine CLBP patients' understanding, feelings and behaviour in response to their diagnostic labels. Semi-structured interviews were conducted with twenty CLBP patients who were recruited from one osteopathic and one pain management clinic in the UK. Sampling, data collection and analysis were driven by a grounded theory approach. Data were analysed through four stages of coding: open, selective, axial and theoretical coding. Data collection and coding continued until data achieved saturation. Results indicated that lack of a clear diagnosis is associated with distress, further treatment seeking and uncertainty. It also influenced participants' perception of their social relationships; having visible evidence and a clear diagnosis gave patients' pain more social credibility. Participants reported feeling guilty about the consequences of their pain to themselves and others, and for failing to recover. Overall, participants' narratives suggest that at least for some, absence of a clear diagnosis has considerable negative implications. The goal of the study was to inform clinicians and policy makers about the

* Correspondence: Danijela Serbic, Department of Psychology, Royal Holloway, University of London, Egham, Surrey, TW20 0EX, United Kingdom. E-mail: danijela.serbic@rhul.ac.uk

impact of diagnosis on CLBP patients' adjustment and emotional burden; findings suggest that legitimising the pain experience is of prime importance to CLBP patients.

Keywords: Chronic low back pain, diagnosis, pain-related guilt

Introduction

Low back pain (LBP) affects about 80% of the adult population over a life span (1), has considerable impact on individuals and accounts for substantial socioeconomic costs (2). When a definitive cause and a clear diagnosis cannot be established patients are often given labels such as non-specific LBP (3). Diagnosis is defined as the 'identification of a disease or condition by a scientific evaluation of physical signs, symptoms, history, laboratory test results, and procedures' (4). However, non-specific LBP is diagnosed by exclusion and is defined as non-specific or musculoskeletal back pain where underlying pathology cannot be found (2). It is often understood as a symptom or a syndrome rather than a diagnosis (5). Diagnostic labelling is defined as 'the act of classifying a patient according to a diagnostic category' (4). In the case of non-specific LBP labelling can be problematic and misleading because non-specific LBP is not a single diagnostic category; it represents a number of different subtypes of back pain (6). Non-specific LBP represents the majority of LBP patients as only in about 5-10% of cases precise causes of back pain can be identified (2).

In the absence of clear physical evidence the meaning of diagnosis becomes ambiguous, and it becomes questionable whether non-specific LBP should be seen as a diagnosis or not. As there is no consensus and clear guidelines in the literature on this issue, but there is sufficient evidence to indicate that the non-specific LBP label is problematic and ambiguous, in this paper we will refer to it as an unclear diagnosis/diagnostic label.

Having no clear physical evidence means that some patients feel that their pain is delegitimised and disbelieved (7). Some patients who lack clear physical evidence to justify their pain experiences also report feeling guilty (7). However, to our knowledge there are no studies specifically investigating pain-related guilt in CLBP patients and no instruments have yet been developed to measure it. Therefore, a secondary aim of this study was to explore pain-related feelings of guilt in CLBP patients, especially in relation to unclear diagnosis. Guilt is a type of emotional distress that is founded on the likelihood that we may be in the wrong, or that others may perceive us that way (8). Guilt is often found to be a feature of depression, and it is recognised that many depressive symptoms are prevalent in chronic pain disorders (9) such as CLBP. It is therefore important to explore if pain- and diagnosis-related guilt is present in CLBP patients.

Methods

Sampling, data collection and data analysis were driven by grounded theory, which is considered a suitable methodology to understand participants' experiences and to produce a theory that explains the phenomenon under study (10). Grounded theory was selected because its systematic and precise procedures for data sampling, collection and analysis should contribute to validity and reliability of findings. We based our theory on the premise (constructivist grounded theory) that multiple and socially constructed realities exist, and concepts are created rather than discovered from data (11).

Recruitment and sample

Grounded theory employs a theoretical purposive sampling which is aimed towards theory construction and data saturation rather than population representativeness. Therefore, we continued with data collection and analysis until saturation was achieved (10). Inclusion criteria were LBP patients seeking treatment, aged over 18 and with a pain duration of at least 3 months (2). Exclusion criteria consisted of any conditions other than musculoskeletal back pain (e.g., rheumatoid arthritis, ankylosing spondylitis, cancer) ascertained by self-report and by examining patients' medical notes with practitioners. Participants were recruited from two clinics in London, UK: a private pain management institution and an osteopathic clinic, selected to achieve a diverse sample with a range of disability levels. Information about participants' diagnosis was obtained from their medical notes and by consulting with practitioners in the participating centres. An information sheet with a short screening questionnaire and opt-in slip were handed out to patients. Patients who fulfilled the inclusion criteria were contacted by the researcher to arrange an interview. Two measures of participants functioning were collected to allow full description of participants' characteristics: (i) Roland Disability Questionnaire (RDQ) (12), which is a reliable measure of low back disability (6); and (ii) Hospital Anxiety and Depression Scale (HADS) (13), which has been widely used in studies of depression and anxiety in medical populations.

Data collection

Semi-structured interviews were based on a schedule including exploration of participants' condition, their understanding of their diagnostic labels, their response to diagnostic labelling, their coping with CLBP and their relationships with others. Because of sensitivity attached to the terminology of guilt we opted not to ask about this directly in the first instance, but it was used as a probe.

All the interviews were conducted by the first author in the participating clinics. Interviews were tape recorded and later transcribed. Length of interview ranged from 9.02 to 34.58 minutes, the average length was 24.45 minutes. This study was approved by the University's Ethics Committee.

Data analysis

Data collection and analysis were carried out simultaneously. All coding was completed by hand. Comparisons of statements and incidents were made within the same interview and then compared with statements and incidents in other interviews. Categories were supported by verbatim quotes from interview transcripts (14, 15).

We combined elements of coding from Glaser (14) and Strauss and Corbin (15) grounded theory in the following way: all interviews were coded, first by using open coding; each transcript was analysed line by line in order to identify key words, phrases and eventually codes (14). Selective coding (14) followed: we selected and employed the most significant and recurrent categories to code large amounts of data. However, Glaser's (14) selective coding does not provide specific procedures for studying relationships between categories and subcategories, for this reason axial coding (15) was also employed. Theoretical coding (14) was the final stage of coding; this was used to bring related categories together. Theoretical categories were intergraded into an interpretative theoretical framework (15), which explains the studied phenomenon by showing how these categories are related (see Figure 1).

Data triangulation

Observer triangulation was achieved by the second author coding 10% of the interviews (blind to the first author's coding); and then by examining codes and categories (against interview transcripts) developed by the first author; this was done throughout the coding process. Additionally, observer triangulation was achieved by an independent auditor, a health psychologist with considerable experience in qualitative research inspecting the coding process and categories developed against the interview transcripts. Theory validity was achieved by: (i) returning to already analysed data to check if any instances could be found that contradict the emerging theory, and (ii) collecting new data (10): five participants with a clear diagnosis were interviewed, four of these five participants experienced a prolonged period of being undiagnosed (between several months and eight years) prior to being given a diagnosis. These cases enabled a direct comparison between absence and presence of a clear diagnosis.

Results

We excluded one participant due to insufficient proficiency in English. Therefore, 20 participants' data were included in the analysis: 12 participants were from an osteopathic clinic, 7 were on a pain management course and 1 pilot participant who fulfilled the inclusion criteria.

The characteristics of the participants are summarised in Table 1. Fifteen out of 20 participants had mechanical non-specific LBP, and the remaining 5 participants had a clear diagnosis (e.g., prolapsed disc). The information from these participants was analysed alongside the remaining 15 participants' data as part of theory triangulation. Four out of these five participants experienced a prolonged period of being undiagnosed (between several months and eight years) prior to being given a clear diagnosis and overall there were no apparent differences in their emerging themes. On a few occasions they were asked to make a direct comparison between undiagnosed and diagnosed state; these instances are clearly flagged in the findings.

Table 1. Characteristics of the participants

		Osteopathic* Clinic	Pain Management Clinic	Pilot	Total
N		12	7	1	20
Male (N)		4	2		6
Female (N)		8	5	1	14
Age (Mean & SD)		50.5 (16.9)	41.1 (8.4)	33	46.4 (14.7)
Pain intensity (Mean & SD) on a scale: 0-10		6.1 (2.6)	6.3 (1.8)	3	6 (2.3)
Pain duration (N)	1-2 years	1	1		2
	2-3 years	1			1
	4-5 years	2	3		5
	5+ years	2	1		3
	10+ years	6	2	1	9
HADS (Mean & SD)	Anxiety	7.9 (4.8)	9.4 (5.0)	8	8.5 (4.7)
	Depression	4.1 (1.7)	8.3 (6.9)	7	5.9 (4.8)
RDQ (Mean & SD)		7.1 (4.4)	10.4 (6.2)	3	8.2 (5.3)

Abbreviations: N-number of participants; SD-standard deviation; HADS- Hospital Anxiety and Depression Scale; RDQ- Roland Disability Questionnaire.

*Two patients from the osteopathic clinic did not complete HADS & RDQ.

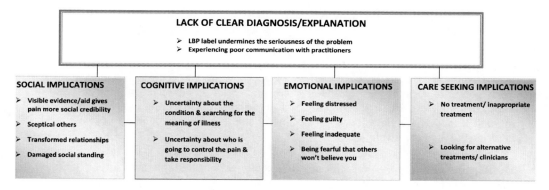

Figure 1. Theoretical framework to represent the implications of lack of clear diagnosis on CLBP patients. (Lines that connect theoretical categories indicate that all of them are related to each other; however the nature and direction of these relationships cannot be established by the use of qualitative methodology).

Structure and characteristics of the theoretical framework

The theoretical framework (see Figure 1) consists of five theoretical categories: Lack of clear diagnosis and explanation about the back pain, Social implications of lack of clear diagnosis, Cognitive implications of lack of clear diagnosis, Emotional implications of lack of clear diagnosis and Implications of lack of clear diagnosis on care seeking. Our findings indicate that all categories are related; however the nature and direction of these relationships cannot be established using qualitative methodology. Theoretical categories consist of two or more first order categories. Theoretical categories are more abstract than first order categories and are used to conceptualise how the categories may be related and amalgamated into the theory (14). We included participant's gender (M-male, F-female) and age with each quotation.

Theoretical categories

Lack of clear diagnosis and explanation about the back pain

Interviews with the participants revealed that the meaning of not having a clear diagnosis can be understood as a prolonged state that impacts on how participants cope with back pain, how they perceive themselves and how they think they are perceived by others. This state does not normally come to existence in a single point of time in which the doctor is either able or unable to deliver a diagnosis to the patient; our findings showed that this is a process characterised by a prolonged search for a diagnosis and an understanding of the experienced symptoms. This theoretical category consists of two first order categories: 'experiencing poor communication with practitioners' and 'LBP label undermines the seriousness of the problem'.

Participants reported several problems relating to their communication with practitioners, such as being given very little advice:

'And I think I've seen about four different consultants by now, not one of them has offered any advice' [F39].

Practitioners want clear and simple explanation from patients about their symptoms; however patients are not always able to produce one, due to the complexity of their symptoms:

'… I mean it wasn't like how are you feeling and how are you coping...It was more like: 'okay so where does the pain go and is it piercing'...a lot of, not technical, but stuff that I didn't really understand, and I tried my best to explain it, considering the pain changed a lot, and it moved around a lot. I just felt pretty stupid because I couldn't pin point and describe my pain very well' [F33].

Participants reported that practitioners use technical and complicated jargon so they are often left puzzled:

'...so they tend to say there is nothing to see, it's obviously mechanical, that's what they always say; what mechanical means you see, I don't know' [F46].

Most participants used the LBP label or just back pain to describe their condition. Participants' accounts indicate that the LBP label undermines the seriousness of the problem, and that it is puzzling to practitioners:

'...cause I know the doctors and GPs and everyone kind of scoffs then, when you say those words [back pain], it means oh well we don't really know' [F33].

It is also assumed to be a short duration problem:

'I know they [new people she meets] won't understand because everybody at some time has back pain and they think it's over in days or weeks, but with mine it hasn't gone away ever; it's always there. I get varying degrees of it' [F39].

This indicates that in general people misunderstand LBP and that they are not sufficiently informed about it:

'… because it's the whole system, it does not lead you to kind of, um…to have this kind of very accurate understanding of it [back pain]' [F35].

Social implications of lack of clear diagnosis

Participants believed that visible evidence and having a more concrete label would give them more credibility, tolerance and sympathy:

'...but if you had something more concrete [in terms of diagnosis] for them to go on, they'd look at you in a completely different light, like oh my God… so if I could say this is a back problem of some proportion, or whatever, then yeah, I would be quite happy to have that'[F39].

Other forms of visible evidence such as carrying a stick, telling others about being on painkillers and having positive results from medical tests is another way of emphasising the seriousness of the condition and gives participants' pain more social credibility. One participant did not receive a clear diagnosis until an MRI scan (eight years later) showed three prolapsed discs. When asked whether having a clear diagnosis now has made any difference, she said:

'Yes, I think so...they have an idea of what that is, so at least it helps in that sense rather than just: 'ohh I've got a bad back'...I feel better for the fact that it sounds awful even though it isn't necessarily that bad, it's kind of stupid' [F46].

Lack of physical evidence and clear diagnosis presents a problem when participants need to justify their pain; participants reported feeling inadequate and being disbelieved by others, especially by managers and work colleagues:

'Yeah, there was no point [in explaining to work colleagues and managers the problem], absolutely no point because everybody else around you wants a diagnosis and when you can't give one you feel like you're a failure yourself' [F39].

The majority of participants acknowledged that they felt, rather than experienced direct scepticism:

'He [the manager] said: 'oh, all you can do is go and see another specialist and see if you can get some kind of firm diagnosis for it'...I don't actually think they believed me in the beginning…I think they just thought I wanted some time off...They didn't turn around and say: 'no, we think you're faking it'; and you know...but you can tell by the way they behave towards you, that they don't believe you' [M54].

Almost all participants reported that they get understanding and support from family members; but their relationships with friends are more problematic. Several participants said that a shift occurs in how friends and other people perceive them and some participants said that having a clear diagnosis would change these perceptions. Participants also reported that these perceptions influenced and changed their relationships with other people and impacted negatively on their social standing:

'It would be brilliant if they had one [diagnosis]...and it would mean my friends would know that I'm not being a rubbish friend...I'd be taken a lot more seriously in many ways' [F33].

Cognitive implications of lack of clear diagnosis

Uncertainty about the condition and searching for its meaning was a prominent category in the study. Managing patients' expectations about what is possible to achieve through consultations with health care practitioners appears to be one way to address this uncertainty. For instance, being informed about the non-specificity of LBP at early stages of the problem may help patients to have more realistic expectations:

'... there's a massive area in there where patients don't initially understand, so I think it should be made clear to patients, right out from the outset. So there is no big expectation that's then dropped through the hole in the middle. So...to start off with, and say: 'look it can't always be diagnosed specifically'...reduce their expectation level...and I think that'll help. Because you're not chasing these ghosts' [M54].

Feeling uncertain about one's condition contributed to feeling helpless:

'I want answers, it can't be right to be in this position for so long, and there must be something that you can do to help me' [F39].

It also contributed to the level of distress:

'It was very, very tough [being in so much pain and not being able to explain to herself and other people what really caused it], it was very depressing; I ended up extremely depressed' [F46].

Participants needed a label that will represent and give a meaning to their experiences:

'I'd rather have an explanation than all this...and I felt the unknown sort of thing, I wasn't very happy with that' [F36].

Having a clear diagnosis would contribute to their wellbeing and self-concept:

'...cause all I wanted was somebody to say this is it, this is what's wrong with you...and just for my own well-being, just to sort of confirm this is it, this is the problem' [F39].

However, for some participants having received adequate explanation regardless of being given a diagnosis made them feel reassured:

'He [the doctor] did not know exactly what it was but it still did not matter because he was showing me, he was explaining a lot more...Yeah I had some sort of reassurance as to say, this is what you've got but we can sort it out, sort of thing; or we can go through procedures...he made me feel better' [F35].

Participants also expressed uncertainty about who is going to take responsibility and control the pain. Having a clear diagnosis and/or understanding of the condition would mean that practitioners may be able to control the pain:

'...so it would be nice to just have one diagnosis and say this is what we think it is, and this is what they're going to do to relieve the pain or to help you' [F38].

Practitioners would also take responsibility for it:

'So you know you've got this problem and this is how they're gonna fix it. That's what's in your mind...you know, who's gonna take responsibility for it, if you like, who's gonna put it in the correct direction' [M54].

Emotional implications of lack of clear diagnosis

Participants reported feeling distressed, feeling inadequate and being fearful that others will not believe their symptoms. These feelings are associated and have been reported with above categories; here we focus specifically on feelings of guilt.

Feelings of guilt were grouped into three subcategories: feeling guilty towards other people, feeling guilty towards yourself and feeling guilty for not getting better.

Feelings of guilt towards other people can be split further into: (i) feeling guilty for what you have done:

'Guilt, always saying sorry to everybody as if it's my fault, you know, didn't know what to say or do, just felt I was just apologising all the time...for my actions...' [M39].

(ii) Feeling guilty for what you cannot do, such as not being able to help and do things with family and friends:

'You feel like you're letting people down, like when you should be able...to be a good friend or be a good employee, then you feel guilty 'cause you can't and it sucks' [F33].

A number of different situations were mentioned from not being able to cook a meal for the family, attend birthdays to not being able to care and provide for children:

'...but I'm not working, I can't do...I feel very guilty with my children' [M34].

Some participants said they were feeling guilty towards their colleagues at work, for instance for not being able to go to work due to back pain:

'...and the pressure on my colleagues and you know you can see the stress in their faces. They have recruited a temp...that's relieved my guilt actually' [F28].

Participants also reported feeling guilty for not meeting friends' expectations and disappointing them:

'Why do you feel guilty for like you should be there but you can't? Also they don't believe that your excuse is real. You feel like you'd done something wrong and you haven't' [F28].

They also said that friends expect them to be the same type of person as before back pain started, and they do not understand that the back pain has brought a change. When friends do understand, for some participants the guilt does not disappear, they reported feeling guilty because others are trying to make allowances and be helpful:

'But then that has a knock down effect as well, that makes me feel guilty as well because they [friends] are making allowances' [F36].

How do participants deal with feelings of guilt related to other people? Some participants reported distancing themselves from other people because they cannot understand their situation.

This seemed to be common behaviour by a number of participants in the study, not only as a reaction to feelings of guilt but to other emotional and social factors discussed above. Other participants tried to say 'no' more often and not feel bad about it, or they simply built a resistance towards guilty feelings over the years:

'...I've kind of given up on guilt...I think just because I got my head into a space where I just don't buy guilt any more. I've spent a lot of my life feeling guilty about one thing or another...and umm...it's just useless so I really don't go there' [M44].

Not all participants reported feeling guilty. About one third of them said they did not experience feelings of guilt. Various reasons were put forward such as experiencing a different kind of feeling instead of guilt, for instance feeling frustrated and anxious rather than guilty, to living alone/not having a family:

'...maybe because I live alone, you know, I don't need to, you know, to do things for other people' [F35].

Some participants also reported feeling guilty towards themselves (personal guilt). Back pain impacts on participants' level of involvement in daily activities and this seems to be related to how they feel about themselves. Participants reported feeling guilty for not living up to their own potential, expectations and values:

'When I had these two crises, I couldn't do anything, even to myself, I couldn't go down to the shops, I couldn't do my work, and I had deadlines to follow...I felt guilty because I wasn't doing what I was supposed to be doing' [F35].

Not being able to provide for themselves appears to be a problem too:

'The guilt is big when it comes to money, and not being able to work, that's really bad, that's horrendous' [F33].

Some participants reported feeling guilty for not getting better and for not being able to give a specific reason for their pain:

'I've beaten myself up on a regular basis, why I can't ...why it's not better, why am I still getting episodes of pain, why hasn't it gone...I feel guilty that I can't tell anybody something concrete, that I cannot give a specific reason. I would have loved the doctor just to have gone 'that's what's wrong with you', and be happy, because then I've got something more concrete to say to everybody' [F39].

However, the fact that the back pain was caused by uncontrollable circumstances made some participants feel less guilty:

'...but if any relief [from guilty feelings], because it's always been put down to my caesarean section. I always say it wasn't like I was just bungee jumping somewhere and then hurt my back' [F38].

Implications of lack of clear diagnosis on care seeking

In many instances participants made links between inappropriate treatment or absence of treatment and absence of physical evidence and clear diagnosis:

'Well you have nothing too serious [GP said], there is no need for physiotherapy...and things like that...but you know, at the time it was really needed' [F35].

Participants also reported waiting for too long for treatment:

'[GP] didn't really explain why I was in so much pain, and he just said I'd have to go on a waiting list which should take about two months to get physiotherapy, and he didn't have any immediate help'[F33].

Several participants expressed confusion about their treatment, and in a number of instances this could be linked to a lack of information and poor communication with practitioners:

'I didn't feel like I was able to ask about the other therapy options...so it's been like confusion I think in terms of what is best for my body, and no-one knows' [F28].

When current treatment does not work many participants reported looking for alternative treatments and seeing private clinicians. This patient explained why she came to see an osteopath:

'When I go to an osteopath I get looked at...it incorporates not just that specific pain, but you know your lifestyle...' [F62].

Discussion

The findings suggest that lack of clear diagnosis and lack of understanding about one's condition affect participants' social, cognitive and emotional functioning. Participants spent much time and effort trying to understand their diagnosis and condition; they invested themselves in this process.

Our findings indicate that uncertainty and a perceptual search for the meaning of the condition are important aspects of LBP, at least for some patients. The ability to find meaning is an important cognitive process and is an essential component of psychological recovery from stressful health related events (16). For the majority of participants, their label provided a poor fit with their experience of the condition and they stated that the LBP label undermined the seriousness of the problem. This is important, because such a fit is necessary for acceptance of the diagnosis (17) and consequent adherence and care seeking. Additionally, it can be difficult to direct attention to non-pain aspects of life if one does not accept the presence of pain. Acceptance of pain is characterised by a willingness to have pain, or other uncomfortable private experiences and it has been linked to better function in several studies (18). The question these findings pose and that needs further investigation is whether acceptance of pain is possible in the absence of an acceptable diagnosis or explanation, and before the very identity of the pain and its causes is accepted?

Participants consistently reported that having visible evidence, such as magnetic resonance imaging (MRI) scan or x- ray positive results, actually serve as a long awaited proof of their symptoms. However, in most cases such tests are negative, and most guidelines now recommend that clinicians should not carry out testing for non-specific LBP. Research on diagnostic approaches for CLBP that has centred on finding biological causes has been recently scrutinised. For instance, the use of early MRI scans has been employed as a means of providing earlier diagnosis and treatment, or reassuring CLBP patients. However, it appears that this leads to an increase in unnecessary surgery and perceptions of poor health (19). In fact, radiological evidence does not support a link between observable disc changes and LBP (20), and the National Institute for Health and Clinical Excellence (NICE) guidelines for CLBP in the UK now recommend against carrying out x-ray and MRI tests in these populations (21). This also means that many patients are simply told that there is nothing wrong with their back, but instead of reassuring them, such statements can result, at least in some patients, in heightened anxiety, seeking further care and examinations and mistrust in clinicians (22). Our findings support these findings.

Findings from this study suggest that the information participants received from practitioners was often conflicting, and this added to the confusion and uncertainty about their condition. This supports findings from other studies, such as McIntosh and Shaw's qualitative study (23), who found that many LBP patients were dissatisfied with the information they received from their GPs about their diagnosis and treatment. Our findings also showed that in the absence of a clear diagnostic label participants put in immense effort in justifying their pain experiences and convincing practitioners and other people (especially work colleagues and managers) that they were not malingering. Patients' perception that others think they malinger is in line with findings from other research, for instance a study (7) explored the meaning of diagnostic tests for people with LBP and found that in the absence of positive test results many patients felt that practitioners did not believe their accounts of pain. Overall, our findings suggest a misunderstanding and lack of communication between patients and practitioners, and that to an extent managing patients' expectations from the onset may help to solve this problem. Participants said that practitioners should provide much clearer and more detailed explanations, and warn patients that a definitive cause and diagnosis may not be possible to establish.

The participants struggle with their pain and they reported that their distress and suffering impact on their relationships with other people, for instance they said they experienced resentment, a sense of isolation and guilt. It also appears that feelings of guilt are closely linked to disbelief and stigma associated with non-specific LBP. For instance, some participants reported feeling guilty for not getting better and for not being able to give a specific reason for their pain. This suggests a link between pain-related guilt and unknown aetiology/lack of physical evidence, but this should be confirmed by comparing reported guilt in pain populations with a clear diagnosis and physical evidence.

While trying to cope with the social and emotional consequences of a lack of clear diagnosis participants appeared to be exposed to uncertainty and confusion about what their symptoms mean, why they persists, and how they should be treated. Overall, our findings seem to suggest that a lack of clear diagnosis impacts on participants' self-management of their back pain. However, this cannot be concluded based on qualitative methodology alone and further research is needed.

Strengths and limitations

To our knowledge, this is the first study that explored pain- and diagnosis-related guilt in CLBP patients. Considering that in the majority of LBP patients clear physical evidence cannot be found, and consequently no clear diagnosis can be given, it is crucial to understand associated emotional states in this group of patients.

A methodological strength of the study is that a great degree of care was taken to carefully tailor and justify every step of the analysis according to already well developed strands of grounded theory. However, several limitations are also indicated.

As the inclusion into the study was limited to persons on the pain management programme and undergoing osteopathy treatment, the findings may not generalise to other LBP populations. In addition, the small sample of volunteers who agreed to be interviewed may have been subject to other biases. Future research should test the developed theory in large and diverse samples of CLBP patients. We acknowledge that participants' accounts may be constructed through social processes and demands of the situation, although we tried to minimise these as much as possible. Most importantly, our findings are limited to patients' perception and their own interpretation of their experiences. Exploring any link, especially causal, between receiving and accepting diagnostic labels and subsequent clinical status and health-related behaviours must be explored quantitatively and prospectively in appropriately large samples.

Implications for patients and clinicians

The findings could be interpreted to suggest that there is a need for a clearer labelling system for musculoskeletal conditions with no apparent biological origin, and for a label that will give a new meaning to CLBP and distance it from the current stereotypical view. However, the labelling issue is clearly problematic; for instance it has been debated whether providing labels which indicate biological origins for conditions that do not seem to have one may strengthen the individual's belief that s/he is ill and encourage disability (24).

In addition, it is important to search for more helpful interactions between practitioners and patients that do not depend on the presence or absence of visible evidence (25). The findings of this study provide supporting evidence to this view and encourage practitioners to consider the importance of diagnosis and labels in CLBP, and better and more acceptable explanations. However, this may present a challenge to practitioners as currently there is no consistency and no clear guidelines for delivering diagnosis, explanation and reassurance for LBP.

Many participants reported feeling guilty and further research should examine if pain- and diagnosis-related guilt is associated with depressive mood. This may have implications for refining therapies, such as cognitive behavioural therapy (CBT) by targeting specific emotional states and cognitive processes. Refining CBT to suit specific groups of patients is one of the most important and urgent priorities (9).

Conclusion

The findings indicate that at least some LBP patients invest heavily in a search for biological causes of their condition, as such causes can rarely be found. Participants reported that they do not want to be classed as psychological cases and that they keep looking for evidence of biological or biomechanical malfunction. Their narratives suggested that many participants experienced difficulties as a result of the lack of understanding and acknowledgement of their suffering by practitioners and other people. Participants identified that these difficulties were linked to a lack of clear diagnostic label; the label that would justify their pain experiences. This poses a challenge to clinicians in the context of uncertainty and further emphasises the importance of clear, acceptable explanations that may replace diagnoses based on physical evidence.

Acknowledgments

We would like to thank all the patients who agreed to participate in this research and the staff at the two participating clinics for their assistance. The study was partly funded by the British College of Osteopathic Medicine, but they had no involvement in the study design, data collection, data analysis and manuscript preparation.

References

[1]   Walker BF, Muller R, Grant WD. Low back pain in Australian adults. Health provider utilization and care seeking. J Manipulat Physiol Ther 2004;27(5):327-35.
[2]   Krismer M, van Tulder M. Low back pain (non-specific). Best Pract Res Clin Rheumatol 2007;21(1):77-91.
[3]   Coste J, Paolaggi JB, Spira A. Classification of nonspecific low back pain. I. Psychological involvement in low back pain: A clinical, descriptive approach. Spine 1992;17(9):1028-37.
[4]   Mosby medical dictionary, 8th ed. St. Louis, MO: Mosby, 2009.
[5]   Cedraschi C, Robert J, Goerg D, Perrin E, Fischer W, Vischer TL. Is chronic non-specific low back pain chronic? Definitions of a problem and problems of a definition. Br J Gen Pract 1999;49(442):358-62.

[6] Waddell G. The back pain revolution, 2nd ed. Edinburgh: Churchill Livingstone, 2004.

[7] Rhodes LA, McPhillips-Tangum CA, Markham C, Klenk R. The power of the visible: the meaning of diagnostic tests in chronic back pain. Soc Sci Med 1999;48(9):1189-203.

[8] Baumeister RF, Stillwell AM, Heatherton TF. Guilt. An interpersonal approach. Psychol Bull 1994;115(2):243-67.

[9] Eccleston C. Role of psychology in pain management. Br J Anaesth 2001;87(1):144-52.

[10] Robson C. Real world research: A resource for social scientists and practitioner-researchers, 2nd ed. Oxford: Blackwell, 2002.

[11] Charmaz K. Constructing grounded theory: A practical guide through qualitative analysis. London: Sage, 2006.

[12] Roland M, Morris R. A study of the natural history of back pain.1. Development of a reliable and sensitive measure of disability in low-back-pain. Spine 1983;8(2):141-4.

[13] Zigmond AS, Snaith RP. The hospital anxiety and depression scale. Acta Psychiatr Scand 1983;67(6):361-70.

[14] Glaser BG. Theoretical sensitivity: Advances in the methodology of grounded theory. Mill Valley, CA: Sociology Press, 1978.

[15] Strauss AL, Corbin JM. Basics of qualitative research: techniques and procedures for developing grounded theory, 2nd ed. Thousand Oaks, CA: Sage, 1998.

[16] Taylor SE. Adjustment to threatening events. A theory of cognitive adaptation. Am Psychol 1983;38(11):1161-73.

[17] Madden S, Sim J. Creating meaning in fibromyalgia syndrome. Soc Sci Med 2006;63(11):2962-73.

[18] McCracken LM, Vowles KE. Acceptance of chronic pain. Curr Pain Headache Rep 2006(10):90-4.

[19] Ash LM, Modic MT, Obuchowski NA, Ross JS, Brant-Zawadzki MN, Grooff PN. Effects of diagnostic information, per se, on patient outcomes in acute radiculopathy and low back pain. Am J Neuroradiol 2008;29(6):1098-103.

[20] Boos N, Rieder R, Schade V, Spratt KF, Semmer N, Aebi M. The diagnostic accuracy of magnetic resonance imaging, work perception, and psychosocial factors in identifying symptomatic disc herniations. Spine 1995;20(24):2613-25.

[21] National Institute for Health and Clinical Excellence. Low back pain. Early management of persistent non-specific low back pain. CG88. London: National Institute for Health and Clinical Excellence, 2009.

[22] Linton SJ, McCracken LM, Vlaeyen JWS. Reassurance: Help or hinder in the treatment of pain. Pain 2008;134(1-2):5-8.

[23] McIntosh A, Shaw CFM. Barriers to patient information provision in primary care: patients' and general practitioners' experiences and expectations of information for low back pain. Health Expectations 2003;6(1):19-29.

[24] Ehrlich GE. Fibromyalgia, a virtual disease. Clinical Rheumatol 2003;22(1):8-11.

[25] Kenny DT. Constructions of chronic pain in doctor-patient relationships: bridging the communication chasm. Patient Educ Couns 2004;52(3):297-305.

In: Pain Management Yearbook 2013
Editor: Joav Merrick

ISBN: 978-1-63117-944-0
© 2014 Nova Science Publishers, Inc.

Chapter 4

Comparison of baseline quality of life scores in patients with bone and brain metastases as assessed using the EORTC QLQ-C30

Michael Poon, MD(C)[1], Liang Zeng, MD(C)[1], Liying Zhang, PhD[1], Ling-Ming Tseng, MD[2], Ming-Feng Hou, MD[3], Alysa Fairchild, MD[4], Vassilios Vassiliou, MD[5], Reynaldo Jesus-Garcia, MD[6], Mohamed A Alm El-Din, MD[7], Aswin Kumar, MD[8], Fabien Forges, PharmD[9,10], Wei-Chu Chie, MD[11], Arjun Sahgal, MD[12], Erin Wong, BSc(C)[1] and Edward Chow, MBBS[1*

[1]Department of Radiation Oncology, Odette Cancer Centre, Sunnybrook Health Sciences Centre, University of Toronto, Toronto, Ontario, Canada
[2]Department of Surgery, Taipei Veterans General Hospital, National Yang-Ming University, Taipei, Taiwan
[3]Department of Gastroenterologic Surgery, Kaohsiung Medical University Hospital, Kaohsiung, Taiwan
[4]Department of Radiation Oncology, Cross Cancer Institute, Edmonton, Alberta, Canada
[5]Department of Radiation Oncology, Bank of Cyprus Oncology Centre, Nicosia, Cyprus
[6]Department of Orthopedic Oncology, Federal University of Sao Paulo, Sao Paulo, Brazil
[7]Department of Clinical Oncology, Tanta University Hospital, Tanta Faculty of Medicine, Tanta, Egypt
[8]Division of Gynaecology and Genitourinary Oncology,

* Correspondence: Professor Edward Chow, MBBS, MSc, PhD, FRCPC, Department of Radiation Oncology, Odette Cancer Centre, Sunnybrook Health Sciences Centre, 2075 Bayview Avenue, Toronto, Ontario, Canada M4N 3M5. E-mail: edward.chow@sunnybrook.ca

Department of Radiation Oncology, Regional Cancer Center, Trivandrum, Kerala, India
[9]Inserm CIE3, Saint Etienne University Hospital, Saint-Etienne, France
[10]Unit of Clinical Research, Innovation, and Pharmacology,
Saint Etienne University Hospital, France
[11]Department of Public Health and Institute of Epidemiology and Preventative Medicine,
National Taiwan University, Taipei, Taiwan
[12]Department of Radiation Oncology, Princess Margaret Hospital,
University of Toronto, Toronto, Ontario, Canada

Abstract

In advanced cancer patients, quality of life (QOL) is often a more meaningful clinical endpoint as patients often have shorter life expectancies and treatment intent is palliative in nature. Since 1993, the European Organization for Research and Treatment of Cancer Core 30 Questionnaire (EORTC QLQ-C30) has been widely used to study cancer-specific health-related quality of life. This study seeks to compare EORTC QLQ-C30 scores in patients with bone and brain metastases. Methods: The EORTC QLQ-C30 was used to assess QOL internationally in patients with bone metastases. A univariate linear regression model (GLM) was applied to detect significant differences between both groups on each QLQ-C30 scale at baseline. To normalize the distribution, natural log-transformations were applied for each C30 summary scale. Results: KPS, gender, marital status, and primary cancer site were found to be significantly different between the two groups (p < 0.005). After accounting for these confounding factors, three EORTC-C30 scales found to be significantly different between patients with bone and brain metastases: physical functioning (p < 0.0001), role functioning (p < 0.0004), and pain scale (p < 0.0001). Bone metastases patients reported worse pain and physical functioning, while brain metastases exhibited greater role functioning deficits. Conclusion: Patients with bone metastases have more pain and reduced physical functioning. However, patients with brain metastases have more severe role functioning deficits. The use of disease-specific assessment modules such as the QLQ-BM22 and QLQ-BN20 will enhance the capture of relevant QOL in these populations.

Keywords: Bone metastases, brain metastases, EORTC, quality of life, EORTC QLQ-C30, palliative care, advanced cancer patients

Introduction

Quality of life (QOL) is a subjective, multidimensional measurement that reflects physical symptoms, functional ability, psychosocial aspects and health perceptions of patients (1). In advanced cancer patients, QOL is often a more meaningful clinical endpoint for clinical trials as due to shorter patient life expectancies; traditional endpoints such as survival are less relevant (2). In most cases, QOL assessments are performed in the form of questionnaires, completed by either the patient themselves, or via proxy. These assessments tools can provide information about patient's responsiveness and effectiveness of treatment (1).

Bone metastases are a frequent complication of advanced cancer. Breast and prostate carcinomas commonly metastasize to bone, occurring in their disease trajectory in up to 70% of patients (3). In addition, 15% to 30% of lung, thyroid, and renal cell carcinomas metastasize to bone (3). Although the exact incidence of bone metastases is unknown, it is estimated that 70% to 85% of cancer patients have bone metastases at the time of autopsy (4). Bone metastases are a common cause of intractable pain as well as skeletal related events (SREs). Traditionally, primary outcomes in clinical trials examining bone metastases have focused on objective endpoints of these SREs, such as pathological fractures, spinal cord compression, analgesic use, or hypercalcemia (5). However, patient's health-related quality of life has recently garnered increased focus (6).

Brain metastases (BN) are the most common intracranial neoplasm in adults. The majority of BN originate from primary lung (40–50%), breast (15–25%) or skin (5–20%) cancer (7,8). BN occurs in 10–15% of patients with advanced cancer (9,10), and depending on the location may cause patients to present with a wide range of neurological symptoms including headaches, focal weakness, mental disturbances, behavioural changes, seizures, speech difficulties, and ataxia (11). While survival and local brain tumour control are important endpoints, quality of life (QOL) is arguably the more relevant given the prognosis of this patient population (12).

Since 1993, the European Organization for Research and Treatment of Cancer core questionnaire (EORTC QLQ-C30) has been widely used in the study of cancer-specific QOL (13, 14). It is an internationally validated questionnaire which is commonly used to assess QOL in advanced cancer patients, such as patients with bone or brain metastases.

This instrument can be administered with relative ease, which can reduce the burden on patients and avoid unnecessary hospital appointments. To date, comparisons with the palliative cancer patient setting among broad patient subgroups have not been made. This study seeks to compare EORTC QLQ-C30 scores in bone and brain metastases patients and delineate how these conditions affect patients' QOL.

Methods

Patients with bone metastases were accrued internationally from March 2010 until January 2011, under the supervision of the EORTC QOL module development group for the development of the bone metastases module (the QLQ-BM22) (6). These patients were recruited from Edmonton, Alberta, Canada; Kaohsiung, Taiwan; Kerala, India; Nicosia, Cyprus; Sao Paulo, Brazil; Taipei, Taiwan; Tanta, Egypt; and Toronto, Ontario, Canada. Patients were required to be aged 18 years with histological confirmation of their primary cancer and radiologic evidence of bone metastases. To be included the patients also had to be cognitively able to complete the questionnaire and must understand the language used in the questionnaire. All EORTC questionnaires were translated into the region's primary language by at least 2 fluent translators to ensure accuracy. Languages used in the current included Arabic, English, French, Greek, Malayalam, Mandarin (Taiwan), and Portuguese (Brazil).

Within the same time period, patients undergoing whole-brain radiotherapy (WBRT), radiosurgery/gamma knife and/ or neurosurgical resection for their brain metastases from Sunnybrook Odette Cancer Centre were approached. To be eligible patients were required to be aged 18 years and speak English with documented single or multiple brain metastases. Both studies received ethics approval from their respective hospital ethics boards.

EORTC QLQ-C30

The QLQ-C30 is a 30-item quality of life instrument validated for the assessment of QOL in patients with advanced cancer (13). It contains five subscales: physical functioning, role functioning, emotional functioning, cognitive functioning and social functioning (13). It also entails six single-item symptom scales (sleep disturbance, constipation, diarrhoea, dyspnoea, appetite loss and financial issues), three symptom scales (fatigue, pain and nausea) and a single global health status scale (13).

Items were rated on a 4 point Likert scale from 1 'not at all' to 4 'very much' with the exception of the last two items assessing overall health and overall QOL which were scored from 1 (very poor) to 7 (excellent). The responses for each scale and single item were translated according to published manuals into scores from 0-100 (14). In symptom scales, a high score is reflective of greater severity. In contrast, on the functional scales and the global QOL scale, higher scores indicate greater functional ability.

Statistical analyses

Descriptive analysis was conducted in all patients, in patients with bone or brain metastases, respectively. The mean, standard deviation (SD), median, and ranges were calculated for continuous demographic variables, and categorical variables were expressed as proportions of patients.

To compare baseline characteristics, between patients with bone metastases and patients with brain metastases, Chi-squared tests were applied for categorical variables and the Wilcoxon rank-sum test was performed for age and KPS. A two-sided p-values of <0.05 was considered statistically significant.

A simple univariate linear regression model (GLM) was applied to detect significant differences between patient groups on each QLQ-C30 scale (after scoring). Each unscored subscales was compared between both patient groups using a Chi-square test. To normalize the distribution, natural log-transformations were applied for each QLQ-C30 summary scale. The outcomes were natural log scales of each QLQ-C30 scale and the independent variable was treated as binary (1=bone metastases, 0=brain metastases). No confounding factors were considered at this step.

The coefficient, standard error (SE) of the coefficient, p-value and mean square error (MSE) of the model were calculated. The MSE refers to the estimate of error variance: residual sum of squares divided by the number of degrees of freedom. Relative to the smaller estimated error variance, MSE was close to zero. Positive coefficient of a group indicated that patients with bone metastases have higher score than patients with brain metastases.

The scored QLQ-C30 results were further analyzed adjusting for confounding factors previously identified in the comparison of demographics between both groups.

To see which QLQ-C30 scales had statistical significant differences between patients with bone and brain metastases, after accounting for the confounders (KPS, gender, married status, and primary cancer site), each confounding factor was treated as a categorical variable. For gender, 1 indicated female and 0 male; for marital status, 1 indicated married and 0 indicated others. Primary cancer site was treated as an unordered categorical variable (breast, lung, prostate, gastrointestinal, renal cell, and other). Simple univariate linear regression analysis was performed.

The outcome was a natural log scale of each C30 scale. The independent variables were the binary variable of group (1=BM, 0=BN) and 4 the confounders. Therefore, the model used was: $ln(C30\ scale) = a + b \times (Group) + c \times (KPS) + d \times (Gender) + e \times (Married) + f \times (Primary\ Cancer\ Site)$. To account for multiple comparisons, a Bonferroni adjusted p-value of p< 0.002 (0.05/30 items) was considered statistically significant. Analyses were performed using Statistical Analysis Software (SAS version 9.2 for Windows) and PROC GLM was applied for modelling.

Results

Table 1. Demographics in Patients with Bone Metastases and in Patients with Brain Metastases

	Total N=444	Bone Metastases N=397	Brain Metastases N=47	p-value *
Age (years)				0.1012
Mean (SD)	58.3 (12.9)	58.0 (13.0)	60.6 (11.9)	
Median (range)	57 (24-95)	57 (26-95)	61 (24 – 86)	
KPS at baseline				<0.0001
Mean (SD)	81.9 (16.9)	83.2 (16.8)	70.4 (13.3)	
Median (range)	80 (30-100)	80 (30-100)	70 (40-100)	
Gender				0.0067
Female	328 (73.87%)	301 (75.82%)	27 (57.45%)	
Male	116 (26.13%)	96 (24.18%)	20 (42.55%)	
Married status				<0.0001
Married	149 (66.82%)	114 (64.77%)	35 (74.47%)	
Widowed	27 (12.11%)	21 (11.93%)	6 (12.77%)	
Single	20 (8.97%)	15 (8.52%)	5 (10.64%)	
Other	27 (12.11%)	26 (14.77%)	1 (2.13%)	
Primary cancer site				<0.0001
Breast	287 (64.64%)	271 (68.26%)	16 (34.04%)	
Lung	48 (10.81%)	31 (7.81%)	17 (36.17%)	
Prostate	45 (10.14%)	45 (11.34%)	0 (0.00%)	
Gastrointestinal	16 (3.60%)	10 (2.52%)	6 (12.77%)	
Renal Cell	11 (2.48%)	9 (2.27%)	2 (4.26%)	
Other	37 (8.33%)	31 (7.81%)	6 (12.77%)	
Patients status				0.1191
Outpatient	404 (91.20%)	364 (91.92%)	40 (85.11%)	
Inpatient	39 (8.80%)	32 (8.08%)	7 (14.89%)	
Previous systemic treatment				0.6047
Yes	154 (69.06%)	123 (69.89%)	31 (65.96%)	
No	69 (30.94%)	53 (30.11%)	16 (34.04%)	

* P-value was obtained by Chi-squared test for categorical variables and Wilcoxon rank-sum test for age and KPS.

A total of 47 patients with brain metastases and 400 patients with bone metastases were enrolled. Among the 400 patients with bone metastases, 3 patients were missing responses for some of the QLQ-C30 items and were excluded from the analysis. Baseline patient characteristics of the two study populations are summarized in Table 1.

Comparison of baseline characteristics

In a comparison of the demographics of both groups, KPS, gender, marital status, and primary cancer site were found to be significantly different between the two groups ($P < 0.005$). In patients with bone metastases the most common primary cancer sites were the breast (68%), followed by the prostate (11%), while in the brain metastases study population the most common primary cancers were of the lung (36%) and breast (34%). A greater proportion of patients with primary breast or prostate cancer and lower proportions of patients with primary lung, gastrointestinal or renal cell sites were seen in bone metastases patients compared to the brain metastases.

The bone metastases patient group also had higher KPS scores, more females, smaller proportions with married status when compared to patients with brain metastases. No significant differences between patient status, gender, age of patients who completed the assessment or proportion of patients whom received previous systemic therapy were found ($p > 0.005$).

Baseline quality of life

Patients with bone metastases reported average functional scores (mean ± standard deviation) ranging from 58.3 to 73.4 (Table 2). Cognitive functioning was found to be the best (highest average score) within this patient population and role functioning the worst (lowest average score). Overall, cognitive and emotional functioning were found to be better than physical, social, or role functioning. Symptom scores ranged between 14.0 ± 21.61 and 49.3 ± 32.46 in the BM patient group. Pain (49.3 ± 32.46), fatigue (46.1 ± 27.83), and insomnia (40.9 ± 33.65) were the most severe symptoms, while nausea/ vomiting and diarrhoea were the least severe with scores of 14.0 ± 21.61 and 10.9 ± 19.80, respectively.

Similar results were seen within patients with brain metastases. This group reported functional scores between 55.1 ± 28.73 (role functioning) and 73.4 ± 23.74 (cognitive functioning). The EORTC QLQ-30 symptom scores ranged between 4.3 ± 16.47 and 44.1 ± 28.36. In this group, fatigue was the most severe symptom (44.1 ± 28.36), followed by insomnia (39.7 ± 27.49). Diarrhoea was the least severe symptom (4.3 ± 16.47). Overall QOL scores were found to be slightly better in patients with brain metastases than patients with bone metastases, with scores of 57.4 ± 18.02 versus 50.3 ± 23.31 respectively.

Table 2. Converted Functional and Symptom Scores between Bone and Brain Metastases Patients at Baseline

		N	Mean	Std	Median	Min	Max
Functional Scales							
Physical Functioning	Group						
	BM-C30	390	63.6	27.90	66.7	0	100
	BN-C30	46	65.8	24.02	66.7	13	100
Role Functioning	Group	396	58.3	35.13	66.7	0	100
	BM-C30						
	BN-C30	46	55.1	28.73	50.0	0	100
Emotional Functioning	Group						
	BM-C30	397	66.2	24.71	66.7	0	100
	BN-C30	47	66.5	24.36	66.7	17	100
Cognitive Functioning	Group						
	BM-C30	397	73.4	23.74	83.3	0	100
	BN-C30	47	73.4	23.74	83.3	17	100
Social Functioning	Group						
	BM-C30	397	61.9	32.14	66.7	0	100
	BN-C30	47	59.2	29.04	66.7	0	100
Global health status / QOL	Group						
	BM-C30	397	50.3	23.31	50.0	0	100
	BN-C30	46	57.4	18.02	58.3	25	100
Symptom Scales							
Fatigue	Group						
	BM-C30	396	46.1	27.83	44.4	0	100
	BN-C30	46	44.1	28.36	38.9	0	100
Nausea / Vomiting	Group						
	BM-C30	397	14.0	21.61	0.0	0	100
	BN-C30	47	14.2	17.71	0.0	0	67
Pain	Group						
	BM-C30	397	49.3	32.46	50.0	0	100
	BN-C30	47	29.8	29.27	33.3	0	100
Dyspnoea	Group						
	BM-C30	395	22.6	26.35	33.3	0	100
	BN-C30	46	17.4	21.93	0.0	0	67
Insomnia	Group						
	BM-C30	397	40.9	33.65	33.3	0	100
	BN-C30	47	39.7	27.49	33.3	0	100
Appetite loss	Group						
	BM-C30	396	29.5	33.15	33.3	0	100
	BN-C30	47	32.6	32.96	33.3	0	100
Constipation	Group						
	BM-C30	396	27.1	31.65	33.3	0	100
	BN-C30	47	27.0	30.80	33.3	0	100
Diarrhoea	Group						
	BM-C30	396	10.9	19.80	0.0	0	100
	BN-C30	47	4.3	16.47	0.0	0	100
Financial Problems	Group						
	BM-C30	396	23.9	30.57	0.0	0	100
	BN-C30	47	29.8	32.03	33.3	0	100

BM-C30: Patients with bone metastases, BN-C30: patients with brain metastases.

Comparison of EORTC QLQ-C30 scores unadjusted for confounders

The findings of the simple univariate linear regression model are summarized in Table 3.

Table 3. Comparing both groups by Univariate Linear Regression Analysis: without accounting for Confounders

At Baseline	Coefficient	SE	p-value *	MSE
Global Health Status	-0.308	0.139	0.0273	0.798
Physical Functioning	-0.198	0.150	0.1853	0.921
Role Functioning	-0.205	0.233	0.3789	2.239
Emotional Functioning	-0.073	0.112	0.5170	0.531
Cognitive Functioning	-0.049	0.104	0.6395	0.456
Social Functioning	-0.165	0.196	0.4015	1.619
Fatigue	0.103	0.176	0.5608	1.282
Nausea / Vomiting	-0.164	0.264	0.5338	2.921
Pain	1.070	0.226	<0.0001	2.142
Dyspnoea	0.315	0.294	0.2832	3.551
Insomnia	-0.236	0.275	0.3901	3.173
Appetite loss	-0.233	0.306	0.4473	3.935
Constipation	-0.035	0.303	0.9079	3.854
Diarrhoea	0.675	0.246	0.0062	2.534
Financial Problems	-0.354	0.301	0.2402	3.800

Natural log-transformation was applied for each C30 scale. MSE = Mean square error;
* Bonferroni adjusted p-value < 0.002 was considered statistical significant.

Only the C30 symptom scale of pain was found to be significantly different (p < 0.0001). Patients with bone metastases had more pain compared to patients with brain metastases (average scale score of 49.3 vs. 29.8). Significant differences between BM and BN in other scales were not seen (p > 0.002).

Comparison of EORTC QLQ-C30 scores adjusting for confounders

After accounting for the confounding factors of KPS, gender, marital status, and primary cancer site, two other scales were found to be significantly different as well (Table 4).

The three EORTC-C30 scales found to be significantly different between patients with bone metastases and patients with brain metastases were physical functioning (p < 0.0001), role functioning (p = 0.0004), and pain scale (p < 0.0001). Patients with brain metastases reported better physical functioning, with an average score of 65.8 compared to 63.6. However, patients with bone metastases are more likely to have better role functioning, with average scores of 58.3 and 55.1 respectively.

As previously seen in the comparison of EORTC QLQ-C30 scores without confounding factor adjustment, patients with bone metastases had more problems on only one symptom scale, pain, compared to patients with brain metastases. Other scales had no significant difference between patient groups after adjusting for confounders (p > 0.002).

Table 4. Comparing both groups by Univariate Linear Regression Analysis: accounting for Confounders

At Baseline	p-value of Group (bone vs. brain)	*p-value of Confounders*				
		KPS	Gender	Married Status	Primary Cancer Site	MSE
Global Health Status	0.0040	0.0004	0.4876	0.2500	0.4287	0.778
Physical Functioning	<0.0001	<.0001	0.2246	0.5015	0.5432	0.631
Role Functioning	0.0004	<.0001	0.0072	0.6439	0.0207	1.589
Emotional Functioning	0.0416	<.0001	0.8024	0.4256	0.5986	0.479
Cognitive Functioning	0.1066	0.0011	0.0157	0.1766	0.0143	0.436
Social Functioning	0.0037	<.0001	0.0057	0.7747	0.2703	1.362
Fatigue	0.1109	<.0001	0.2296	0.9093	0.9650	1.102
Nausea / Vomiting	0.8496	0.4646	0.0638	0.8062	0.2882	2.924
Pain	<0.0001	<.0001	0.9134	0.5854	0.5589	1.816
Dyspnoea	0.5150	0.0544	0.5112	0.0198	0.9200	3.542
Insomnia	0.9222	0.0047	0.8198	0.4667	0.1865	3.095
Appetite loss	0.3281	<.0001	0.4048	0.4850	0.1238	3.554
Constipation	0.4674	<.0001	0.9498	0.2227	0.7708	3.625
Diarrhoea	0.0132	0.4190	0.9807	0.2575	0.9102	2.544
Financial Problems	0.4677	0.0001	0.3495	0.0851	0.0004	3.463

Natural log-transformation was applied for each C30 scale. MSE = Mean square error;
* Bonferroni adjusted p-value < 0.002 was considered statistical significant.

Following analysis, the confounders of gender and married status were no longer significant; primary cancer site was only significant associated with financial problems. KPS was still significantly related to all C30 scales, except for nausea/vomiting, dyspnoea, and diarrhoea.

Discussion

Quality of life is an important endpoint, especially in advanced cancer patient clinical trials. To our knowledge, this is the first study to compare baseline EORTC QLQ-C30 baseline scores of patients with brain metastases to patients with bone metastases. After adjusting for confounding factors (KPS, gender, marital status, and primary cancer site), patients with bone metastases were found to have significantly greater pain than those with brain metastases. These patients also had significantly better role functioning. In comparison, patients with brain metastases functioned better physically than those with bone metastases. Other scores were not found to be significantly different. This may be a result of how both patient groups experience these symptoms and have similar functional difficulties.

Localized pain commonly presents itself in bone metastases patients, occurring in 75% of patients (15). Therefore, the significantly greater pain in bone metastases patients found upon analysis was expected. It is for this reason, in a study of QOL with bone metastases, thirty-nine of all forty-seven studies measured the intensity and frequency of bony pain (16). Similarly, reduced physical functioning was expected in patients with bone metastases. Along with SREs, decreased mobility and spinal instability are common symptoms that manifest over the course of bone disease (17,18). These symptoms would equate to higher raw scores of items 1-5 of the QLQ-C30, indicating reduced physical functioning, as patients would be unable to do strenuous activity and would have reduced ambulatory capabilities.

The clinical presentation of brain metastases is similar to that of any intracranial mass lesions. Two thirds of patients with brain metastases develop neurological symptoms during the course of their illness (19). Signs and symptoms of brain metastases can be divided into a "generalized" category and a "focal" variety. Typically, generalized symptoms refer to symptoms secondary to cerebral edema and/or increased intracranial pressure; this includes symptoms such as headaches, nausea/vomiting, and cognitive problems (20). The "focal" variety, which frequently results from localized compression or destruction of brain tissue, usually manifests as weakness, numbness, speech disturbance, or seizures (20). It was expected that the domain of cognitive functioning would be different in patients with bone and brain metastases. Although cognitive functioning was the most impacted, our analysis shows no such indication, with similar scores in both patient groups. The similar cognitive functional deficits experienced by both patient groups may be resulting from different symptoms. In patients with bone metastases, deficits may be caused by pain, which can limit cognitive aspects such as concentration (21, 22). On the QLQ-C30, this could result in a similar score to what brain metastases patients experience because of dizziness or other neurological symptoms. Although more validation is necessary and compliance issues need to be minimized, specific modules tailored to symptoms of brain metastatic disease such as the FACT-BR or EORTC QLQ-BN20 should be employed to accurately distinguish the root of difficulties experienced (23,24). This would limit the ambiguity and focus assessments on issues of importance to patients.

A similar conclusion can be drawn from how lower role functioning was found in patients with brain metastases. From only the two role functioning items in the QLQ-C30, it is difficult to pinpoint why patients are unable to perform their regular daily activities. It is likely a result of the aforementioned generalized and focal symptoms, in particular fatigue and nausea/ vomiting (25). However, in the analysis, no significant differences in these symptom scales were found between brain and bone metastases patients. Nonetheless, this difference may still be a result of fatigue and nausea due to the heterogeneity in patients' understanding of these symptoms (26). Patients can refer to nausea as a brief episode lasting mere seconds or a prolonged period of symptoms that can last hours or days (27). In many cases, nausea episodes are ambiguous and symptoms can be mistaken or confused by patients. Future studies should seek to evaluate how individual symptoms correlate and affect patients' ability to maintain their norm activities.

This study is primary limited as patients are selected for inclusion by their reason for referral. This means that in the patient populations, patients were not excluded if they had other illnesses or metastases so long as the reason for their referral was for treatment of their brain or bone metastases. If a patient required palliative radiotherapy for painful bone metastases but also had brain metastases for which they previously were treated, they would be included solely in the bone metastases group, which may confound our findings. Heterogeneity within the two subgroups is also likely to be present. While patient status was accounted for, we are unable to comment as to where patients were on the continuum of disease trajectory. This may potentially influence our analysis as symptoms experienced by patients increase in severity with reduced survival. The patient population size was also vastly different, with almost eight times the patient population in the bone metastases group than the brain metastases group. Perhaps within a larger brain metastases population, more significant differences between these two subgroups would be exhibited.

In conclusion, the difficulties bone and brain metastases patients experience are different in several ways. Patients with bone metastases have more pain and reduced physical functioning. However, patients with brain metastases have more severe role functioning deficits. With use of the QLQ-C30, it is also found that there is ambiguity regarding the root of patient issues. Future studies that require more comprehensive disease-specific findings should include disease-specific assessment modules such as the QLQ-BM22 and QLQ-BN20. Important domains such as the minimal clinically important difference should also be established in individual subgroups of patients to assist in clinical trial design.

Acknowledgments

We thank the generous support of Bratty Family Fund, Michael and Karyn Goldstein Cancer Research Fund, Joseph and Silvana Melara Cancer Research Fund, and Ofelia Cancer Research Fund.

Conflict of interest statement: Nil

References

[1]   Chow E, Hoskin P, van der Linden Y, Bottomley A, Velikova G. Quality of life and symptom end points in palliative bone metastases trials. Clin Oncol (R Coll Radiol) 2006;18(1):67-9.

[2]   Zeng L, Chow E, Zhang L, Tseng LM, Hou MF, Fairchild A, et al. An international prospective study establishing minimal clinically important differences in the EORTC QLQ-BM22 and QLQ-C30 in cancer patients with bone metastases. Support Care Cancer 2012 May 6.

[3]   Mundy GR. Metastasis to bone: causes, consequences and therapeutic opportunities. Nat Rev Cancer 2002;2(8):584-93.

[4]   Soni MK, Cella D. Quality of life and symptom measures in oncology: an overview. Am J Manag Care 2002;8(18 Suppl):S560-73.

[5]   Major PP, Cook R. Efficacy of bisphosphonates in the management of skeletal complications of bone metastases and selection of clinical endpoints. Am J Clin Oncol 2002;25(6 Suppl 1):S10-8.

[6]   Chow E, Nguyen J, Zhang L, Tseng LM, Hou MF, Fairchild A, et al. International field testing of the reliability and validity of the EORTC QLQ-BM22 module to assess health-related quality of life in patients with bone metastases. Cancer 2012;118(5):1457-65.

[7]   Schouten LJ, Rutten J, Huveneers HA, Twijnstra A. Incidence of brain metastases in a cohort of patients with carcinoma of the breast, colon, kidney, and lung and melanoma. Cancer 2002;94(10):2698-2705.

[8]   Barnholtz-Sloan JS, Sloan AE, Davis FG, Vigneau FD, Lai P, Sawaya RE. Incidence proportions of brain metastases in patients diagnosed (1973 to 2001) in the Metropolitan Detroit Cancer Surveillance System. J Clin Oncol 2004;22(14):2865-72.

[9]   Chamberlain MC. Brain metastases: a medical neuro-oncology perspective. Expert Rev Neurother 2010;10(4):563-73.

[10]   Sperduto PW, Chao ST, Sneed PK, Luo X, Suh J, Roberge D, et al. Diagnosis-specific prognostic factors, indexes, and treatment outcomes for patients with newly diagnosed brain metastases: a multi-institutional analysis of 4,259 patients. Int J Radiat Oncol Biol Phys 2010;77(3):655-61.

[11]   Posner JB. Management of central nervous system metastases. Semin Oncol 1977;4(1):81-91.

[12]   Caissie A, Nguyen J, Chen E, Zhang L, Sahgal A, Clemons M, et al. Quality of Life in Patients With Brain Metastases Using the EORTC QLQ-BN20+2 and QLQ-C15-PAL. Int J Radiat Oncol Biol Phys 2012;83(4):1238-45.

[13]   Aaronson NK, Ahmedzai S, Bergman B, Bullinger M, Cull A, Duez NJ, et al. The European Organization for Research and Treatment of Cancer QLQ-C30: a quality-of-life instrument for use in international clinical trials in oncology. J Natl Cancer Inst 1993;85(5):365-76.

[14]   Fayers P, Aaronson N, Bjordal K, Groenvold M, Curran D, Bottomley A editors. The EORTC QLQ-C30 scoring manual (3rd edition). Brussels: European Organisation for Research and Treatment of Cancer, 2001.

[15]   Wagner G. Frequency of pain in patients with cancer. Recent Results Cancer Res 1984;89:64-71.

[16]   Tharmalingam S, Chow E, Harris K, Hird A, Sinclair E. Quality of life measurement in bone metastases: A literature review. J Pain Res 2008;1:49-58.

[17]   Nielsen OS, Munro AJ, Tannock IF. Bone metastases: pathophysiology and management policy. J Clin Oncol 1991;9(3):509-24.

[18]   Goetz MP, Callstrom MR, Charboneau JW, Farrell MA, Maus TP, Welch TJ, et al. Percutaneous image-guided radiofrequency ablation of painful metastases involving bone: a multicenter study. J Clin Oncol 2004;22(2):300-6.

[19]   Cairncross JG, Kim JH, Deck MD, Posner JB. Radiation therapy of brain metastases. Trans Am Neurol Assoc 1979;104:252-5.

[20]   Shaffrey ME, Mut M, Asher AL, Burri SH, Chahlavi A, Chang SM, et al. Brain metastases. Curr Probl Surg 2004;41(8):665-741.

[21]   Kenefick AL. Pain treatment and quality of life: reducing depression and improving cognitive impairment. J Gerontol Nurs 2004;30(5):22-9.

[22]   Padilla GV, Ferrell B, Grant MM, Rhiner M. Defining the content domain of quality of life for cancer patients with pain. Cancer Nurs 1990;13(2):108-15.

[23]   Lien K, Zeng L, Nguyen J, Cramarossa G, Cella D, Chang E, et al. FACT-Br for assessment of quality of life in patients receiving treatment for brain metastases: a literature review. Expert Rev Pharmacoecon Outcomes Res 2011;11(6):701-8.

[24]   Leung A, Lien K, Zeng L, Nguyen J, Caissie A, Culleton S, et al. The EORTC QLQ-BN20 for assessment of quality of life in patients receiving treatment or prophylaxis for brain metastases: a literature review. Expert Rev Pharmacoecon Outcomes Res 2011;11(6):693-700.

[25]   Bower JE, Ganz PA, Desmond KA, Rowland JH, Meyerowitz BE, Belin TR. Fatigue in breast cancer survivors: occurrence, correlates, and impact on quality of life. J Clin Oncol 2000;18(4):743-53.

[26]   Olver I, Molassiotis A, Aapro M, Herrstedt J, Grunberg S, Morrow G. Antiemetic research: future directions. Support Care Cancer 2011;19(Suppl 1):S49-55.

[27]   Dennis K, Maranzano E, De Angelis C, Holden L, Wong S, Chow E. Radiotherapy-induced nausea and vomiting. Expert Rev Pharmacoecon Outcomes Res 2011;11(6):685-92.

In: Pain Management Yearbook 2013
Editor: Joav Merrick

ISBN: 978-1-63117-944-0
© 2014 Nova Science Publishers, Inc.

Chapter 5

Asymptomatic presentation of lung and bone metastases in a patient with breast cancer

Michael Poon, MD(C)*, Emily Chen, BSc(C), Linda Probyn, MD, Liang Zeng, BSc(C), Natalie Lauzon, MRTT, Lori Holden, MRTT and Edward Chow, MBBS

Rapid Response Radiotherapy Program, Department of Radiation Oncology, Odette Cancer Centre, Sunnybrook Health Sciences Centre, University of Toronto, Toronto, Ontario, Canada

Abstract

Bone metastases are often one of the first signs of disseminated disease, especially in patients with breast cancer. It has been found that up to 79% of patients experience severe pain in the period before palliative therapy. This case describes a fifty year old female, who clinically presents with numerous pulmonary nodules yet remains asymptomatic. Despite multiple pelvic osteolytic lesions and progressive deterioration, the patient reports no pain, can bear weight, has good exercise tolerance and is not short of breath. This report highlights that clinical symptoms do not always reflect computer tomography imaging features or the extent of disease and metastases. Imaging features seen do not necessarily equate to the amount of pain experienced by patients.

Keywords: Asymptomatic, bone metastases, imaging features, breast cancer

---

* Correspondence: Professor Edward Chow MBBS, MSc, PhD, FRCPC Department of Radiation Oncology, Odette Cancer Centre, Sunnybrook Health Sciences Centre, 2075 Bayview Avenue, Toronto, ON Canada. E-mail: Edward.Chow@sunnybrook.ca

Introduction

Metastases are typically associated with clinical manifestations indicative of patients' health. Bone metastases are often one of the first signs of disseminated disease, especially in patients with breast cancer (1). In these patients, treatment intent is typically palliative aimed towards reducing pain, preventing fractures, maintaining activity and possibility prolonging survival.

In this report, we present the case of a middle aged woman whose radiological imaging reveal multiple pelvic and lung metastases associated with breast cancer, yet remains asymptomatic and painless.

Case report

A 50 year old female patient breast cancer patient was seen in Rapid Response Radiotherapy Program at the Odette Cancer Centre, Sunnybrook Hospital on September 29, 2011, presenting with multiple pulmonary nodules (see figure 1). In spite of these numerous pulmonary nodules, the patient was asymptomatic. The patient was noted to have been in Hong Kong for two weeks with her mother, whom was recently diagnosed with tuberculosis. Queries were raised as to whether pulmonary nodules were from infectious origins or were suspected lung metastases consistent with breast cancer. As such, a CAT scan guided biopsy of one of the pulmonary lesions was ordered. A whole body bone scan was ordered in search of possible bony lesions as well.

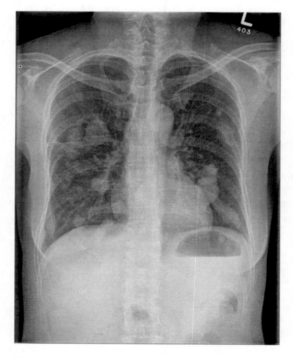

Figure 1. X-ray of chest (May 2012) showing the multiple pulmonary nodules.

The whole body bone scan completed October 18, 2011 showed bilateral ischial uptake (increased ischial tuberosity) and a subsequent follow-up CT identified multiple lytic lesions in her pelvis. This included a permeative destructive lesion in the right ischial tuberosity with mixed lytic and sclerotic components and bony expansion with a small amount of extraosseous soft tissue. A prominent lytic lesion involving the left ischial tuberosity extending into the posterior acetabular column with patchy areas of sclerosis was also found. This was consistent with metastases given the clinical history of breast cancer. Further deterioration was seen with a cortical breech at the inferior margin compatible with pathologic fracture and degenerative changes to the lower lumbar spine and sacroiliac joints. The core biopsy from the right lower lobe lung nodules was positive for breast malignancy, and was both estrogen and progesterone positive indicating possible response to hormone therapy.

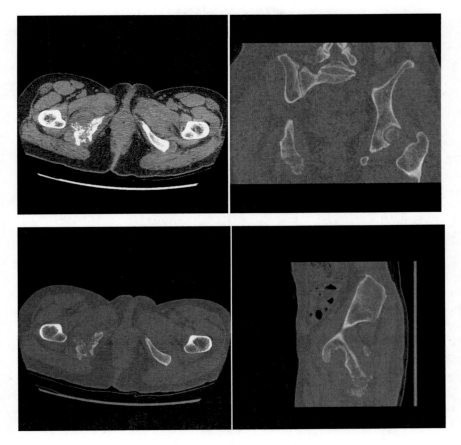

Figure 2. Multiple views of pelvic CT scan (April 2012) illustrating a permeative destructive lesion in the right ischial tuberosity with mixed lytic and sclerotic components.

Yet again, the patient remained totally asymptomatic, denying any pain, even when ambulating or bearing weight. She had good exercise tolerance and was not short of breath either. While X-ray scans did not portray a need for prophylactic surgery, the patient proceeded with prophylactic radiation treatment as the lesion was in a weight bearing area.

The patient received a prescribed dose of 30 Gy in 10 fractions and tolerated the treatment very well. There were no reports of episodes of pain flares, nausea or vomiting. The patient was restarted on Tamoxifen as of November 2011 and was tolerating it well. Previously, she stated she had only taken Tamoxifen for a short period of time due to liver discomfort. Clodronate was started December 2011.

Despite treatment, progressive osteolysis of the bone metastasis in the pelvis was shown on the repeat CAT scan April 2012 (Figure 2). Even with the deterioration shown on the scans, she remained completely asymptomatic and was feeling better than she had been in a long time. Unfortunately, the tumour was progressing with increased size of lung lesions in conjunction with some new lytic bony lesions.

Discussion

In the progression of metastatic disease, symptoms indicating deterioration of health are expected as part of a patient's normal disease trajectory. Diagnosis of bone metastases in breast cancer patients is typically associated with increased morbidity (2). These bone metastases clinically manifest as pain and can lead to many issues including skeletal related events such as spinal cord compression and use of radiation (2). It has been found that up to 79% of patients experience severe pain in the period before palliative therapy (3).

However, despite progressive deterioration and a worsening of her condition seen in imaging, this patient remained asymptomatic. She denied experiencing pain or discomfort, uncharacteristic of her physical state.

The imaging of this patient revealed extensive metastases. Multiple pulmonary nodules and lytic lesions were discovered without the expected clinical symptoms of coughing, dyspnea, or fatigue. For this reason, diagnostically, it is important to recognize clinical symptoms do not always reflect computer tomography imaging features or extent of disease. Imaging features seen do not necessarily equate to if pain is experienced or the severity of pain experienced by patients. A comprehensive assessment of patient symptoms is required.

There is a lack of consensus regarding the optimal treatment of asymptomatic patients with bone metastases. This contention arises from how treatment of bone metastases is primarily palliative in nature.

Among others, the aims of treatment are to relieve pain, improve function, and better quality of life (4). Therefore without clinical signs of distress, an optimal course of action requires careful consideration of a patient's immediate and future prognosis. Whether to actively observe or to opt to treat requires relative risk to benefit assessment and forethought towards potential treatment side effects.

Some investigators have recommended a no-treatment policy for asymptomatic patients (5). In this case, radiotherapy was ordered prophylactically as lesions were located in a weight bearing area of the pelvis. This was performed in the hopes of delaying the osteolytic progression of bone metastasis. Because of the primary being breast cancer, the patient was put on the respective systemic therapy.

Conclusion

Use of diagnostic imaging is extremely important, but is not always reflective of patients' clinical symptoms. Imaging features do not necessarily equate to pain response. Bone and lung metastases can sometimes present atypically as asymptomatic.

Acknowledgments

We thank the generous support of Bratty Family Fund, Michael and Karyn Goldstein Cancer Research Fund, Joseph and Silvana Melara Cancer Research Fund, and Ofelia Cancer Research Fund.

References

[1]   Nielsen OS. Palliative treatment of bone metastases. Acta Oncol 1996;35 Suppl 5:58-60.
[2]   Roodman GD. Mechanisms of bone metastasis. N Engl J Med 2004;350(16):1655-64.
[3]   Janjan N. Bone metastases: approaches to management. Semin Oncol 2001;28(4 Suppl 11):28-34.
[4]   Nielsen OS. Palliative radiotherapy of bone metastases: there is now evidence for the use of single fractions. Radiother Oncol 1999;52(2):95-6.
[5]   Nielsen OS, Munro AJ, Tannock IF. Bone metastases: pathophysiology and management policy. J Clin Oncol 1991;9(3):509-24.

In: Pain Management Yearbook 2013
Editor: Joav Merrick

ISBN: 978-1-63117-944-0
© 2014 Nova Science Publishers, Inc.

Chapter 6

Prophylaxis with radiation treatment after surgery to the cervical spine for established heterotopic ossification

Gemma Cramarossa, MD(C), Emily Chen, BSc (C),
Liang Zeng, BSc (C), Cyril Danjoux, MD, Kevin Higgins, MD,
Nicholas Phan, MD, Richard Aviv, MD, Natalie Lauzon, MRTT,
Kristopher Dennis, MD and Edward Chow, MBBS[*]
Odette Cancer Centre, Sunnybrook Health Sciences Centre,
University of Toronto, Toronto, Ontario, Canada

Abstract

Radiation treatment for prophylaxis of heterotopic ossification following surgery has not been comprehensively described in sites other than the pelvis. The present case describes a 54 year old male with previous spinal cord injury at the C5-C6 level who was experiencing dysphagia caused by the presence of osteophytes from heterotopic ossification. The osteophytes in that area of previous trauma were indenting the posterior pharyngeal wall at the C3-C4 and C4-C5 spinal levels, as evidenced by a CT scan. They were resected, followed by a single radiation dose of 8 Gy the following day. Since then, the patient has been feeling well with no difficulty in swallowing. Further studies are necessary to confirm that radiation is effective at preventing or at least decreasing the risk for heterotopic ossification after surgery to remove osteophytes in sites outside the pelvis.

Keywords: Osteophyte, cervical spine, radiation, heterotopic ossification

[*] Correspondence: Professor Edward Chow MBBS, MSc, PhD, FRCPC, Department of Radiation Oncology, Odette Cancer Centre, Sunnybrook Health Sciences Centre, 2075 Bayview Avenue, Toronto, ON, Canada M4N 3M5. E-mail: Edward.Chow@sunnybrook.ca

Introduction

Heterotopic ossification (HO) is the abnormal formation of bone in soft tissue outside the skeleton (1,2). It may be caused by a number of factors including central nervous system disorders, injury, bone or joint surgery or hereditary causes (1-3). Radiation treatment is often prophylactic in nature and there are few reports on successful irradiation for established HO outside the pelvis. Of these reports, all cases were established HO in the pelvis which were treated with single or multiple fractions (4,5). Although radiation treatment for prophylaxis of HO has been reported to be successful in many studies after bone and joint surgery to the pelvis, little is known about whether it is effective in the cervical spine and what the optimal dose of radiation would be. A single case report by Lo et al. in 1996 reported excision of an osteophyte in the C3-C4 region of the spine and administration of a single radiation dose of 6 Gy the following day (6). Recurrence of the osteophyte was reported, however noted to be less prominent.

The present case is a middle-aged quadriplegic who underwent surgery after the presence of osteophytes were discovered in his C spine and he subsequently received radiation treatment to the area to prevent the reformation of HO.

Case report

A 54 year old male was injured in a car accident 20 years ago which required a C5-C6 decompression and fusion as a consequence of a cervical spine fracture, resulting in quadriplegia. The patient has ankylosing spondylitis. He began to experience worsening dysphagia over a few months, beginning around May 2011. Initially he began to find it difficult to swallow pills, however he could still eat solid foods including meat and vegetables. By August 2011, he required a liquefied diet. He had been referred to the Rapid Response Radiotherapy Program (RRRP) at the Odette Cancer Centre, Sunnybrook Hospital for a consultation regarding lower back pain in May of 2011, but this treatment was put on hold as dysphagia became a more pressing concern.

In June of 2011, flexible nasopharyngoscopy was performed which confirmed the effects of osteophytes at the C3-C4 and C4-C5 spinal levels. The osteophyte around C3-C4 was quite large and was evidently causing an indentation in the patient's posterior pharyngeal wall, pushing the epiglottis anteriorly. A CT scan of the neck was ordered at the end of June which clearly displayed the prominent osseous overgrowths in the area. Overgrowth of the anterior longitudinal ligament was seen at inferior C3 and superior C4, with osteophytes extending 1 cm anterior to the C4 body proper. The displacement of the posterior pharyngeal mucosa was notable (Figure 1). The osteophyte at the level below, C4-C5, was smaller. A CT scan of the thoracic and lumbar spine revealed osteophytes in these areas as well, however they were not causing any pressing issues.

Those involved in the patient's care reasoned that the osteophyte slowly progressed over the years and was presenting a concern now because of the size it had reached and the area it was infringing upon. Surgical resection involving anterior cervical decompression and drilling of C3-C4 and C4-C5 osteophytes was performed on August 30, 2011 with no complications. An awake-tracheotomy was required because of the airway narrowing. The following day, he received a single radiation treatment of 8 Gy post-surgery to prevent osseous regrowth in that cervical spine region.

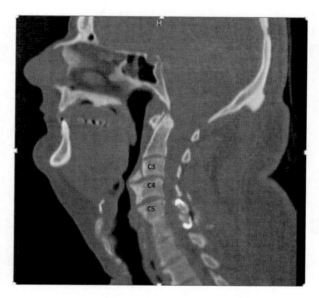

Figure 1. CT scan prior to resection of osteophytes. Narrowing of the pharynx is evident. A plain X-ray in October did not show any abnormal osseous growth and alignment of the cervical spine was normal. The patient was seen again at the RRRP in May 2012 and reported that he was no longer having problems with dysphagia. A CT scan in May showed minor C3-C4 and C4-C5 marginal osteophytes that appear stable (Figure 2). This imaging confirms that the difference between pre- and post-treatment is evident. Further follow-up imaging should continue to monitor whether the osteophytes remain stable and if heterotopic ossification reoccurs.

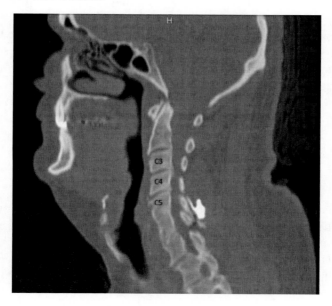

Figure 2. CT scan approximately 8 months after treatment. Minor osteophytes visible at C3-C4 and C4-C5.

Discussion

Heterotopic ossification may present following bone or joint surgery or as a consequence of central nervous system (CNS) injury (1-3). In patients undergoing surgery due to HO, as in this case report, there may be an increased risk of HO following surgery. Other risk factors include ankylosing spondylitis and osteoarthritis, as reported in studies involving surgery to the hip (7-10).

The incidence of HO in patients with spinal cord injuries is between 20% and 25%, likely a result of immobilization (3). The incidence of clinically significant HO is low following hip surgery, however radiographic evidence is present in approximately 56% of patients (11). Since the patient presented with HO and ankylosing spondylitis as well as a history of spinal cord injury, he was at high risk for recurrence of HO.

Due to the limited literature on radiation treatment for established HO as well as irradiation for HO in non-pelvic regions of the body, the patient's physicians discussed whether radiation treatment would be appropriate as well as what dose they deemed to be safe and effective. It was agreed given this patient's likelihood of developing post-surgery HO that radiation would be offered. The single case report by Lo et al. stated that a single dose of 6 Gy was given to their patient, who was also experiencing dysphagia, the day after C3-C4 osteophytes were removed (6). Follow-up studies revealed recurrence of the osteophyte. Taking this case into consideration, as well as other studies which reported a single dose of 8 Gy as effective for prophylaxis of HO in the hip, the decision to give a higher dose of 8 Gy was made in the hopes of preventing reoccurrence (12-13).

Further studies on radiation treatment for established HO and for the prophylaxis of HO in non-pelvis areas must be conducted to collect data on success rates as well as conclusively determine the optimal dose fractionation. Current literature may be lacking not only due to the low incidence of this phenomenon, but also may be due to unsuccessful radiation treatment which is not reported as often as successful results. Another reason for the limited literature may be due to lack of follow-up as these patients are rarely followed long term by radiation oncologists and surgical follow-up is variable. The patient in this report is not currently experiencing dysphagia or other related symptoms, however this finding is reported less than a year after treatment. Further studies should be conducted to assess if and how long after resection and radiation treatment clinically significant osteophytes may reappear in the cervical spine.

Conclusion

Radiation treatment may be effective for preventing reoccurrence of heterotopic ossification in the cervical spine. The potential benefit of irradiation must be weighed against the potential risk of creating a radiotherapy-induced malignancy. Radiation should be considered for patients at high risk of HO and the literature on the subject must be expanded in order for physicians to be informed when making radiation treatment decisions following surgery for established HO.

Acknowledgments

We thank the generous support of Bratty Family Fund, Michael and Karyn Goldstein Cancer Research Fund, Joseph and Silvana Melara Cancer Research Fund, and Ofelia Cancer Research Fund.

References

[1]   McCarthy EF, Sundaram M. Heterotopic ossification: a review. Skeletal Radiol 2005;34:609-19.

[2]   Vanden Bossche L, Vanderstraeten G. Heterotopic ossification: a review. J Rehabil Med 2005;37:129-36.

[3]   Garland DE. A clinical perspective on common forms of acquired heterotopic ossification. Clin Orthop Relat Res 1991;13-29.

[4]   Schaeffer MA, Sosner J. Heterotopic ossification: treatment of established bone with radiation therapy. Arch Phys Med Rehabil 1995;76:284-6.

[5]   Jang SH, Shin SW, Ahn SH, Cho IH, Kim SH. Radiation therapy for heterotopic ossification in a patient with traumatic brain injury. Yonsei Med J 2000;41:536-9.

[6]   Lo TCM, Pfeifer BA, Smiley PM, Gumley GJ. Case report: radiation prevention of heterotopic ossification after bone and joint surgery in sites other than hips. Br J Radiol 1996;69:673-7.

[7]   De Lee J, Ferrari A, Charnley J. Ectopic bone formation following low friction arthroplasty of the hip. Clin Orthop 1976;121:53–9.

[8]   Michelsson JE, Rauschning W. Pathogenesis of experimental heterotopic bone formation following temporary forcible exercising of immobilized limbs. Clin Orthop 1983;176:265–72.

[9]   Ekelund A, Brosjo O, Nilsson OS. Experimental induction of heterotopic bone. Clin Orthop 1991;263:102–12.

[10]   Kjaersgaard-Andersen P, Ritter MA. Prevention of formation of heterotopic bone after total hip arthroplasty. J Bone Joint Surg Am 1991;73:942–7.

[11]   Thomas BJ. Heterotopic bone formation after total hip arthroplasty. Orthop Clin North Am 1992;23:347–58.

[12]   Board TN, Karva A, Board RE, Gambhir AK, Porter ML. The prophylaxis and treatment of heterotopic ossification following lower limb arthroplasty. J Bone Joint Surg Br 2007;89:434-40.

[13]   Pellegrini VD Jr, Konski AA, Gastel JA, Rubin P, Evarts CM. Prevention of heterotopic ossification with irradiation after total hip arthroplasty: radiation therapy with a single dose of eight hundred centigray administered to a limited field. J Bone Joint Surg Am 1992;74:186-200.

In: Pain Management Yearbook 2013
Editor: Joav Merrick

ISBN: 978-1-63117-944-0
© 2014 Nova Science Publishers, Inc.

Chapter 7

Good surgical outcome and long survival in a patient with occipitocervical instability requiring occiput to C3 fixation

Michael Poon, MD(C), Michael Ford, FRCSC, Liang Zeng, MD(C),
Monique Christakis, FRCPC, Emily Sinclair, MRTT,
Natalie Lauzon, MRTT, Marko Popovic, BHSc(C)
*and Edward Chow, MBBS**

Rapid Response Radiotherapy Program, Department of Radiation Oncology,
Odette Cancer Centre, Sunnybrook Health Sciences Centre, University of Toronto,
Toronto, Ontario, Canada

Abstract

Spinal metastases in the occipitocervical junction typically present with pain secondary to neck instability. Non-traumatic upper cervical instabilities are quite rare and are usually connected to C1 or C2 metastasis, rheumatoid polyarthritis, infection or congenital malformations. In many cases, these instabilities are symptomatic and can cause bilateral or quadrilateral limb paresthesias, sharp neck pain or upper back pain. Occipitocervical fixation is typically required for the treatment of these conditions. Commonly, rigid constructs are employed where plates are typically fixed into place with screws or wires. This report presents the case of a breast cancer patient who had neck instability and extensive left C1 destruction. Surgical stabilization from the patient's posterior occiput to C3 was performed with excellent results. The patient regained ambulatory function, with

* Correspondence: Professor Edward Chow MBBS, MSc, PhD, FRCPC Department of Radiation Oncology, Odette Cancer Centre, Sunnybrook Health Sciences Centre, 2075 Bayview Avenue, Toronto, ON Canada. Email:Edward.Chow@sunnybrook.ca

no intra-operative or post-operative complications. Exceptional survival was observed as well, with an improvement in quality of life, for 47 months to date.

Keywords: Occipitocervical instability, occipitocervical fixation, oncology

Introduction

The third most common site of metastasis is the skeletal system, following lung and liver (1). It has been found that upon autopsy, vertebral body metastases have been found in over one third of all cancer patients (1). Metastases to this region may cause the loss of vertebral body structural integrity due to metastatic destruction and produce instability (1). For this reason, treatment of spinal metastases around the atlanto-axial region is required. However, flexion, extension, lateral bending, and rotation must be limited while accounting for poor bone quality and possible pannus (2). In many cases, these unique biomechanical and anatomical characteristics complicate occipitocervical stabilization procedures (3).

Patients with spinal metastases in the occipitocervical junction typically present with pain secondary to neck instability. Occipitocervical fixation is required for the treatment of upper cervical instabilities not related to trauma. Plates are typically fixed into place with screws or wires. However, this type of fixation is counter-indicated in the treatment of patients with osteoporosis or significant thinning of the occipital bone (4). Non-traumatic upper cervical instabilities are quite rare and are usually connected to C1 or C2 metastasis (as was the case with this patient), rheumatoid polyarthritis, infection or congenital malformations (4,5). We document the case of a woman with breast cancer who presents with cervical instability in her neck, whom by employing a rigid fixation construct has regained ambulatory function and has exceeded survival expectations.

Case report

A 70 year old female patient with breast cancer presented in the Rapid Response Radiotherapy Program (RRRP) at the Odette Cancer Centre, Toronto, Canada on May 16, 2008 with severe neck pain for consideration of radiation treatment. Pathology revealed that the tumor was an invasive ductal carcinoma, both estrogen and progesterone positive but negative for HER2/NEU. The sentinel lymph node biopsy at that time showed 1 of the 2 intramammary lymph nodes was positive for metastatic cancer. By recommendation of the surgeon, since one of the two sentinel lymph nodes was positive for tumor cells, a complete axillary lymph node dissection was planned. However, because of a complicating infection, the procedure was postponed. Upon the patient's full recovery, the possibility of carrying out the initial surgery with subsequent palliative radiotherapy was revisited.

An x-ray taken subsequent to her visit to RRRP indicated that the patient had an unstable neck. Review of the x-ray showed occipitocervical instability secondary to left C1 lateral mass destruction, causing the loss of ambulatory ability. An orthopedic surgeon was consulted with regard to how to treat the patient as well as viability of surgical intervention.

The patient was promptly scheduled for an occipital cervical fusion up to C3 on the posterior aspect of her cervical spine.

The patient underwent surgery to stabilize from her posterior occiput to C3 in June 2008. The right lateral mass of C1 and the right pars of C2 were noted to be destroyed by tumour on the computer tomography (CT) scan (see figure 1). No attempt was made to place instrumentation into those sites. Lateral mass screws were inserted into the left lateral mass of C1 and at C3; a pars screw was inserted at C2. The occipital plate was applied and a rod was appropriately contoured and fixed to the screws. Excellent purchase was obtained in C3 secondary to fairly large osteophytes with good quality sclerotic bone. Additional adjuvant fixation was carried out using an interspinous cable through the spinous processes of C2 and C3 around the rods of the construct. Polymethyl methacrylate (PMMA) bone cement was laid onto the posterior cervical spine and up onto the skull to further reinforce the construct. Intraoperative x-rays demonstrated the implants were in good position (see figure 2). There were no intraoperative complications and the patient was transported to the recovery room in good condition. Neural monitoring signals were intact throughout the procedure.

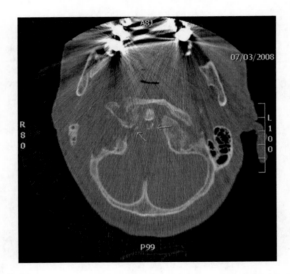

Figure 1. Cervical spine CT (July 2008) before surgery showing the destruction of the right lateral mass of C1 and the right pars of C2.

The patient returned to the RRRP on July 31, 2008. The results of her surgical stabilization were excellent; she reported that she was able to walk again. Post-operative radiation of 2000 cGy in 5 fractions was delivered to her neck and it was suggested that she should discuss the possibility of systemic treatment. For the last two years, she had been on tamoxifen. Since she had her stabilization, she has experienced mild stiffness in her neck but there is no pain in her neck nor radiating down her arms. She denies any paresthesias or weakness in the arm.

The patient is now 3-4 years post-occiput to C3 fusion for metastatic disease. The patient is doing extremely well. She is no longer taking pain medications and has managed to gain weight. She has developed some stiffness but still reports no pain or neurological symptoms.

X-ray shows minor degenerative listhesis that is stable below her construct with no other significant change (see figure 3). There is no evidence of any recurrence of tumor.

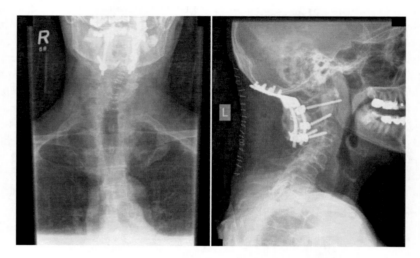

Figure 2. Intra-operative x-ray of cervical spine and occipitocervical (July 2008) demonstrating the implants to be in good position.

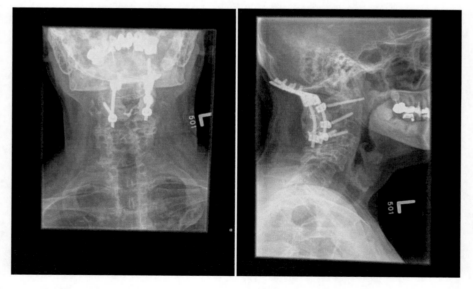

Figure 3. X-ray of cervical spine and occipitocervical construct (May 2012) 4 years post occipitocervical stabilization showing stable, minor degenerative listhesis below her construct with no other significant changes.

Discussion

Non-traumatic upper cervical instabilities are quite rare and are commonly connected to C1 or C2 metastasis. In many cases, these instabilities are symptomatic and can cause bilateral or quadrilateral limb paresthesias, sharp neck pain or upper back pain (6).This need for arthrodesis has buoyed various methods for occipitocervical fixation. As Garrido et al. (5) found, clinical complications rates are significantly lower in patients treated with rigid occipitocervical fixation methods (10%) compared to non-rigid (48%). In this case, a rigid internal fixation construct was used as it provides immediate stability and eliminates the need for poorly tolerated external fixators. The results were very positive; the patient regained ambulatory function with no intraoperative or post-operative complications to report.

In a retrospective study by Fourney et al. (3) of patients with C-1 or C-2 metastases that underwent surgery at the University of Texas MD Anderson Cancer Center between 1994 and 2001, the mean follow-up period was found to be 8 months. This study sought to review surgical strategies to stabilize the spine and advocated the use of posterior stabilization of the spine, citing the durable pain relief and preservation of ambulatory status (3). This result acquiesces with the similar outcome the patient presented experienced. However, through Kaplan-Meier analysis, the median survival was only reported to be 6.1 months (3). In the patient presented, not only was a good surgical outcome seen but much longer survival as well.

This exceptional survival was observed, with an improvement in quality of life, for 47 months to date. This far surpasses the median survival of 6.1 months previously expected from literature.

This case adds to the literature advocating the use of posterior stabilization of the spine and avoidance of poorly tolerated external fixators. In the 4 years post-occiput to C3 fusion, occipitocervical stabilization has provided pain relief and preservation of the patient's ambulatory status, improving the quality of her life.

Acknowledgment

We thank the generous support of Bratty Family Fund, Michael and Karyn Goldstein Cancer Research Fund, Joseph and Silvana Melara Cancer Research Fund, and Ofelia Cancer Research Fund. We thank Ms. Stacy Yuen for the secretarial support.

References

[1] Ratliff JK, Cooper PR. Metastatic spine tumors. South Med J 2004;97(3):246-53.

[2] Bongartz EB. Two asymmetric contoured plate-rods for occipitocervical fusion. Eur Spine J 2004;13(3):266-73.

[3] Fourney DR, York JE, Cohen ZR, Suki D, Rhines LD, Gokaslan ZL.Management of atlantoaxial metastases with posterior occipitocervical stabilization. J Neurosurg 2003;98(Suppl 2):165-70.

[4] Paquis P, Breuil V, Lonjon M, Euller-Ziegler L, Grellier P. Occipitocervical fixation using hooks and screws for upper cervical instability. Neurosurgery 1999;44(2):324-31.

[5] Garrido BJ, Myo GK, Sasso RC. Rigid versus nonrigid occipitocervical fusion: a clinical comparison of short-term outcomes. J Spinal Disord Tech 2011;24(1):20-3.

[6] Cook C, Brismee JM, Fleming R, Sizer PS, Jr. Identifiers suggestive of clinical cervical spine instability: a Delphi study of physical therapists. Phys Ther 2005;85(9):895-906.

In: Pain Management Yearbook 2013
Editor: Joav Merrick
ISBN: 978-1-63117-944-0
© 2014 Nova Science Publishers, Inc.

Chapter 8

Peer mentorship teaches social tools for pain self-management: A case study

*David Goldenberg, BS[1], Laura A Payne, PhD[*2],*
Loran P Hayes, BA[3], Lonnie K Zeltzer, MD[2],
and Jennie CI Tsao, PhD[2]

[1]Geisel School of Medicine at Dartmouth, Hanover, New Hampshire
[2]UCLA Pediatric Pain Program, David Geffen School of Medicine,
Los Angeles, California
[3]Department of Psychology, University of Utah, Salt Lake City, Utah,
United States of America

Abstract

Pain in children can become chronic and disabling, associated with high degrees of social isolation from schooling absences, physical limitations that prevent participation in social settings, and difficulties forming self-identity. This lack of social support network impairs social coping skills and can lead to worsening pain symptoms. Objective: In this case study, we describe a new program to disrupt the cycle of social isolation and chronic pain by emphasizing social coping skills via peer mentorship. The program aimed to utilize peers who have learned to self-manage their own chronic pain to assist patients with social coping skills to reduce isolation caused by chronic pain conditions. Study Group: Children and adolescents with chronic pain. Methods: This case describes the experience of a 17 year-old, African American boy with diffuse chronic body pain as a participant ("the mentee") in the program; his mentor was a 19 year-old girl with chronic pain associated with rheumatoid arthritis. The mentor received six hours of training and

* Correspondence: Laura A Payne, PhD, Pediatric Pain Program, David Geffen School of Medicine at UCLA, 10833 Le Conte Ave, 22-464 MDCC, Los Angeles, CA 90095-1752 United States. E-mail: LPayne@mednet.ucla.edu

she mentored the patient in 10 weekly sessions. Results: The mentee connected very well with his mentor through sharing similar pain experiences. He demonstrated improvements in positive affect, sleep, social coping, and perception of bodily pain on a variety of quantitative measures. Qualitative data from interviews also suggested that the mentee learned important social coping skills through peer mentorship. Conclusions: A peer mentoring approach to chronic pain may help alleviate social isolation in adolescents and result in improvements in a number of associated symptoms.

Keywords: Children, chronic pain, peer mentorship, social coping

Introduction

Chronic pain is recognized as an important and common condition estimated to occur in 25-45% of children (1,2). While some of these patients function effectively in educational and social settings, many are unable to control their pain, often resulting in excessive medication use, psychological problems such as depression and anxiety, sleeplessness, and impaired functioning in a variety of environments. Aside from the possibility of pain continuing into adulthood, chronic pain can have lasting consequences. It is well documented that impaired functioning in children with chronic pain is associated with psychological and social distress (3-5) as well as lower quality of life (3,6-9)

In particular, children with chronic pain often experience difficulties in social settings and subsequently experience higher degrees of social isolation than do healthy children. Forty percent of children with unexplained chronic pain problems were found to have social impairments (7). Because of absences in schooling, physical problems, and differences in self-identity, children with chronic pain have difficulties relating to peers and forming social connections (10). These children are often unable to discuss their pain with peers, and feel isolated because they have not encountered anyone with similar experiences (10).

Social functioning impairments are important because of the significant role of sociability in both physical and mental health. Access to social support may buffer the harmful effects of stress by enhancing coping. Additionally, social support networks have an influence on well-being regardless of stress level (11,12). Social withdrawal has been shown to lead to higher rates of depression in children (13). Furthermore, children without social support from peers also appear to have higher instances of chronic pain, and poorer recovery from pain conditions. Feelings of being an outsider and loneliness are associated with increased back pain and headache in school-age children (14). Social isolation also moderates the relationship of chronic pain and depression in patients with juvenile idiopathic arthritis, so that patients with higher levels of social isolation experiences higher depression with the same level of pain (15).

Social coping is an adaptive tool to reduce the negative impact of chronic pain through social relationships (16,17). Given the role of social support in the association of pain and mood, it is no surprise that social coping is an effective and necessary strategy for pain self-management. Children with chronic juvenile arthritis (18) and headaches (3) need increasing amounts of social coping in order to control pain and maintain quality of life. Social coping was found to be one of the most common means of pain coping among girls with chronic pain (16).

There appears to be a cyclical relationship where pain leads to deficient social networks and social isolation (10), which in turn leads to diminished social coping and increased mental and physical pain (14,15). Yet inadequate formation and utilization of social interventions for childhood pain are recognized as among the biggest obstacles to optimal pain management in children (19). An intervention focused on promoting social connection, reducing isolation, and learning pain self-management from a peer has the potential to disrupt this cycle and may help improve the quality of life for children with chronic pain.

We present a case study as an illustrative example of a new program that seeks to facilitate engagement in pain self-management skills via peer mentoring. By enhancing social contact, this program aims to interrupt this cycle of deficient pain coping and thereby enhance daily functioning, improve mood, and facilitate better sleep habits. The techniques emphasized in the Peer Mentor Program (PMP) are novel because they are taught through a social medium from a peer who has been through similar experiences as the patient. The purpose of teaching pain self-management in a social peer environment was to give patients firsthand experience utilizing social relationships to self-manage pain.

Case study

The mentee

The mentee was a 17 year old African American adolescent boy in the 12th grade with diffuse chronic pain that had been constant for almost one and a half years. Pain was localized to the lower back, leg above knee, head, neck, and around scapula edge. This pain first started when he became ill with flu-like symptoms for three weeks. He experienced recurrent bouts of illness throughout the following year that seemed to increase during stressful times. He also had great difficulty with sleep onset and sleep maintenance throughout the night. As a result of sleep problems, he was tired throughout the day and lacked energy. Prior to enrolling in the PMP, he had tried physical therapy and medication, but neither was effective in controlling pain nor establishing normal sleep schedules. He was treated successfully by the UCLA Pediatric Pain Program for fibromyalgia seven years prior to this study, and that specific pain had since resolved. At that time he received biofeedback and physical therapy, both of which were useful in managing fibromyalgia, but they had not been tried yet for his most recent pain condition.

Social relationships. The mentee had a close group of friends but, at times, felt uncomfortable in large groups. He got along with most people and was well-liked by peers, but did not feel comfortable discussing his pain with his peers. His pain prevented him from seeing friends as much as he would like, although he tried to see them once every week. Most of his social activities were sedentary due to chronic pain. He preferred to stay home when having pain flare-ups. He reported that his friends tried to be supportive, but he felt that they did not really understand the pain he was experiencing and how it affected him. His pain prevented him from interacting with peers because it limited his physical abilities, and also affected his mood. Additionally, sleep difficulties drained him of energy to spend with friends and family. He was also limited in his ability to travel.

School/hobbies. The mentee had attended the same school since kindergarten. He had extensive hobbies and interests, including teaching an after school class to elementary school students and being president of a local club. He was also involved with the school newspaper, wrote his own blog, and was passionate about photography. He volunteered with community service in foreign countries. He was very ambitious and academically driven. However, pain interfered with his education by causing extensive school absence and impaired concentration on studies. He also expressed his difficulty concentrating on exams because of his pain. Despite his chronic pain, the mentee was able to keep up his grades and perform in school.

The mentor

The mentor was a 19 year old university student who was diagnosed with juvenile arthritis when she was three years old. Three years prior to the PMP, she started to experience a constant headache that did not diminish with any treatment. She experienced no relief from medication, became incapacitated, and missed 10 weeks of school. She was seen at the UCLA Pediatric Pain Program and began therapies such as Iyengar yoga, acupuncture, and various medications to control pain and promote sleep. Using techniques learned from these therapies, she had learned to control her pain and to lead as normal a life as possible.

Mentor training

The mentor received six hours of instruction from doctoral-level research personnel before working with the assigned mentee. A written training manual included information on chronic pain conditions and strategies for pain self-management; specific goals for the peer relationship; guidance for teaching material about pain and pain-related behaviors; techniques based on cognitive-behavioral approaches to chronic pain to reinforce positive thinking and guide negative statements; tips for building interpersonal relationships; managing contentious issues (i.e., depression, suicidality, or other potential emergencies), and ending the relationship after 10 weeks of mentorship. The mentor was specifically instructed to educate the mentee about pain and accompanying behaviors, emotions, and thoughts, as well as provide an opportunity to discuss the mentee's own personal pain experience, and enhance confidence in his ability to manage his condition, while challenging negative thoughts and beliefs formed throughout his care. The mentor was also trained to draw from her own pain experiences to create an open environment where the mentee could feel comfortable discussing any apprehensions about his conditions and the recommended treatments, and to encourage the mentee to adhere to the treatment plan of prescribed therapies. She was specifically trained to be supportive, but not dogmatic.

Intervention: The Peer Mentor Program (PMP)

The mentor and mentee met for 10 sessions of 20-30 minutes over a period of nine weeks without missing any sessions. Phone calls were monitored by trained research personnel on a secure conference call line and no contact between the mentee and the mentor took place outside of the PMP phone sessions. Sessions were recorded and analyzed to determine the progress of the mentee-mentor relationship and gain insight into how the pair interacted. Both mentee and mentor had access to a slide presentation during each session so that specific information could be easily reviewed and explained (see additional details below). The intervention was developed by the UCLA Pediatric Pain Program team (LAP, JCIT, & LKZ) and was based on cognitive behavioral principles. The mentee was informed that he would be excluded from the study if he missed two consecutive or three of the 10 total sessions for non-emergency reasons; the mentor was only permitted to miss two sessions in total.

Measures

Several quantitative measures were utilized to examine changes in functioning over the course of the study. Qualitative interviews were also conducted by trained research personnel before and after the PMP to obtain data on how the mentee responded to the program. All of the following measures were given at baseline and four-month follow-up:

The Pittsburgh Sleep Quality Index (PSQI) is a measure to determine sleep quality and disturbance during the previous month (20). The Health Beliefs Scale (HBS) is a proprietary measure designed to assess the patience's confidence in treatments offered through the UCLA Pediatric Pain Program. The Positive and Negative Affect Schedule for Children (PANAS-C) is a 27-item questionnaire that has two global measures: positive affect and negative affect (21).

The Child Health Questionnaire (CHQ) is a multidimensional test to assess different components of physical and psychosocial health (22). Items on multi-item subscales (behavior, self-esteem, general health perceptions, and bodily pain) are averaged to attain raw scores which are then transformed into a 0-100 continuum for each subscale. Higher scores indicate better health and functioning (e.g., less pain). Two single-item subscales (global health and global behavior) are also transformed into a 0-100 continuum. The single-item subscale of change in health is treated as a categorical variable representing respondents' perceived change in health over the previous year. The CHQ is among the most widely used measures for children; reliability and validity tests have been extensive.

The Pain Coping Questionnaire (PCQ) is a measure that uses eight subscales to determine three overarching coping strategies used to control emotions associated with pain. We were particularly interested in the change of social coping skills. The seeking social support subscale consists of 5 items rated on a 1 (never) to 5 (very often) scale. Item responses are averaged to obtain the subscale score, with higher scores indicating greater use of that coping strategy. The PCQ has demonstrated reliability and validity (17).

Structure and content of the PMP sessions

The mentor would generally begin each session by asking for updates about how the mentee had been progressing with pain and then move on to the scheduled agenda for the week. Material was presented in a Powerpoint slide presentation that was available to both mentee and mentor. Throughout the session, the mentor would give personal anecdotes regarding how the slide presentations related to both her life and the mentee's day-to-day pain experience. The mentor would then conclude the session by asking the mentee if he had questions about the material and giving advice on how to incorporate the information into his own life.

Session one was an introduction to pain management in general and a chance for the mentee to get to know the mentor. The mentee and the mentor both gave the histories of their conditions, and explained their different experiences with pain. Session two provided information about the Complimentary Alternative Medicine (CAM) techniques offered through the UCLA Pediatric Pain Program. The mentee discussed his inhibitions about different approaches as well as his previous success with biofeedback controlling fibromyalgia seven years prior. Session three described the bidirectional nature of pain and mood and emphasized how controlling mood can reduce pain and vice versa. In this session, the mentee related a story about how he went to a concert and it distracted him from his pain. The mentor described how distractions are an effective means of controlling pain, and used this idea as a theme throughout several other sessions. In Session four, the mentee discussed his own behaviors when experiencing pain and how to modify these behaviors in order to reduce pain. The mentee described that when he felt pain he would usually lay down by himself although he acknowledged that, while it helped initially, after extended periods it made his pain worse. The mentor again reminded him of the value of maintaining an active lifestyle and focusing on continuing activities he enjoys. Session five described that pain can lead to negative thoughts that could affect mood, behaviors, and subsequent pain. The mentor recommended changing thoughts through distractions – to focus on positive thoughts and realize that negative thoughts are often exaggerated. Session six taught relaxation techniques to cope with chronic pain and reduce flare-ups. In this session, the mentor recommended to stop "stressing about stressing" and emphasized that worrying about stress will increase it. Session seven stressed the importance of prioritizing aspects of life and working on strategies to continue interests despite pain or other problems. Session eight addressed managing sudden increases in pain. The mentee learned techniques from biofeedback in the past to help relax during a pain flare-up and found it very helpful. However, he acknowledged that during current pain flare-ups he tried to force himself to keep working and felt that he did not have sufficient time to do the relaxation techniques. The mentor advised him to take time from his work to relax so that he could be more efficient. Session nine reviewed material from all previous sessions, and Session ten was reserved for feedback about the program and discussion about any progress made. Session nine generated conversation about previous techniques learned and reinforced key ideas that were brought up in previous sessions. The mentee explained that he had been doing biofeedback, aquatherapy, and talk therapy; all of which were helpful in relaxing, but biofeedback was the most effective of his techniques. Session nine was a very personal session because both participants expressed that they had really connected and understood each other. In this session, the mentee recounted how he used techniques to deal with a pain flare up. Instead of agonizing alone at home or pushing himself to continue to work while experiencing the pain, the mentee utilized the advice presented in Session eight and decided to get coffee with a friend. He was able to effectively resume his work after using these new social skills to self-manage his pain.

Results

The mentee reported considerable improvements in sleep over the course of the mentorship program. Prior to the study he reported that he would sleep 4-5 hours and take 60-70 minutes to fall asleep, while at the 4 month follow-up, he reported sleeping on average 5-6 hours and taking only 30-45 minutes to fall asleep. He improved on 5 of 8 PSQI domains of sleep including duration, sleep disturbance, overall sleep, sleep quality, need for medication to sleep, and global sleep score. However, he remained at the highest level for sleep latency, and had decreases in sleep efficiency and daytime dysfunction.

On the HBS, the mentee reported large increases in ratings of the techniques utilizing social coping skills on 4-month follow-up compared to baseline. He rated "Talk therapy" and "Talking with someone else who had pain" to help "a lot" from "a little" (2 to 4 on 5-point scale).

In addition to improvements on sleep and the perceived utility of social interactions, the mentee also showed great improvements on global mood measures. The PANAS-C negative affect subscale decreased from 36 to 22, while the positive affect subscale improved from 19 to 39.

The mentee also reported improvement across different measures of health. The CHQ showed improvements in global health [0 to 30], behavior [73 to 82], global behavior [85 to 100], self-esteem [30 to 55], general health perceptions [20 to 25], and change in health [2 to 3]. Bodily pain was also substantially improved at follow-up compared to baseline [40 to 20].

The mentee reported higher levels of social coping on the PCQ. His measure increased on the seeking social support subscale [2 to 3].

During the qualitative interviews, the mentee reported that he felt very comfortable with the mentor and felt that he was able to relate to her better than any other person he knows:

> "I don't think really anyone else truly understands, like, what I've been dealing with for the past couple of months and the past year, so it's nice to have someone who gets where I am coming from and also can provide constructive feedback for how to go about dealing with it."

The mentee found that the PMP was able to help him self-manage his pain because the mentor was going through similar situations and was able to provide feedback tailored directly to his experiences:

> "I think [the program] was really helpful. The peer mentor was really knowledgeable, and a lot of her issues with pain were really reflective of mine. So she was able to give me really concrete, salient advice for better ways to deal with my pain. And also she was a similar age group as me so she knew how my peer group would act, and the way I would approach situations with my friends and parents. I thought it was really helpful."

In Session ten, the mentee described how he used a technique he learned through the PMP to deal with a pain flare-up. Instead of internalizing pain, he decided to get coffee with a friend and distract himself from the pain. The mentee attributed this new technique to advice he learned from the mentor. The very nature of the mentor relationship taught the mentee how to talk to somebody else about his pain. He became more comfortable interacting with others and developed a new social tool to confront his pain. This allowed him to be productive throughout the rest of the day.

> Mentee: "I did what we talked about yesterday. Like if I wasn't feeling well. I left to get coffee with a friend after we met which was nice and then I went home and I was really efficient so that definitely helped."
> Mentor: "Good! So instead of not getting anything done, you had fun and got work done. Good! That's great, good to hear."

Utilizing social relationships to deal with his pain was the most useful technique that the mentee learned from the peer mentorship program.

> "I tend to, when I am not feeling well, to stay at home and wallow in how I am not feeling well or to try and get through my work even though it was kind of pointless, and [she taught] that I can go out and do something relaxing and then come back and do my work."

In addition to the gains in social pain self-management that the mentee learned, the program had an additional benefit – the peer mentor also learned new techniques to deal with her own pain. The mentorship relationship worked both ways, and after hearing the success the patient was having with biofeedback the mentor, the mentor became inspired to start biofeedback for herself.

> Mentor: "Continue with what works... I've been thinking about trying biofeedback and I just haven't gotten around to doing it, you know it sounds like it's been helping you a lot so I'm thinking about it more and more."
> Mentee: "Yeah – biofeedback has been really helpful."
> Mentor: "I should try it, I really should. I'll talk to my doctor about it next time I see her. (laughs) See! Your experience helps me too!"

Discussion

This case presents the results of a new intervention to help pediatric patients cope with chronic pain. The PMP benefited the patient through the instruction of social tools to increase overall affect, sleep patterns, and improve his perception of bodily pain; it imparted and reinforced information that is essential for pain self-management in a cost and time efficient manner; additionally, mentorship also helped break the cycle of social withdrawal often seen in chronic pain. By reinforcing new social tools to deal with the pain, the mentee was able to reduce the crippling nature of pain flare-ups through social interaction. Instead of inwardly projecting the isolation and physical impairments inherent in the pain, the mentee was able to cope with these issues by discussing them with friends and family. We observed, through quantitative psychological measures (PANAS-C and CHQ) that increasing social coping facilitated increases in overall positive affect as well as a decreases in negative affect in our patient. Sleep habits also improved considerably with increases in total amount of sleep and decreases in time needed to fall asleep. Improvement in sleep was reflected in higher scores in the majority of measures of the PSQI, including the global sleep score.

Most importantly, perception of bodily pain improved on the CHQ, reflecting that the pain was not as debilitating as it was prior to the mentorship.

Throughout the mentorship, the mentee learned important information that is critical to self-manage pain. It is often not possible to sufficiently teach and enforce strategies for pain management in the traditional patient visit because of limited time, and a shortage of healthcare professionals.

By pairing patients with each other in a mentoring relationship, it is possible to utilize an otherwise untapped resource to improve the care of this common condition.

Ultimately, the most important role this intervention plays is disrupting the cycle of social isolation and chronic pain. Children with chronic pain will withdraw from their peers because of both physical limitations and psychological insecurities (10).

Our case suggests that these children believe that nobody else completely understands their daily struggles, and are hesitant to describe their isolation. This lack of social connection deprives the patient of important social coping mechanisms to deal with their chronic pain, which, in turn, leads to a greater perception of the pain, more isolation and so forth. By pairing the patient with a peer who has been through and overcome many of the same issues and challenges, it is possible to increase social coping and break the cycle of pain and social disconnection.

Acknowledgments

This research was supported by a grant from the National Institute of Child Health and Human Development (5R21HD057421; PI: Lonnie K. Zeltzer).

References

[1] Perquin CW, Hazebroek-Kampschreur AAJM, Hunfeld JAM, Bohnen AM, van Suijlekom-Smit LWA, Passchier J, et al. Pain in children and adolescents: A common experience. Pain 2000;87(1):51-8.

[2] Roth-Isigkeit A, Thyen U, Raspe HH, Stoven H, Schmucker P. Reports of pain among german children and adolescents: An epidemiological study. Acta Paediatr 2004;93(2):258-63.

[3] Bandell-Hoekstra I, Abu-Saad HH, Passchier J, Frederiks CMA, Feron FJM, Knipschild P. Coping and quality of life in relation to headache in dutch schoolchildren. Eur J Pain 2002;6(4):315-21.

[4] Kashikar-Zuck S, Goldschneider KR. Powers SW, Vaught MH, Hershey AD. Depression and functional disability in chronic pediatric pain. Clin J Pain 2001;17(4):341-9.

[5] Reid GJ, Lang BA, McGrath PJ. Primary juvenile fibromyalgia: Psychological adjustment, family functioning, coping, and functional disability. Arthritis Rheum 1997;40(4):752-60.

[6] Hunfeld JAM, Perquin CW, Duivenvoorden HJ, Hazebroek-Kampschreur A, Passchier J, van Suijlekom-Smit LWA, et al. Chronic pain and its impact on quality of life in adolescents and their families. J Pediatr Psychol 2001;26(3):145-53.

[7] Konijnenberg AY, Uiterwaal C, Kimpen JLL, van der Hoeven J, Buitelaar JK, Graeff-Meeder ERD. Children with unexplained chronic pain: Substantial impairment in everyday life. Arch Dis Child 2005;90(7):680-6.

[8]   Nodari E, Battistella PA, Naccarella C, Vidi M. Quality of life in young italian patients with primary headache. Headache 2002;42(4):268-74.

[9]   Powers SW, Patton SR, Hommel KA, Hershey AD. Quality of life in childhood migraines: Clinical impact and comparison to other chronic illnesses. Pediatrics 2003;112(1):E1-5.

[10]   Walco GA, Dampier CD. Chronic pain in adolescent patients. J Pediatr Psychol 1987;12(2):215-25.

[11]   Cohen S, Wills TA. Stress, social support, and the buffering hypothesis. Psychol Bull 1985;98(2):310-57.

[12]   Kawachi I, Berkman LF. Social ties and mental health. J Urban Health 2001;78(3):458-67.

[13]   Boivin M, Hymel S, & Bukowski WM. The roles of social withdrawal, peer rejection, and victimization by peers in predicting loneliness and depressed mood in childhood. Dev Psychopathol 1995;7(4):765-85.

[14]   Brattberg G. The incidence of back pain and headache among swedish school-children. Qual Life Res 1994;3:S27-31.

[15]   Sandstrom MJ, Schanberg LE. Brief report: Peer rejection, social behavior, and psychological adjustment in children with juvenile rheumatic disease. J Pediatr Psychol 2004;29(1):29-34.

[16]   Lynch AM, Kashikar-Zuck S, Goldschneider KR, Jones BA. Sex and age differences in coping styles among children with chronic pain. J Pain Symptom Manag 2007;33(2):208-16.

[17]   Reid GJ, Gilbert CA, McGrath PJ. The pain coping questionnaire: Preliminary validation. Pain 1998;76(1-2):83-96.

[18]   Sawyer MG, Whitham JN, Roberton DM, Taplin JE, Varni JW, Baghurst PA. The relationship between health-related quality of life, pain and coping strategies in juvenile idiopathic arthritis. Rheumatology 2004;43(3):325-30.

[19]   Craig KD, Lilley CM, Gilbert CA. Barriers to optimal pain management in infants, children, and adolescents social barriers to optimal pain management in infants and children. Clin J Pain 1996;12(3):232-42.

[20]   Buysse DJ, Reynolds CF, Monk TH, Berman SR, Kupfer DJ. The pittsburgh sleep quality index - A new instrument for psychiatric practice and research. Psychiat Res 1989;28(2):193-213.

[21]   Laurent J, Catanzaro SJ, Joiner TE, Rudolph, KD, Potter KI, Lambert S, et al. A measure of positive and negative affect for children: Scale development and preliminary validation. Psychol Assessment 1999;11(3):326-38.

[22]   Landgraf JM, Ware JA. Child health questionnaire (CHQ): A user's manual. Boston, MA: Health Act, 1999.

In: Pain Management Yearbook 2013
Editor: Joav Merrick

ISBN: 978-1-63117-944-0
© 2014 Nova Science Publishers, Inc.

Chapter 9

Pain relief through palliative radiation therapy in a patient with cervical spine bone metastases

Rehana Jamani, BSc(C)[1], Liang Zeng, MD(C)[1],
Linda Probyn, MD[2], Natalie Lauzon, MRTT[1], Lori Holden, MRTT[1],
Nemica Thavarajah, BSc(C)[1], Erin Wong, BSc(C)[1]
and Edward Chow, MBBS[1]*

[1]Rapid Response Radiotherapy Program, Department of Radiation Oncology,
[2]Department of Medical Imaging, Sunnybrook Health Sciences Centre,
University of Toronto, Toronto, Ontario, Canada

Abstract

In up to 75% of cases, prostate cancer metastasizes to the bone, often to the spine. Metastatic destruction often leads to a loss of vertebral body structural integrity, thus leading to instability. As a result of instability, patients often experience intense pain. Radiation therapy is generally known to provide pain relief and tumour control for patients with bone metastases; however, it does not improve bone stability. We present with a prostate cancer patient with bone metastases to the cervical spine (C-spine) leading to basilar invagination. The result of this was limited neck motion and severe pain. The metastases were treated with external beam radiation. At the most recent follow-up, the patient had regained neck movement and had experienced significant pain relief.

Keywords: Spinal metastases, pain relief, palliative radiation oncology

* Correspondence: Professor Edward Chow MBBS, MSc, PhD, FRCPC, Department of Radiation Oncology, Odette Cancer Centre, Sunnybrook Health Sciences Centre, 2075 Bayview Avenue, Toronto, ON Canada. E-mail: Edward.Chow@sunnybrook.ca

Introduction

Metastasis to the bone is common in patients with advanced prostate cancer, occurring in up to 75% of patients (1). In particular, vertebral body metastases are generally found in more than one third of autopsied cancer patients (2). The median survival of patients with prostate cancer metastatic to the bone is 12-53 months (1).

There are multiple treatment options for spinal metastases including surgery and radiotherapy. Indications for surgery include spinal instability from pathological fracture, neurological compression, and disease or pain unresponsive to radiotherapy, chemotherapy, or hormone therapy. In cases where a patient is unable to undergo an open surgical procedure (for example due to co-morbidities), minimally invasive approaches are available. Vertebroplasty and kyphoplasty are two such options for the treatment of spinal instability. By improving a patient's spinal instability, the goal is to reduce their pain level (1).

Radiation therapy is known to be effective in providing pain relief, and in most cases of vertebral body metastases, is the first therapy considered (3). Metastatic destruction often leads to a loss of vertebral body structural integrity, thus leading to instability (2). Pain is often the first symptom that presents in patients with spinal metastases, often as a result of instability (4). Radiation therapy is generally known to provide pain relief and tumour control for patients with bone metastases; however, it does not improve bone stability (3). Previous research has shown that as many as one-third of patients treated with radiotherapy experience total pain relief, independent of primary cancer or lesion type, and a further one-third experience some level of pain relief (1). The following case demonstrates the effectiveness of radiation therapy as a method of pain relief for a patient with spinal metastases.

Case report

A sixty-seven year old male patient with prostatic adenocarcinoma and painful bone metastases was seen in the Rapid Response Radiotherapy Program (RRRP) at the Odette Cancer Centre (OCC), Toronto, Canada. The patient presented with limited neck rotation, difficulty with lateral flexion, and pain in the bilateral hip area. Previous scans showed multiple spots of metastatic disease including the skull base involving the clivus, the cervical spine (C1), and the bilateral femora. A single 8 Gy fraction of radiation was given to the area after plain films showed no risk of fracture in the femora. The patient was referred to be seen in the orthopedic clinic regarding the disease in the skull base and cervical spine and was prescribed a soft collar.

CT scans completed after the patient's appointment in the RRRP showed basilar invagination (figures 1 and 3). As such, the orthopedic surgeon recommended posterior occipitocervical instrumented fusion followed by post-operative radiotherapy to stabilize the patient. The patient declined the surgical approach and chose instead to begin with radiation treatment.

The patient received 20 Gy in 5 fractions to the cervical spine in May 2012 and was seen post-treatment in the Fracture Clinic. Surgery was once again offered as an option to address stability. Due to the decrease in pain from the radiation treatment and the higher risks associated with surgery post-radiation, the patient opted to remain with the nonsurgical approach.

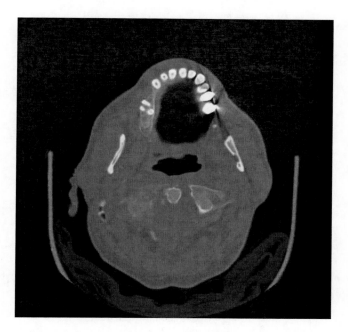

Figure 1. Axial CT image through the C1 level on bone window (W3000, L600) pretreatment demonstrating a predominately lytic lesion in the right C1 lateral mass.

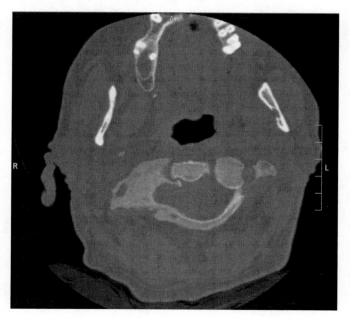

Figure 2. Axial CT image through the C1 vertebra on bone window (W3000, L600) post-treatment demonstrating increased sclerosis of the lesion involving the C1 lateral mass.

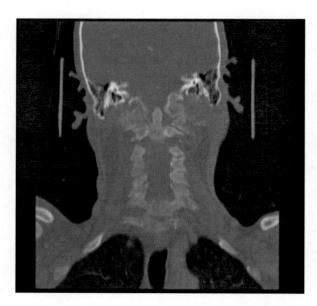

Figure 3. Coronal CT image on bone window (W3000, L600) pretreatment demonstrating a predominantly lytic lesion with the right C1 lateral mass with lateral displacement and mal-alignment between the C1 and C2 lateral masses.

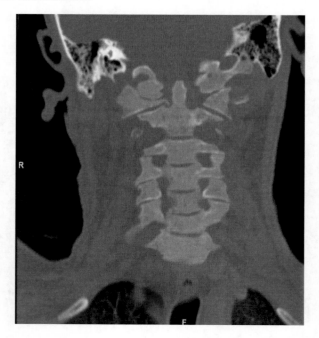

Figure 4. Coronal CT image on bone window (W3000, L600) post-treatment demonstrating increased sclerosis of the C1 lateral mass laterally displacing and mal-alignment between the C1 and C2 lateral masses is unchanged.

The patient was last seen on July 13, 2012 in the Bone Metastases Clinic (BMC) at the OCC with the repeat imaging (Figures 2 and 4). He no longer had pain associated with neck movement and as such, no longer required the use of a collar. It was decided that due to the positive response to radiation, no further treatment was needed for the neck at present. The patient will continue to be followed closely.

Discussion

Non-traumatic upper cervical instabilities are uncommon. They generally occur as a result of rheumatoid poly-arthritis, complex congenital malformations, or C1 or C2 metastasis, as seen in this patient (5). Cervical instabilities often cause symptoms such as bilateral or quadrilateral limb paresthesias, upper back pain, or sharp neck pain (6). Uncontrolled cancer-related pain occurs in over 70% of patients with metastases (7).

The need to treat bone metastases with radiotherapy is indicated by pain, risk for pathological fracture, or spinal cord compression. Due to the lower tolerance to radiation of the spinal cord, radiotherapy doses administered to spinal metastases are often palliative. The treatment is intended to cause tumour regression and ideally alleviate symptoms for the long term (7). Localized external beam radiotherapy aims to relieve symptoms, restore function, and stop disease progression. This has shown to be an effective treatment modality for patients with bone metastases. Previous studies have shown that 80-90% of such patients treated with various fractionations of radiotherapy have experienced pain relief (3).

In addition, it has been shown that prostate cancer patients are likely to experience a decrease in pain early post-treatment. Radiation is an effective option for patients with metastases to the cervical spine as studies have shown that the location of vertebral metastases (cervical, lumbar, or thoracic) does not impact patient response to the treatment (8).

This case demonstrates the effectiveness of radiotherapy as a method of relieving pain and restoring mobility. In the two months since radiation treatment to the cervical spine, the patient has experienced substantial pain relief and has regained the function of his neck, significantly improving his overall quality of life.

Acknowledgments

We thank the generous support of Bratty Family Fund, Michael and Karyn Goldstein Cancer Research Fund, Joseph and Silvana Melara Cancer Research Fund, and Ofelia Cancer Research Fund. We thank Ms Stacy Yuen for secretarial assistance.

References

[1]   Nguyen J, Chow E, Cramarossa G, Finkelstein J, Goh P. Handbook of Bone Metastases for healthcare professionals. Toronto: Odette Cancer Centre, Sunnybrook Health Sciences Centre, 2011.

[2]   Ratliff JK, Cooper PR. Metastatic spine tumors. South Med J 2004;97(3):246-53.

[3]   Chow E, Wu J, Barnes ET. Cancer drug discovery and development. Bone metastases: Experimental and clinical therapeutics. Totowa: Humana Press, 2005:323-36.

[4]   Katagiri H, Takahashi M, Inagaki J, Kobayashi H, Sugiura H, Yamamura S, Iwata H. Clinical results of nonsurgical treatment for spinal metastases. Int J Radiat Oncol Biol Phys 1998;42(5);1127-32.

[5]   Paquis P, Breuil V, Lonjon M, Euller-Ziegler L, Grellier P. Occipitocervical fixation using hooks and screws for upper cervical instability. Neurosurgery 1999;44(2):324-31.

[6]   Cook C, Brismee JM, Fleming R, Sizer PS Jr. Identifiers suggestive of clinical cervical spine instability: a Delphi study of physical therapists. Phys Ther 2005;85(9):895-906.

[7]   Janjan NA. Radiation for bone metastases. Cancer 1997;80:1628-45.

[8]   Nguyen J, Chow E, Zeng L, Zhang L, Culleton S, Holden L, Mitera G, Tsao M, Barnes E, Danjoux C, Sahgal A. Palliative response and functional interference outcomes using the brief pain inventory for spinal bony metastases treated with conventional radiotherapy. Clin Oncol (R Coll Radiol) 2011;23(7):485-91.

In: Pain Management Yearbook 2013

Editor: Joav Merrick

ISBN: 978-1-63117-944-0

© 2014 Nova Science Publishers, Inc.

Chapter 10

Single fraction palliative radiation treatment in the treatment of bone metastases with soft tissue mass

Nicholas Lao, Michael Poon, BSc(C), Linda Probyn, MD, Marko Popovic, BHSc(C), Ronald Chow, Natalie Lauzon, MRTT and Edward Chow, MBBS*

Rapid Response Radiotherapy Program, Department of Radiation Oncology, Odette Cancer Centre, Sunnybrook Health Sciences Centre, University of Toronto, Toronto, Ontario, Canada

Abstract

Pain associated with bone metastases can substantially decrease the quality of life (QOL) in cancer patients; single or multiple fraction radiation treatment is commonly used to treat uncomplicated bone metastases. However when the bone metastasis is associated with soft tissue mass, we tend to deliver multiple radiation treatments. We present a case report involving a 56-year old female breast cancer patient presenting with a right femur bone metastasis with soft tissue mass. The patient was treated with a single 8 Gy fraction of radiation and responded well to the treatment with good pain relief and shrinkage of the soft tissue mass.

Keywords: Single fraction radiotherapy, bone metastases, soft tissue mass, quality of life, breast cancer

* Correspondence: Professor Edward Chow MBBS, MSc, PhD, FRCPC Department of Radiation Oncology, Odette Cancer Centre, Sunnybrook Health Sciences Centre, 2075 Bayview Avenue, Toronto, ON Canada. E-mail: Edward.Chow@sunnybrook.ca

Introduction

Bone metastases occur in up to 85% of breast cancer patients [1]. For these patients, pain is a common symptom [2]. Palliative treatments for bone metastases are aimed at reducing pain experienced by the patient and improving their overall quality of life (QOL) [3].

Treatment options include single or multiple fraction radiotherapy for pain. Debate exists in the literature on which one is optimal for palliative cancer patients [2]. When the bone metastasis is associated with soft tissue mass, we tend to deliver multiple radiation treatments.

In this report, we present the case of a middle-aged woman with primary breast cancer who developed a right femur bone metastasis with soft tissue mass lesion and was treated with a single 8 Gy of radiation.

Case report

In November of 2008, a 56-year old female with a right breast carcinoma was referred to the Odette Cancer Centre, Sunnybrook Hospital. Breast lumpectomy and sentinel node biopsy were performed and positively identified the cancer as an invasive ductal carcinoma. The lesion was of high-grade and measured 2.3 cm. It was also found to be ER/PR negative and HER-2 negative. One sentinel lymph node was removed and found to be negative for metastatic disease. The biopsy also revealed perineural invasion without invasive tumor necrosis.

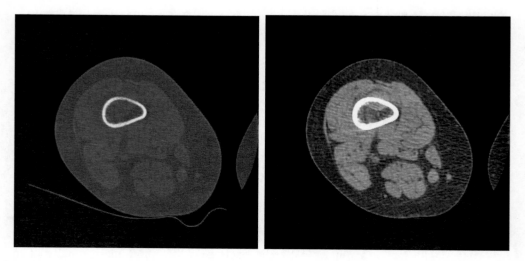

Figure 1. Axial CT images through the right femur pre-radiation treatment on soft tissue and bone windows demonstrating a cortical-based soft tissue mass at the anterior femur with endosteal, intramedullary and extraosseous components compatible with metastases from breast carcinoma with permeative change of the cortex.

An abdominal ultrasound performed showed no evidence of metastatic disease within the liver. She began four cycles of chemotherapy with good tolerance.

Radiotherapy of 5000 cGy was delivered in 25 fractions to the right breast and completed in March of 2009. Afterwards, the patient developed shingles for which she received Calamine Lotion and antiviral medications. In April 2012, the patient developed local recurrence and was treated with mastectomy and lymph node dissection. There were at least seven lymph nodes found involved with extranodal extension. The tumor itself and measured 0.6 x 0.1 cm. The patient was at a very high risk of distant metastases. In June 2012, the patient was referred to the Bone Metastases Clinic after a painful lesion of 4-5 cm developed in her right distal femur. A computed tomography (CT) scan showed that the lesion was both intramedullary and extramedullary and primarily soft tissue without definite evidence of cortical breach (Figure 1). No prophylactic fixation was needed as there was no significant loss of structural bone. She received a single 8 Gy.

A post-radiation CT scan was performed on the right femur. The soft tissue mass had substantially decreased in size, and new endosteal and periosteal bone had formed in the femur (Figure 2). The patient also reported substantial pain relief.

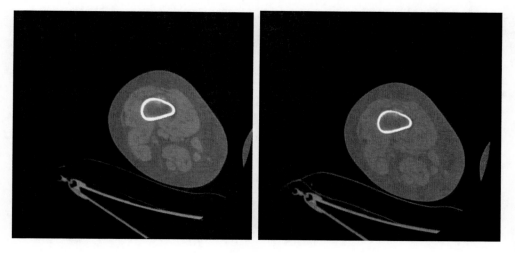

Figure 2. Axial CT images through the right femur post-radiation treatment on soft tissue and bone windows and sagittal reformatted image on bone windows demonstrating a decrease in size of the soft tissue mass in the intramedullary and extraosseous components with residual permeative change of the cortex and periosteal reaction related to a treatment response.

Discussion

Radiation is a common treatment for pain in patients with bone metastases. Treatments in Canada usually consist of multiple fractions or a single fraction [4]. In this case, the patient received a single 8 Gy radiation to her right femur and experienced good pain relief as well as a good response in the post-radiation CT scan.

These responses indicate the efficacy of single fraction radiation to bone for the palliative treatment of bone metastases in both reducing pain and shrinking the soft tissue mass.

Acknowledgments

We thank the generous support of Bratty Family Fund, Michael and Karyn Goldstein Cancer Research Fund, Joseph and Silvana Melara Cancer Research Fund, and Ofelia Cancer Research Fund. We thank Stacy Yuen for secretarial assistance.

References

[1]   Verbeeck A. Bone metastases from breast cancer: Guidelines for diagnosis. A case report from the chiropractic office. J Manipulat Physiol Ther 2004; 27(3): 211-5.

[2]   Badzio A, Senkus-Konefka E, Jereczek-Fossa B, Adamska K, Fajndt S, et al. 20 Gy in five fractions versus 8 Gy in one fraction in palliative radiotherapy of bone metastases. A multicenter randomized study. NOWOTWORY J Oncol 2003;53(3):261-4.

[3]   Hartsell W, Scott C, Bruner D, Scarantino C, Ivker R, et al. Randomized trial for short-versus long course radiotherapy for palliation of painful bone metastases. J Natl Cancer Institute 2005;97(11):798-804.

[4]   Kachnic L, Berk L. Palliative single-fraction radiation therapy: How Much more evidence is needed? J Natl Cancer Institute 2005;97(11):786-8.

In: Pain Management Yearbook 2013
Editor: Joav Merrick

ISBN: 978-1-63117-944-0
© 2014 Nova Science Publishers, Inc.

Chapter 11

Palliative radiotherapy in the treatment of lung metastases or advanced lung cancer

Jasmine Nguyen, MBBCh(C), Dominic Chu, MBBCh(C),
Gillian Bedard, BSc(C), Erin Wong, BSC(C), Flo Jon, MRTT,
Cyril Danjoux, MD, Elizabeth Barnes, MD, May Tsao, MD,
Lori Holden, MRTT, Edward Chow, MBBS
and Natalie Lauzon, MRTT*

Rapid Response Radiotherapy Program, Department of Radiation Oncology,
Odette Cancer Centre, Sunnybrook Health Sciences Centre,
University of Toronto, Toronto, Ontario, Canada

Abstract

External beam radiotherapy (EBRT) given to advanced lung cancer patients undergoing palliative care is intended to relieve the symptoms that disrupt a patient's overall Quality of Life (QOL). This treatment, however, may also pose unwanted toxicities and side effects. This report presents five cases in which patients have been diagnosed with advanced lung cancer or lung metastases and were subsequently treated with external beam radiotherapy. In an attempt to assess the efficacy of the treatment, diaries were given to the patients to fill out at baseline, during treatment and 10 days after treatment. The diary collected data on the medications taken by the patient and evaluated the perceived severity of the following acute toxicity symptoms: coughing, hemoptysis, dysphagia, chest pain and dyspnea. In addition, the patients completed QOL questionnaires, European Organization for Research and Treatment of Cancer (EORTC)

---

* Correspondence: Ms. Natalie Lauzon BSc, MRTT Department of Radiation Therapy, Odette Cancer Centre, Sunnybrook Health Sciences Centre, 2075 Bayview Avenue, Toronto, ON Canada. Email: Natalie.Lauzon@Sunnybrook.ca

Quality of Life Questionnaire Core 15 Palliative (QLQ-C15-PAL) along with the EORTC QLQ-Lung Cancer (QLQ-LC13). Four of the patients had a generally improved or stabilized QOL, while one felt intensified symptoms and a worsened QOL. The information gathered from these assessments can provide clinicians with a greater understanding of the experience of EBRT through the patients' perspective and can therefore guide future modifications in EBRT treatment.

Keywords: External beam radiotherapy, lung cancer, lung metastases, quality of life, EORTC QLQ-C15-PAL, EORTC QLQ-LC13

Introduction

Lung cancer often presents itself as an incurable and non-remediable disease as it is usually identified in its advanced stages or has metastasized to other regions of the body (1). Patients often face numerous and debilitating symptoms such as anxiety, fatigue, weakness, loss of appetite, dyspnea, cough, and hemoptysis (2). In order to help these patients, palliation of these symptoms is provided through chemotherapy, surgery, or radiotherapy. This report examines specifically external beam radiotherapy (EBRT), which is effective in controlling some of the symptoms (2), however, the effects of the treatment itself need to be examined.

This case series examines five patients with advanced lung cancer who were referred to a palliative outpatient clinic and were thereby treated with EBRT. In this report, we attempt to decipher whether or not the benefits of such a treatment outweigh its toxicities with regards to five advanced lung cancer patients with the use of an acute toxicity symptoms evaluation diary and the European Organization for Research and Treatment of Cancer (EORTC) Quality of Life Questionnaire Core 15 Palliative (QLQ-C15-PAL) in conjunction with the EORTC QLQ-Lung Cancer (QLQ-LC13).

Case report

Case #1

The first patient is an eighty-year-old female who was diagnosed with primary bladder cancer metastatic to the lungs and was referred due to dyspnea and hemoptysis. Consequently, the patient was treated with palliative EBRT with 20Gy/5fr. At the baseline point prior to treatment, the patient took neither medications nor oxygen for her lung symptoms. However, she experienced slight hemoptysis and mild shortness of breath, which she found to moderately interfere with her daily activities. According to the EORTC QLQ-C15-PAL and the EORTC QLQ-LC13, she noticed nausea, trouble sleeping, fatigue, mild tension, tingling on her hands/feet and slight depression.

During treatment, she no longer experienced hemoptysis. She briefly experienced dyspnea and chest pain, but for the last 2 days of treatment, the patient was symptom free. Over the course of the treatment, her diary entries had suggested that she found her symptoms to be in a better state than at baseline and that they did not interfere with her daily activities. On the last day of treatment, the patient was re-administered the EORTC QLQ-C15-PAL along with the EORTC QLQ-LC13 surveys, which showed that her fatigue and dyspnea had increased during the prior week, however, she no longer experienced tingling on her hands/feet, hemoptysis and had lessened nausea. All other evaluated symptoms remained the same.

After treatment, the patient did not take any pain medication. She had encountered slight coughing and reacquired her slight dyspnea until both symptoms went away 5 days post-treatment. She was briefly symptom free, but later encountered dysphagia until the last assessment. Within those 10 days, the patient noted that her symptoms had improved and had not been interfering with her daily activities.

Case #2

The second patient is a sixty-nine-year-old male who was diagnosed with primary lung cancer that metastasized to the brain. He was referred to the clinic for chest pain and was then treated with palliative EBRT with 20Gy/5fr. At baseline, the patient noted on the diary that he took neither medications nor oxygen and noticed no acute toxicity symptoms (coughing, hemoptysis, dysphagia, chest pain and dyspnea); however, on the first day of treatment, he took the EORTC QLQ-C-15-PAL and the EORTC QLQ-LC-13 and noted that he had experienced slight coughing and slight hemoptysis. He also claimed he had an excellent QOL (7/7).

Out of the four consecutive days of treatment, the patient did not take any pain medications. The patient experienced a sustained cough and a brief, mild hemoptysis. Overall, none of the symptoms seemed to have interfered with his daily activities.

For the 10 days following the radiation treatment that were followed-up on the diary, the patient did not take any pain medications and felt only slight coughing urges. The patient was re-assessed a month later and only noted a slight cough. During that time, the patient, again, ranked his QOL as excellent.

Case #3

The third patient is a forty-eight-year old female who was diagnosed with primary lung cancer metastatic to bone and was referred due to her superior vena cava obstruction. The patient was subsequently treated with EBRT with 20Gy/5fr. At baseline, the patient noted in her diary that she did not take any oxygen but took Advil as a pain medication. She also felt slight coughing as well as slight dyspnea; however, the symptoms did not seem to interfere with her daily activities. A day before the treatment, the patient noted that she also had had slight pain and severe depression on the EORTC QLQ-C15-PAL, and graded her quality of life at a 4/7. According to the EORTC QLQ-LC13, she also seemed to notice slight coughing and a little pain in her arms/shoulders and neck.

During treatment, she noticed slight dyspnea, mild chest pain, nausea, tiredness, and cough. She also still claimed that her symptoms were in a better state than before treatment. On the last day of treatment, she noted a much-worsened dyspnea, increased fatigue, and nausea; however, she no longer noticed any pain on her body nor depression.

After treatment, the patient started taking Dexamethasone alongside Advil. She experienced a brief cough, intensified dyspnea, dysphagia, and increased chest pain. On all 10 days, the patient noted that her symptoms post-treatment were worse than before treatment and that all the symptoms strongly interfered with her daily activities. She completed the EORTC QLQ-C15-PAL and the EORTC QLQ-LC13 again which showed that all the symptoms remained the same since she last completed the questionnaires, except she felt a worsened lack of appetite, pain in her neck, trouble swallowing, and a sore throat/tongue. In addition, the pain in her arms/shoulders, chest and the tingling in her hands and feet seemed to have disappeared. At that time, she also graded her quality life to be 3/7, which was slightly worse than at baseline.

Approximately a month after the treatment started, the patient again took the EORTC-QLQ-C15-PAL and the EORTC QLQ-LC13 and noted that the dyspnea, cough and soreness in her mouth/tongue had improved, while her nausea, tension, fatigue, dysphagia, and chest pain had worsened. The pain in her neck seemed to have moved to her back and she felt slightly depressed. In the same entry, the patient also claimed that she took Tylenol 3 as a pain medication. Finally, she considered her quality of life to be at a 1/7, implying that it was much worse than it was at baseline.

Case #4

The fourth patient is a sixty-year-old female who was diagnosed with primary ovarian cancer metastatic to the lung, was referred for mild coughing and slight hemoptysis. She was thereby treated by EBRT with dosage of 30 Gy/10 fr.

At baseline, the patient was experiencing slight hemoptysis and a moderate cough which only required non-narcotic medication. She did not use any pain medications or take oxygen, and her symptoms seemed to only slightly affect her daily activities. At baseline, she also completed the EORTC QLQ-C15-PAL, which conveyed that she had slight fatigue, trouble sleeping, quite a bit of pain, slight constipation, mild tension and mild depression. Prior to treatment, she completed the EORTC QLQ-LC13, which showed that she also had slight hair loss and a noticeable amount of pain in her groin.

Over the course of the treatment, the patient did not take any pain medications. Her hemoptysis became slightly worse at the start of treatment, but improved back to baseline (as measured by her diary) by the 3rd day of treatment. Her coughing also improved by the same time. Throughout her treatment, the patient noted that her symptoms did not interfere with her daily activities in any way except for the days in which her hemoptysis worsened. On the last day of treatment, The EORTC QLQ-LC13 showed that the pain in her groin moved to her abdomen but was of a lesser extent, while other complaints had not exacerbated except for the nausea, constipation, tension, and depression, all of which improved. Overall, she ranked her quality of life 1 grade higher on this test than on the one at baseline, for a score of 7/7.

By the third day post-treatment, the hemoptysis stopped as recorded in her diary. Only by the 6th day after treatment did the patient start noticing an improvement in her acute toxicity symptoms compared to the start of treatment. Approximately a week after the radiation treatment ended, the patient took the EORTC QLQ-C15-PAL again, which revealed that there was an improvement in all complaints except for that of fatigue. She also re-took the EORTC

QLQ-LC13, which showed a great progression in her abdominal/groin pain, while the hair loss and coughing still persisted. She also maintained her abstinence from pain medications.

Case #5

The fifth patient is a 78-year-old male who was diagnosed with primary lung cancer, metastatic to other parts of the lung and was referred due to coughing and hemoptysis. He was treated with EBRT with dosage of 20 Gy/5 fr to the lower lobes of the lung. At baseline, his diary entry showed that he had a slight cough accompanied by slight hemoptysis. He also took the EORTC QLQ-C15-PAL, which portrayed that he was very weak and fatigued, had much trouble with short walks, lacked appetite, had constipation and was quite depressed. He graded his quality of life a 4/7. Lastly before treatment, he took the EORTC QLQ-LC13, which only showed that he was experiencing a large amount of coughing.

Over the entire course of treatment, coughing was apparent and the patient took neither medication nor oxygen. He developed hemoptysis and slight dyspnea, which were both alleviated near the end of treatment. During the days that he felt hemoptysis and slight dyspnea, he noted that his symptoms were in a worse state than at baseline, however after both of the symptoms had subsided, he claimed that his symptoms were in the same state as before treatment. On the last day, the patient repeated the EORTC QLQ-C15-PAL and the EORTC QLQ-LC13 surveys, which presented an improvement in his cough and hemoptysis. However, the tests also displayed a slight regression in his dyspnea and the emergence of slight dysphagia. In addition, the patient considered his quality of life to be the same as it was at baseline point.

After treatment, he still abstained from pain medications and initially felt better with no noted symptoms. However, he experienced a brief cough and dyspnea within the first few days post-treatment, as well as significant dysphagia near the end of the diary entries.

Approximately a month after the treatment had ended, the patient repeated the EORTC QLQ-C15-PAL and the EORTC QLQ-LC13, which showed that he became slightly tense and quite depressed. He also perceived his cough to be much worse, however, both his dyspnea and dysphagia seemed to have improved. Again, the patient saw no change in his quality of life.

Discussion

Emphasis on palliation is imperative in the treatment of advanced lung cancer patients in light of the incurable nature of the disease as well as the symptom burden it carries. Keeping that in mind, all treatments should ideally foster benefits and lighten that burden and should therefore have no acute toxicities. This report focuses on only EBRT as the treatment of choice, which functions by prompting tumor regression and thus attempting to alleviate most of the patients' lung symptoms (3). However, EBRT is also known to bear acute toxicities, the most common being: coughing, hemoptysis, dysphagia, chest pain and dyspnea, all of which can potentially introduce a diminished QOL post-treatment as they may often conflict with the lung cancer patients' pre-treatment symptoms, which most commonly consist of: fatigue, pain, appetite loss, dyspnea and chest pain (4).

Out of the common pre-treatment symptoms mentioned above, coughing and fatigue were found to be the most prominent, both affecting four out of five patients. The two symptoms were followed by dyspnea and pain, which were apparent in three of five patients. Lastly, appetite loss seemed to have been a pre-treatment symptom for only one patient. These findings are consistent with those of Langendijk et al., who found that the most common pre-treatment symptom is fatigue, followed by cough, dyspnea, pain, and appetite loss respectively (4).

A notable trend was found when assessing the patients while they received their treatment. Coughing was apparent as a pre-treatment symptom in the third, fourth and fifth patient, and persisted as an acute treatment toxicity as well. It had also slightly developed within the first and second patient who had no initial complaints of coughing. These findings are coherent with those of Sundstrom et al. who discovered that a mere 20% of patients with advanced non-small-cell lung carcinoma (NSCLC) found that their cough progressed after receiving radiotherapy (5), implying that only one out of five patients find radiotherapy to be effective in improving their cough. However, Sundstrom et al. also contradicts this idea in the same study as they discovered that clinicians found that cough was improved amongst 40-55% of NSCLC patients within their sample size (5). This contrast presents the highly scrutinized discrepancy between patient-assessed and clinician-assessed symptoms – thus, the fact that all assessments were subjective to the five patients may have presented a limitation to this report.

The second most common acute toxicity during treatment was hemoptysis, which was present in four of the five patients. However, hemoptysis was found to be temporary and merely lasted for a maximum of three days during treatment time. Hemoptysis is then followed by dyspnea and dysphagia, the latters of which affected three patients. Dyspnea was shown to disappear eventually in two of its three cases. Dysphagia, on the other hand, persisted in all three of its cases, which is in parallel with the findings of Falk et al. who found that dysphagia was the most common adverse effect amongst patients over a time span of over a year post-treatment (6).

Furthermore, post treatment assessments showed that in general, overall symptoms had subsided and that overall QOL had increased; three of five cases showed symptom palliation, one displayed no change in QOL but the emergence of a slight cough and lastly, another case showed an actual decline with the appearance of many acute toxicities post-treatment. All patients who experienced hemoptysis during treatment did not experience it within the ten days post-treatment and symptoms such as coughing, dyspnea, pain, and lack of appetite tended to improve or disappear completely. An exception was the third patient, who had a slight improvement in some symptoms, such as dyspnea, cough, and soreness in the throat, but symptoms such as nausea, fatigue, dysphagia, chest and back pain, and depression exacerbated. The extent of her pain post-treatment led her to replace her use of Advil and Dexamethasone with Tylenol 3. The significance of these findings is still controversial, in that different studies have found that patients have taken to EBRT in different ways. Sundstrom et al. (5) found that up to 90% of patients will benefit from the effects of EBRT in reducing cough and hemoptysis, while Falk et al. (6) found no statistically significant evidence that palliative thoracic radiotherapy had any beneficial effect to thoracic symptoms such as cough, hemoptysis, or dyspnea. However, the post-treatment symptoms found in this case study cannot be considered definitive as they were only assessed over the course of ten days. A longer analysis of the patients' symptoms post-treatment may have yielded different results, which is justified by Auchter et al. (7) who have shown that overall toxicity scores in patients with advanced NSCLC have been seen to initially reduce post-treatment, but then increase past baseline thereafter, implying that EBRT benefits may only be temporary.

Within this case series, we found that it could not be found definitive that the change in the patients' symptom burden was a direct product of the EBRT as our sample size was far too small thus; a conclusion could not be drawn regarding the actual effects of EBRT within this patient population. In addition, EBRT specifically targets local pulmonary symptom control. With this, we could not surmise that the persistence or alleviation of systemic symptoms such as nausea, fatigue, loss of appetite or constipation was a consequence of the treatment but rather, it can be hypothesized that such symptoms may have been due to the extra-thoracic spread of their disease. Ultimately, this case report highlights the necessity for further, more rigorous clinical trials to provide more in-depth and accurate evaluation of the toxicities and effects of EBRT within this patient population.

Acknowledgments

We thank the generous support of Bratty Family Fund, Michael and Karyn Goldstein Cancer Research Fund, Joseph and Silvana Melara Cancer Research Fund, and Ofelia Cancer Research Fund.

References

[1]	Mallick I, Sharma SC, Behera D. Endobronchial brachytherapy for symptom palliation in non-small cell lung cancer-Analysis of symptom response, endoscopic improvement and quality of life. Lung Cancer 2007;55(3):313-8.

[2]	Bezjak A. Palliative therapy for lung cancer. Semin Surg Oncol 2003;21(2):138-47.

[3]	Janjan NA. Radiation for bone metastases. Cancer 1997;80:1628-45.

[4]	Langendijk JA, Ten Velde GPM, Aaronson NK, De Jong JMA, Muller MJ, Wouters EFM. Quality of life after palliative radiotherapy in non-small cell lung cancer: A prospective study. Int J Radiat Oncol Biol Phys 2000;47(1):149-55.

[5]	Sundstrom S, Bremnes R, Aasebo U, et al. Hypofractionated palliative radiotherapy (17 Gy per two fractions) in advanced non-small-cell lung carcinoma is comparable to standard fractionation for symptom control and survival: a national phase III trial. Am J Clin Oncol 2004;22(5):801-10.

[6]	Falk SJ, Girling DJ, White RJ, et al. Immediate versus delayed palliative thoracic radiotherapy in patients with unresectable locally advanced non-small cell lung cancer and minimal thoracic symptoms: Randomised controlled trial. BMJ 2002;325(7362):465-8.

[7]	Auchter RM, Scholtens D, Adak S, Wagner H, Cella DF, Mehta MP. Quality of life assessment in advanced non-small-cell lung cancer patients undergoing an accelerated radiotherapy regimen: Report of ECOG Study 4593. Int J Radiat Oncol Biol Phys 2001;50(5):1199-206.

Submitted: September 02, 2012. *Revised:* October 05, 2012. *Accepted:* October 14, 2012.

In: Pain Management Yearbook 2013
Editor: Joav Merrick

ISBN: 978-1-63117-944-0
© 2014 Nova Science Publishers, Inc.

Chapter 12

Radiation therapy alone for established heterotopic ossification

Erin Wong, BSc (C)[1], Gemma Cramarossa, BHSc (C)[1],
Gillian Bedard, BSc(C)[1], Linda Probyn, MD[2], Lori Holden, MRTT[1],
Edward Chow, MBBS[1] and Natalie Lauzon, MRTT[1]*

[1]Rapid Response Radiotherapy Program, Department of Radiation Oncology,
Odette Cancer Centre, Sunnybrook Health Sciences Centre
[2]Department of Medical Imaging, Sunnybrook Health Sciences Centre,
University of Toronto, Toronto, Ontario, Canada

Abstract

There are limited therapeutic treatment options for established heterotopic ossification. The most common treatment option is surgical resection of the bone formed followed with prophylactic radiation treatment to prevent reoccurrence. However, this presents an issue when a patient is not a surgical candidate: how is established heterotopic ossification treated then? Here, we present the case of a 55-year-old male with extensive heterotopic ossification in the pelvis area causing significant pain. Since this patient was not a surgical candidate, his options were limited. A single dose of 8 Gy of radiation was prescribed to the painful area and this patient experienced significant pain relief despite no interval radiological change in the established heterotopic ossification. Further studies should be conducted to assess and understand the efficacy of radiation to palliate pain caused by heterotopic ossification.

Keywords: External beam radiotherapy, therapeutic radiation, heterotopic ossification, pain relief, bone formation

* Correspondence: Ms. Natalie Lauzon BSc, MRTT Department of Radiation Therapy, Odette Cancer Centre, Sunnybrook Health Sciences Centre, 2075 Bayview Avenue, Toronto, ON Canada. Email: Natalie.Lauzon@Sunnybrook.ca

Introduction

Heterotopic ossification, or heterotopic bone formation, is a complication that can be brought about by trauma, central nervous system injuries, operations, fractures or can also occur as a result of a genetic disorder (1-3). It is a condition characterized by the formation of bone outside of the skeleton, occupying space in soft tissue (4). This bone formation can occur in areas such as the skin, muscles, and walls of vessels (5). Although the initial establishment of heterotopic ossification can be asymptomatic, with progression of this bone formation, there are instances in which it can lead to severe pain (2,6).

There are certain risk factors for the development of heterotopic ossification such as gender and past medical history. Those particularly at risk are males, patients that have had a previous history of heterotopic ossification and patients that suffer from paraplegia due to a spinal cord injury (1,6).

In terms of heterotopic ossification prevention, radiation has been recognized as a useful prophylactic treatment after hip surgery (7). There has also been evidence for its role as a prophylactic treatment in other joints such as knee and elbow or the spine (6,8). In general, this is a clinically accepted prophylactic treatment after resection of heterotopic ossification (9).

It has also been suggested through a few case reports that radiation alone may have a role as a therapeutic treatment for established heterotopic ossification, hence, not only as a prophylactic treatment. In two case reports, Schaeffer et al. and Jang et al., both reported an increase in mobility and a reduction of pain in patients with established heterotopic ossification treated with therapeutic radiation (10,11).

In the following case, a 55-year-old quadriplegic male experienced significant pain, which corresponded to areas of heterotopic ossification. Radiation treatment alone was given to the area of pain in hopes of palliation.

Case report

A 55-year-old male has been a C5 quadriplegic secondary to a motor vehicle accident in 1994. Due to the accident, he underwent an anterior cervical spine decompression and fusion at C5-6 because of a cervical spine fracture. He was referred to the Rapid Response Radiotherapy Program (RRRP) at Sunnybrook Odette Cancer Centre in 2011 due to dysphagia caused by heterotopic ossification at the C3-4 and C4-5 level. Of concern were the osteophytes at the C3-4 level, which the orthopedic surgeons felt was operable. Thus in August 2011, the patient proceeded with a C3-4 anterior cervical decompression and drilling followed by a prophylactic radiation treatment of 8 Gy in one fraction post-surgery.

This patient was then seen again in the RRRP in May of 2012 and reported no pain at the C3-5 area and no dysphagia. However, at this time, this patient had pain in the pelvic region, which corresponded with heterotopic ossification imaged on a recent CT scan. This heterotopic ossification was deemed inoperable by two different orthopedic surgeons. Since there was previous evidence from literature that radiation may be used as a therapeutic option for pain caused by heterotopic ossification, we offered this patient a single 8 Gy of radiation to the pelvic region extending to the proximal bilateral femurs to palliate the pain.

From May 11, 2012, the pre-radiation CT scan of the spine, abdomen and pelvis showed extensive bilateral heterotopic ossification in the hip regions, sacroiliac joints and anterior and medial portion of the proximal femurs (Figures 1 and 2). An aspect of ossification was seen in both the left and right iliac wing measuring 20cm and 15cm respectively.

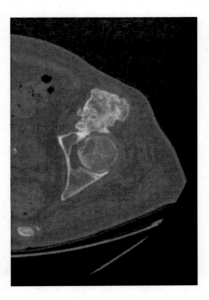

Figure 1. Axial CT scan through the pelvis prior to the therapeutic radiation treatment showing extensive heterotopic ossification anterior to the left hip.

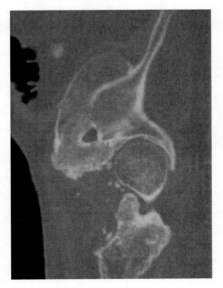

Figure 2. Sagittal reformatted CT scan through the left hip prior to the therapeutic radiation treatment showing prominent heterotopic ossification extending from the left ilium and proximal femur anterior to the hip.

On the left, there was a bulk of ossification anterior to the hip extending from the iliac ossification (Figure 1). Treatment to the pelvic region and bilateral femurs was delivered on May 24, 2012 (Figure 3).

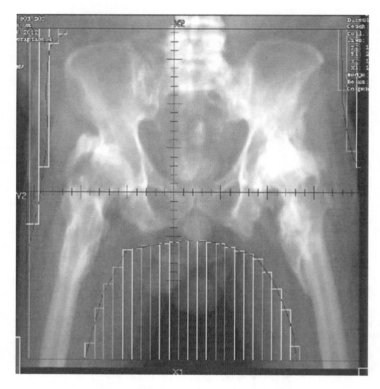

Figure 3. Digitally Reconstructed Image (DRR) representing radiation treatment volume, treated anteriorly and posteriorly for 800 cGy in 1 fraction, delivered on May 24th, 2012.

On September 12, 2012, post-radiation CT scans from the head and neck to bilateral femurs were ordered for comparison. These CT scans showed similar extensive heterotopic ossification along the same regions as noted in May of 2012 (Figures 4 and 5) with no interval change in comparison to the scans from May 11, 2012.

The patient completed a pain diary, daily at the end of each day, to track his pain post-radiation for twenty days. This diary tracked the patient's pain score out of 10, whether the pain was better, worse or the same in comparison to before radiation and the pain medications the patient took that day. As recorded in the pain diary, the patient experienced an increase in pain from the first day after radiation to the seventh day after radiation. At the eighth day after treatment, the patient began noticing some pain relief, with a decrease in pain score from 7/10 to 4/10 with no change in regular pain medication. From the eighth day and onwards, the patient's pain relief fluctuated with some days better than others, but towards the fifteenth day after treatment, pain relief occurred more consistently and at the twentieth day post-radiation, the patient recorded a pain score of 2-3/10 for most of the day. The patient was seen 4 months post-treatment on September 20, 2012. At this follow-up, the patient reported that this pain relief has been consistent and he expressed that he believes the radiation has provided palliation of pain for his extensive heterotopic ossification.

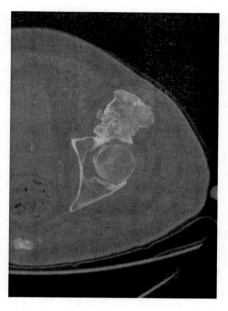

Figure 4. Axial CT scan through the pelvis post-therapeutic radiation treatment showing extensive heterotopic ossification anterior to the left hip as seen previously.

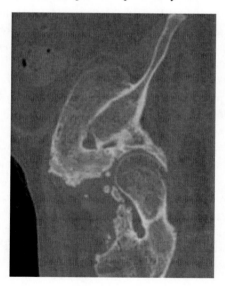

Figure 5. Sagittal reformatted CT scan through the left hip post-therapeutic radiation treatment showing prominent heterotopic ossification extending from the left ilium and proximal femur anterior to the hip as seen previously.

Discussion

In the current body of literature, the utilization of radiation for heterotopic ossification has only been established as a prophylactic treatment, mainly after bone surgery. While the available therapeutic treatment for established heterotopic ossification is severely limited, surgical resection is traditionally the only option (2,3,6,7). This leaves few options for patients that are not surgical candidates. There exists a few cases as reported by Schaeffer et al. (10) and Jang et al. (11) on the usage of radiation as a therapeutic treatment, giving hope to those with established heterotopic ossification.

Schaeffer et al. reported two cases in which patients experienced decrease range of motion and significant pain in the hip and elbow due to the formation of heterotopic ossification in these joints. This pain was palliated and greater range of motion was seen post-radiation treatment in both patients (11). It should be noted that for the aforementioned patients, a dose fractionation schedule of 20 Gy in 10 fractions was used. Similarly, Jang et al. reported on the usage of the 20 Gy in 10 fractions on a patient that developed heterotopic ossification in both hips post-brain trauma. This patient also reported decreased pain and increased activity after the therapeutic radiation treatment (10).

In the current case, this patient suffered from quadriplegia secondary to a motor vehicle accident. It has been suggested that paraplegia is a risk factor for the development of heterotopic ossification, which may explain the extensive formation of heterotopic ossification in this patient that lead to significant pain (1). Based upon the evidence from Schaeffer et al. (10) and Jang et al. (11), we recommended a single dose of radiation as a therapeutic treatment for heterotopic ossification for the palliation of the pain. Despite having no interval radiological change in the heterotopic ossification formed, the patient experienced significant pain relief after radiation. During the twenty days post-treatment, the patient may have experienced a pain flare due to the radiation, as seen in the initial seven days in which he experienced increased pain. Once this increased pain subsided, pain relief was experienced, similar to other radiation-induced pain flare process. The efficacy and mechanism by which radiation acts as a therapeutic treatment for the abnormal formation of bone is still an area of uncertainty. The mechanism for the therapeutic usage of radiation for heterotopic ossification is hypothesized to be due to the stopping of osteoblastic stem cell formation thus preventing continuous bone formation which may be the cause of pain (11).

This case study and the two others that preceded it reveals an area of study that requires further investigation, however this does add to the body of literature supporting the use of radiation alone as a therapeutic treatment for heterotopic ossification. Therefore, radiation may be a possible treatment option to palliate the pain in patients with heterotopic ossification who are experiencing significant pain yet are not surgical candidates. It can be further suggested that a single dose of 8 Gy radiation may be effective in this usage. Further research should be conducted to establish the efficacy of radiation as a therapeutic treatment for heterotopic ossification as well as determining the most effective dose fractionation schedule.

Acknowledgments

We thank the generous support of Bratty Family Fund, Michael and Karyn Goldstein Cancer Research Fund, Joseph and Silvana Melara Cancer Research Fund, and Ofelia Cancer Research Fund.

References

[1]   Shehab D, Elgazzar AH, Collier BD. Heterotopic ossification. J Nucl Med 2002;43(3):346-53.

[2]   Pakos EE, Ioannidis JP. Radiotherapy vs. nonsteroidal anti-inflammatory drugs for the prevention of heterotopic ossification after major hip procedures: a meta-analysis of randomized trials. Int J Radiat Oncol Biol Phys 2004;60(3):888-95.

[3]   Balboni TA, Gobezie R, Mamon HJ. Heterotopic ossification: Pathophysiology, clinical features, and the role of radiotherapy for prophylaxis. Int J Radiat Oncol Biol Phys 2006;65(5):1289-99.

[4]   Baird EO, Kang QK. Prophylaxis of heterotopic ossification - an updated review. J Orthop Surg Res 2009;4:12.

[5]   McCarthy EF, Sundaram M. Heterotopic ossification: a review. Skeletal Radiol 2005;34(10):609-19.

[6]   Lo TC. Radiation therapy for heterotopic ossification. Semin Radiat Oncol 1999;9(2):163-70.

[7]   Vavken P, Castellani L, Sculco TP. Prophylaxis of heterotopic ossification of the hip: systematic review and meta-analysis. Clin Orthop Relat Res 2009;467(12):3283-9.

[8]   Mishra MV, Austin L, Parvizi J, Ramsey M, Showalter TN. Safety and efficacy of radiation therapy as secondary prophylaxis for heterotopic ossification of non-hip joints. J Med Imaging Radiat Oncol 2011;55(3):333-6.

[9]   Vanden Bossche L, Vanderstraeten G. Heterotopic ossification: a review. J Rehabil Med 2005;37(3):129-36.

[10]   Jang SH, Shin SW, Ahn SH, Cho IH, Kim SH. Radiation therapy for heterotopic ossification in a patient with traumatic brain injury. Yonsei Med J 2000;41(4):536-9.

[11]   Schaeffer MA, Sosner J. Heterotopic ossification: treatment of established bone with radiation therapy. Arch Phys Med Rehabil 1995;76(3):284-6.

Submitted: November 07, 2012. *Revised:* December 20, 2012. *Accepted:* December 31, 2012.

SECTION TWO: MORE PAIN

In: Pain Management Yearbook 2013
Editor: Joav Merrick

ISBN: 978-1-63117-944-0
© 2014 Nova Science Publishers, Inc.

Chapter 13

Urinary symptoms in patients with low back pain

Laurence Girard, Neil Baum, MD, and David Mobley, MD*

Harvard University, Cambridge, MA, Department of Urology, Tulane Medical School, New Orleans, Louisiana and Department of Urology, Cornell College of Medicine, Houston, TX, United States of America

Abstract

Chronic back pain is defined as back pain that lasts for more than 7-12 weeks. Other clinicians have defined it as pain that lasts longer than the expected period of healing, and acknowledge that chronic pain may not have well-defined underlying pathological causes. Patients with the symptom of low back pain may have urinary symptoms such as urinary incontinence, urinary frequency, urgency, nocturia, and urinary retention. In this review we looked at the evaluation and treatment of urinary problems in the patient presenting with chronic low back pain primarily focusing on the neurologic causes of low back pain. These symptoms impact a patient's quality of life and can be a cause of embarrassment, reclusive life style, and even depression. Most patients can be helped with an outpatient evaluation and treatment is available for nearly all those unfortunate patients who suffer from urinary symptoms and chronic low back pain.

Keywords: Pain, low back pain, urology

Introduction

Scientific inquiry of low back pain problem demonstrates its socioeconomic importance in most industrialized societies (1). One of the major causes of pain, disability and cost to

---

* Correspondence: Clinical Associate Professor Neil Baum, MD, Department of Urology, Tulane Medical School, 3525 Prytania, New Orleans, LA, United States. E-mail: doctorwhiz@gmail.com.

individuals as well as to society is low-back pain. Nearly 85% of the American population will experience low-back pain at one point in their lives (2). In the majority of cases, low-back pain will resolve in six weeks. Chronic back pain is defined as back pain that lasts for more than 7-12 weeks. Other clinicians have defined it as pain that lasts longer than the expected period of healing, and acknowledge that chronic pain may not have well-defined underlying pathological causes. Patients with the symptom of low back pain may have urinary symptoms such as urinary incontinence, urinary frequency, urgency, nocturia, and urinary retention (3). Herein we review the evaluation and treatment of urinary problems in the patient presenting with chronic low back pain primarily focusing on the neurologic causes of low back pain.

Physiology of voiding

It is important to understand the physiology of voiding under normal conditions to understand what problems can develop in patients with urinary symptoms. Voiding usually begins when a voluntary signal is sent from the cerebral cortex in the brain to initiate urination and will continue until the bladder is empty (4).

Bladder afferent signals ascend the spinal cord to the periaqueductal gray, where they project both to the cerebrum and pontine micturition. After a voluntary signal to initiate voiding occurs, neurons in the pontine micturition center discharge, which causes excitation of the sacral 2,3, and 4 preganglionic neurons. The firing of the neurons in the pontine micturition center causes the detrusor to contract and as a result, an increase in intravesical pressure develops.

The pontine micturition center also causes inhibition of Onuf's nucleus and results in the relaxation of the external sphincter (5). The relaxation of the external urinary sphincter results in urine being released from the urinary bladder. Once urination is complete, the storage function of the bladder starts all over again until the bladder fills to capacity and then the normal cycle repeats itself. The filling phase of the bladder is under sympathetic control and voiding phase is under parasympathetic and voluntary control.

Incidence of voiding symptoms in patients with chronic low back pain

Although the incidence of urinary symptoms in patients with low back pain has been difficult to document, there are studies that report 78% of women with low back pain have urinary incontinence and signs of dysfunctional pelvic floor muscles (6).

In a group of women with degenerative spinal disorders 12.6% out of 214 patients had urinary incontinence. A higher risk of developing incontinence was found in women with radicular weakness (7).

Neurologic Causes

Voiding dysfunction is common in patients with low back pain, but is frequently overlooked as the back pain remains the point of concentration. The etiologies of voiding dysfunction and urinary incontinence includes obstruction, post-surgical conditions, neurological disorders, overdistention of the bladder, inflammatory, or infectious, pharmacological, psychogenic, learned voiding dysfunction, detrusor myopathy and urethral sphincter or urethral incompetence (8). Neurologic causes include caudaequina syndrome, herniated discs, spinal stenosis, multiple sclerosis, diabetes, Parkinson's disease and seizure disorders.

CaudaEquina Syndrome

Caudaequina syndrome (CES) is a neurologic cause which is usually associated with a, space-occupying lesion within the canal of the lumbosacral spine (9). The syndrome is characterized by varying patterns of low back pain, sciatica, lower extremity sensorimotor loss, bowel, bladder and sexual dysfunction. The caudaequina nerve roots provide the sensory and motor innervation to the lower extremities, the pelvic floor and the rectal and urinary sphincters. In a fully developed CES, multiple signs of sensory disorders may appear. The pathophysiology remains unclear but may be related to damage to the nerve roots composing the caudaequina and especially the sacral 2,3 and 4 nerve roots that affect bladder and bowel control.

Another explanation of CES occurs from direct mechanical compression and venous congestion with ischemia. Early diagnosis is often challenging because the initial signs and symptoms are frequently subtle. Classically, the full-blown syndrome includes urinary retention, saddle anesthesia, (see figure 1) bilateral lower extremity pain, numbness, and weakness in the lower extremities. A decrease in rectal tone may be a relatively late finding and this may account for the greater frequency of urinary symptoms than rectal or fecal problems.

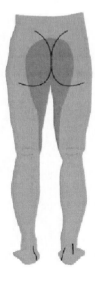

Figure 1. Saddle anesthesia.

Multiple etiologies can cause CES. Among them, non-neoplastic compressive etiologies such as herniated lumbosacral discs, spinal stenosis, and spinal neoplasms play a significant role in the development of the CES. Non-compressive etiologies of the CES include ischemic insults, inflammatory conditions, spinal arachnoiditis and other infectious etiologies.

There are three types of CES that physicians should be aware. The first type is rapid onset of symptoms of back pain, sciatica, with weakness of the lower extremities without a previous history of back problems. The second type is acute bladder dysfunction with a history of low back pain and sciatica. The third is chronic backache and sciatica with gradually progressing CES. Within these groups, CES may be complete or incomplete and its onset may be either acute within hours or gradual and insidious over weeks or months (10).

Early signs and symptoms of a developing postoperative CES are often attributed to common postoperative complaints after back surgery. Therefore, a high index of suspicion is necessary in the postoperative spine patient with back and/or leg pain refractory to medication, especially in the setting of urinary retention. Surgical exploration is warranted if a mass lesion is demonstrated on imaging studies or if symptoms progress and the etiology of the symptoms is not clear based on available information (11). The most common treatment option for CES is spinal decompression (12). Failure to decompress the nerves may result in permanent damage and the possibility of permanent urologic complications.

Herniated Disc

Lumbar disc herniation is a common condition with a generally favorable prognosis. Herniated lumbar disc occurs when the intervertebral disc material (nucleus pulposus or annulus fibrosis) exits beyond the intervertebral disc space. The highest prevalence is among people aged 30-50 years, with a male to female ration of 2:1. Lower urinary tract dysfunction related to herniated disk can raise complex diagnostic and management problems. The two main clinical situations encountered are first, lower urinary tract dysfunction in a context of pain and weakness in the lower extremities, and back pain, and secondly, lower urinary tract dysfunction representing the only clinical sign of herniated disk with no other alteration of the neurological examination. Regardless of the neurological signs, urologic assessment is essential to characterize any lower urinary tract dysfunction and determine the modalities of long-term surveillance (13).

Spinal stenosis

Spinal stenosis is the narrowing of the central lumbar spinal canal, lateral recess, or foramina. Clinically, this narrowing produces neurovascular compression that may lead to pain and urinary symptoms. Lumbar spinal stenosis may be classified by etiology, congenital or acquired, or by symptom complex (radiculopathy, neurogenic claudication, or mechanical back pain). Spinal stenosis can also be classified radiographically, by the location of the stenosis (for example, central canal, lateral recess, or intervertebral foramen) or by the presence of deformity such as spondylolisthesis or scoliosis. Overlap occurs in these schemes of classification in that central stenosis with the sac compression typically leads to neurogenic claudication, whereas lateral recess compression is associated with compression of an individual nerve root and, therefore, radiculopathy. Because radiographic changes associated with stenosis are very common with aging, understanding the pathophysiology of lumbar spinal stenosis is critical in the assessment and management of related symptom complexes.

Spinal stenosis is most common in men and women over 50 years old. The spine is narrowed in one or more of three parts in people with spinal stenosis. The first is the space at the center of the spine. The second is the canal where nerves branch out from the spine. The third is the space between vertebrae. The narrowing puts pressure on the spinal cord and nerves and can cause pain, urinary symptoms and erectile dysfunction in men (14).

Medication causes

Drugs that are often used in patients with low back pain can cause urinary symptoms. Voiding and storage of urine can be affected by the pharmacologic actions of many drugs.

The detrusor muscle that contracts to empty all urine can affect storage and expulsion of urine in two ways. First, if the bladder contracts too often or too strongly, the bladder pressure will overcome the closed urethral sphincter and incontinence may occur. Therefore, medications that stimulate the detrusor muscle or cause involuntary contraction of that muscle will cause incontinence. Examples of medications that stimulate the detrusor muscle include bethanechol and Valrubicin, a chemotherapeutic agent used to treat bladder cancer.

A second effect of the detrusor muscle is relaxation. If drugs such as antihistamines, benzodiazepines, tricyclic antidepressants, inhibit bladder contractions, the bladder will continue to fill and become over-distended and the patient will not be able to urinate and develops urinary retention.

Antiseizure medicines such as thioridazine, chloropromazine (Thorazine®), haloperidol (Haldol®), and clozapine (Clozaril®) also are known to have an alpha-blocker effect and are especially associated with nighttime urinary loss.

Anti-anxiety and muscle relaxant drugs of the benzodiazipine class such as Valium®, Xanax® and Klonopin® also weaken the external urethral sphincter muscle so if there is already some compromise of the external urethral sphincter, incontinence may occur. Diuretic drugs, such as furosamide or hydrocholorothiazide, or even by just consuming excessive amounts of water, or polydipsia, may produce urinary symptoms of frequency, urgency, or incontinence.

Any medication that decreases bowel motility, such as those given for irritable bowel syndrome, may produce problems with urination. Anti-Parkinson drugs and some antihypertensive drugs also block the bladder detrusor. Medications causing incomplete bladder emptying include hyoscyamine, oxybutinin, benztropine, trihexyphenidyl, pindolosp and disopyramide.

Another type of medication that can cause urinary incontinence is soporifics such as the benzodiazepines. Only a small percent of people with incontinence have a problem with eneuresis. However, sedatives may pose a problem for those with incontinence at night. As an alternative, individuals should decrease their fluid and especially their caffeine consumption in the evening.

Opioids

Opioids are commonly used to treat moderate to severe pain especially in patients with chronic low back pain. Some of the most commonly used opioids include morphine, oxycodone and the opiod like drug, tramadol (15) and all of the drugs have side effects of urinary symptoms. Urinary retention is the anticholinergic side effects of opioids and can be secondary to opioid-induced constipation (16).

SSRIs

Patients with chronic back pain frequently use or take anti-depressant medication. Urinary incontinence is one of the side effects listed for serotonergic antidepressants. Exposure to SSRIs is associated with an increased risk for developing urinary incontinence, which can be explained pharmacologically. Approximately 15 out of 1,000 patients treated with an SSRI developed urinary incontinence. Users of Setraline are at the highest risk for urinary incontinence (17).

Dietary Causes

Diet and drinking excessive quantities of water can exacerbate incontinence. Drinking alcoholic beverages can significantly worsen urinary incontinence because alcohol has a direct effect on the detrusor. Alcohol also reduces bladder control and acts as a diuretic while causing dehydration. It actually interferes with the neurological signals from the brain to the bladder, resulting in an increased likelihood that a patient will have a problem of incontinence. Spicy foods such as hot peppers can also increase urinary incontinence acting as an irritant to the lining of the bladder. Acidic foods such as orange juice, cranberry juice, soda and other citrus beverages can have an effect similar to spicy food. Carbonated beverages are particularly deleterious as the carbon dioxide released from the carbonated fluids may irritate the bladder. Excess urine production associated with increased fluid consumption can also be associated with urinary incontinence. Excess urine production may not cause incontinence, per-se, alcohol also reduces bladder control and acts as a diuretic while causing dehydration. It actually interferes with the neurological signals from the brain to the bladder, resulting in an increased likelihood that a patient will have a problem of incontinence. Spicy foods such as hot peppers can also increase urinary incontinence acting as an irritant to the lining of the bladder. Acidic foods such as orange juice, cranberry juice, soda and other citrus beverages can have an effect similar to spicy food. Carbonated beverages are particularly deleterious as the carbon dioxide released from the carbonated fluids may irritate the bladder (18).

Excess urine production associated with increased fluid consumption can also be associated with urinary incontinence. Excess urine production may not cause incontinence, but if there is a weakened continence mechanism, or muscle relaxation due to other medications or due to anatomical weaknesses of the sphincter, then the increased production of urine will overwhelm the impaired detrusor and urethra and may result in incontinence urine leakage.

Caffeine

Caffeine is also considered a bladder irritant and also has the effect of increasing urine output as it serves as a weak diuretic. Caffeine can promote urgency and frequency of urination. Individuals with lower urinary tract symptoms should avoid or be cautious about consuming caffeine-containing foodstuffs.

Obesity

Obesity is an established, but modifiable risk factor for urinary incontinence (19). Obesity is a contributing factor to back pain. Being overweight or obese (BMI >30) can significantly contribute to symptoms associated with osteoporosis, osteoarthritis, rheumatoid arthritis, degenerative disc disease (DDD), spinal stenosis, and spondylolisthesis.

Smoking

Smoking increases the prevalence of lower urinary tract symptoms. Patients with chronic back pain often have comorbidities, including social habits such as tobacco and alcohol abuse. The similarity in the odds ratio between current and former smokers suggests that changes caused by smoking occur early. The decreased risk of lower urinary tract symptoms after the cessation of smoking suggests that the process is reversible (20).

Evaluation of patients with chronic low back pain

The voiding diary is the easiest method of understanding the voiding issues in a patient with chronic low back pain and urinary symptoms (21,22). Most diaries consist of a chart that records fluid intake, voiding and incontinence episode. This is easy to do, although difficult to motivate patients to keep a diary for more than 1-2 days. The test is helpful in distinguishing polyuria, urinary frequency, urinary incontinence and nocturia. It is imperative to perform a urinalysis in all patients with chronic back pain who present with any urinary symptom. If there is evidence of a urinary tract infection, a urine culture is indicated. The urinalysis can also be helpful to detect the presence of glucose, protein, blood, bacteria, all of which can be implicated in the cause of urinary symptoms in patients with chronic low back pain.

Voiding urodynamic study

Urodynamic studies are considered the gold standard for diagnosing urinary symptoms in patients with chronic back pain. The etiology of urinary symptoms associated with low back pain can be determined urodynamically assessing the pressure-flow relationship during bladder filling and voiding.

Urodynamic testing includes procedures that evaluate how well the bladder, sphincters and urethra, are storing and releasing urine. Most of these studies focus on the urine's ability to hold and empty intravesical contents. This is a relatively non-invasive study conducted in the doctor's office can further elucidate the cause of the urinary symptoms in patients with chronic low back pain.

Cystoscopy

If there is a question of intravesical pathology, a cystoscopy is often recommended.

Management of urinary symptoms in patients with chronic low back pain

Nearly all patients with back pain and urinary symptoms begin with conservative management. Pelvic floor muscle training and Kegel exercises, which strengthen muscles that control urination, are often helpful in men and women with mild to moderate urinary symptoms and low back pain. Biofeedback is also an option that involves the insertion of a sensor inserted into the vagina or rectum to aid in muscle identification of the muscles responsible for continence. Many clinicians begin by recommending a trial of bladder control training.

Limiting fluids to no more than 6-8 cups per day while the patient is learning to control their bladder can also helpful for those patients with mild incontinence. Bladder control training is particularly helpful with symptoms of overactive bladder or urgency. Biofeedback involves using electrodes to convert muscle potentials into auditory or visual signals. Patients learn to increase or decrease voluntary muscle activity. Conservative behavioral and biofeedback treatments are safe and effective interventions that should be more readily available to patients as a first-line treatment for voiding dysfunction. Patient education has a favorable success rate and makes the patient more responsible and encourages the patient to take ownership in the treatment.

Weight loss

Significant weight gain can weaken pelvic muscle tone, leading to urinary incontinence. Losing weight through healthy diet and exercise is important. Patients should be referred to weight loss clinics or bariatric physicians who can assist if there is morbid obesity that may also have urinary symptoms as a complication of the weight gain. Some patients with chronic low back pain have difficult exercising.

Low impact exercises might be more appropriate for patients with low back pain such as swimming, elliptical machines, or other low impact exercises like aqua jogging to augment a weight loss program.

Smoking cessation

Smoking cessation can also be helpful for the treatment of urinary inconinence. The results of smoking cessation are XYZ. Varenicline is the most recently approved drug for smoking cessation and has been prescribed widely. Varenicline was approved by the Food and Drug Administration (FDA) in May 2006, and in five years 8.9 million patients received 21.8 million prescriptions for this drug from outpatient retail pharmacies in the United States (23). Varenicline was associated with significantly higher abstinence rates than the nicotine patch (24).

Medications

There is a variety of medications used to treat urinary incontinence. The main categories of (change to just "the medications") medications used in conjunction with behavioral techniques include anticholinergics, topical estrogen, imipramine, duloxetine, and recently the beta-3 agonist, mirabergron. Anticholenergics are medications that relax the detrusor and therefore may be helpful for urge incontinence. Several drugs fall under this category including oxybutynin, tolterodine, darifenacin, fesoterodine, solifenacin, and trospium. Side effects of these types of medications include constipation, dry mouth, blurred vision and flushing. Another treatment option is applying low-dose, topical estrogen in the form of vaginal cream, ring or patch and may help tone and rejuvenate tissues in the vaginal and urethra areas. This can reduce some of the symptoms of incontinence. Imipramine, a tricyclic antidepressant, can be used to treat mixed - urge and stress - incontinence. Imipramine has a dual mechanism of action which includes an anticholinergic effect as well as alpha stimulation of the internal urinary sphincter located at the bladder neck. As a result there is a decrease in detrusor pressure and an increase contraction of the bladder neck with an increase in urethral resistance.

Dluoxetine is an antidepressant sometimes used to treat stress incontinence although it is not approved by FDA in the U.S. for this condition.

Mirabegron first-in-class selective β(3)-adrenoceptor agonist that improves symptoms associated with OAB by enhancing storage function and relaxing the urinary bladder. Mirabegron has been approved the United States for the indication of urgency, urinary frequency and urge urinary incontinence associated with OAB. In phase III clinical trials mirabegron at doses of 50 or 100 mg for 12 weeks significantly decreased the mean number of incontinence episodes and micturition episodes per 24 hours, and was safe and well tolerated (25).

Overactive bladder (OAB) is a chronic syndrome with debilitating symptoms that negatively affect health-related quality of life. Although anticholinergic agents have been first-line treatment for OAB for many years, the efficacious pharmacologic management of this condition has been compromised by concerns regarding tolerability. Anticholinergic agents prevent involuntary contractions of the bladder detrusor muscle by preventing acetylcholine from binding to the M2 and M3 muscarinic receptor subtypes. Anticholinergics are not tissue specific, and their use for treatment of OAB has been associated with side effects such as dry mouth, constipation, and blurred vision. Recent studies with extended-release formulations and newly developed receptor subtype-specific anticholinergic agents demonstrate that side effects are typically mild to moderate and generally tolerable, seldom leading to patient withdrawal. By incorporating patient-initiated dose adjustment into the protocol, the physician can effectively manage adverse events associated with OAB without compromising efficacy. Recent dose-adjustment data with extended-release oxybutynin suggest that, given some control in the process, patients are willing to tolerate certain side effects in exchange for symptom relief (26).

Anticholinergic medications also may have an adverse effect on the central nervous system. Muscarinic receptors in the brain play an important role in cognitive function, and there is growing awareness that antimuscarinic OAB drugs may have adverse central nervous system (CNS) effects, ranging from headache to cognitive impairment and even rare episodes of psychosis. The blood-brain barrier (BBB) plays a key role in protecting the CNS, but it is penetrable. The lipophilic tertiary amines, particularly oxybutynin, are more likely to cross the BBB than the hydrophilic quaternary amine, trospium chloride, which have few adverse CNS effects. In 2008 the US products label for oral oxybutynin were modified to include the potential for anticholinergic CNS events and a warning to monitor patients for adverse CNS effects. Even modest cognitive impairment in the elderly may negatively affect a patient's independence. Selection of an antimuscarinic OAB drug with reduced potential for CNS side-effects is advisable (27).

All available drugs are efficacious for OAB treatment, and clinically relevant differences among them have not been proven consistently. Moreover, age, gender, and the type of OAB (dry vs. wet) seem to lack clinically relevant impact on the efficacy of OAB treatment. The various drugs are similar in tolerability, with the exception of more dry mouth and central nervous effects with slow-release oxybutynin. Knowledge of the pharmacokinetic properties of the individual substances is important in order to choose the appropriate therapy for each patient.

Urecholine for weakness of the detrusor muscle

Urecholine (bethanechol) is a cholinergic agent which is structurally and pharmacologically related to acetylcholine. It acts by producing the effects of stimulation of the parasympathetic nervous system. It increases the tone of the detrusor muscle, sometimes producing a contraction sufficiently strong to initiate micturition and empty the bladder. This is indicated for short-term use in patients with decreased bladder contractions or bladder pressure. A significant drawback to this medication is that the dosage of urecholine required for effective bladder emptying is likely to cause intolerable side effects.

Alpha-blockers for outlet obstruction

Men over the age of 50 years with chronic low back pain often have associated bladder outlet obstruction due to an enlarged prostate. Alpha-blockers are commonly used for the treatment of outlet obstruction in men.

Minimally invasive treatments

Intermittent catherization
Intermittent catherization is used for patients who are unable to empty their bladder and who have the motor skills to perform the procedure. Evacuating the bladder at regular intervals protects the kidneys from infection and damage. It also lowers the risk of over distension the bladder and eliminates the need for using an indwelling catheter, which can be associated with more risks and complications.

Sacral nerve stimulation
Sacral nerve stimulation (SNS) has been used for severe urge incontinence, overactive bladder and urinary retention that have not been successfully managed with other treatment modalities. With SNS an electrical stimulator is inserted under the skin above the buttocks. The stimulator is attached to electrodes that transmit impulses to the sacral 2,3, or 4 nerves, which are the nerves that play a role in bladder storage and emptying. Sacral nerve stimulation is reasonably safe and effective treating refraction urinary urge incontinence or urinary retention.

Posterior nerve stimulation (PTNS)
PTNS is an effective minimally invasive option for treatment of patients with complaints of urge incontinence. Patients treated with PTNS have improvement in both subjective as well as objective parameters. PTNS is the least invasive form of neruomodulation used to treat overactive bladder and can be used as primary therapy. Most of the research on PTNS has been for the treatment of overactive bladder and/or urge incontinence (28).

Surgery

There are several surgical options to ameliorate urinary symptoms associate with low back pain including spinal decompression. Urinary improvement can be anticipated in patients successfully undergoing neurosurgical or orthopedic procedures but a detailed discussion of the surgical back is beyond the scope of this paper.

Conclusion

Patients with chronic low back pain often have urinary symptoms. These symptoms impact a patient's quality of life and can be a cause of embarrassment, reclusive life style, and even depression. Most patients can be helped with an outpatient evaluation and treatment is available for nearly all those unfortunate patients who suffer from urinary symptoms and chronic low back pain.

References

[1]   Nachemson AL. Newest knowledge of low back pain. A critical look. Clin Orthopaedics Relat Res 1992;279:8-20.

[2]   Midelton K, Fish D. Lumbar spondylosis: clinical presentation and treatment approaches. Curr Rev Musculoskelet Med 2009;2(2): 94-104.

[3]   Eliasson K, Elfving B., Nordgren B, et al. Urinary incontinence in women with low back pain. Man Ther 2008;13(3):206-12.

[4]   DasGupta R, Kavia R, Fowler C. Cerebral mechanisms and voiding function. BJU Int 2007;99(4): 731-4.

[5]   Chancellor M, Yoshimura N. Neurophysiology of stress urinary incontinence. Rev Urol 2004; 6(suppl 3): S19-S28.

[6]   Eliasson K, Elfving B, Nordgren B, et al. Urinary incontinence in women with low back pain. Man Ther 2008;13(3):206-12.

[7]   Riggo D, Kolarovski B, Luptak K, et al. Urinary incontinence in degenerative spinal disease. Acta Chir Orthop Traumatol Chech 2011;78(1):67-70.

[8]   Dorfinger A, Monga A. Voiding dysfunction. Curr Opin Obstet Gynecol 2001;13(5):507-12.

[9]   Levis J. CaudaEquina syndrome. West J Emerg Med 2009;10(1):20.

[10]   Gardner A, Gardner E, Morley T. Caudaequina syndrome: A review of the current clinical and medico-legal position. Eur Spine J 2011;20(5): 690-7.

[11]   Spector L, Madigan L, Rhyne A, et al. CaudaEquina syndrome. J Am Acad Orthop Surg 2008;15(8):471-9.

[12]   Spector L, Madigan L, Rhyne A, et al. Caudaequina syndrome. J Am Acad Orthop Surg 2008;16(9):471-9.

[13]   Jordon J, Konstantinou K, O'Dowd J, et al. Herniated lubmar disc. Clin Evid 2011;2011pii:1118.

[14]   National Institute of Arthritis and Musculoskeletal and Skin Diseases. What is spinal stenosis? June 2009.

[15]   Becker D. Pain management: Part 1: Managing acute and postoperative dental pain. Anesth Prog 2010;57(2):67-9.

[16]   Chau D, Walker V, Pai L, et al. Opiates and elderly. Use and side effects. Clin Interv Aging 2008;3(2):273-8.

[17]   Movig K, Leufkens H, Belitser S, Lenderink A, et al. Selective serotonin reuptake inhibitor-induced urinary incontinence. Pharmacoepidemiol Drug Saf 2002;11(4):271-9.

[18]   Miline J. Behavioral therapies for overactive bladder: making sense of the evidence. J Wound Ostomy Continence Nurs 2008;35(1):93-101.

[19]   Subak L, Wing R, West D, et al. Weight loss to treat urinary incontinence in overweight and obese women. N Engl J Med 2009;360(5):481-90.

[20]   Koshimaki J, Hakama M, Huhtala H et al. Association of smoking with lower urinary tract symptoms. J Urol 1998;159(5):1580-2.

[21]   Harkaway R, Bergner D, Altman D, et al. Measurement characteristics of a voiding diary for use by men and women with overactive bladder. Urology 2003;61(4):802-9.

[22]   Nygaard I, Holocomb R. Reproducibility of the seven-day voiding diary in women with stress urinary incontinence. Int Urogynecol J Pelvic Floor Dysfunct 2000;11(1):15-7.

[23]   US Department of Food and Drug Administration. FDA Drug Safety Communication: Safety review update of Chantix (varenicline) and risk of neuropsychiatric adverse events. Accessed 2012 Dec 01. URL: http://1.usa.gov/nHPMJ6

[24]   Hsueh C, Hsueh K, Chou M, et al. A comparison of the effectiveness of varenicline and transdermal nicotine patch in outpatients following a standardized smoking cessation program in Southern Taiwan. Eval Health Prof 2012 Dec 4.

[25]   Gras J. Mirabegron for the treatment of overactive bladder. Drugs Today (Barc) 2012;48(1):25-32.

[26]   Staskin D, Macdiarmid S. Using anticholinergics to treat overactive bladder: the issue of treatment tolerability. Am J Med 2007;119 (3 Suppl 1):9-15.

[27] Kay G, Aboui-Donia M, Messer W, et al. Antimuscarinic drugs for overactive bladder and their potential effects on cognitive function in older patients. Rev Urol 2007;9(4): 191-6.

[28] Onal M, Ugurlucan F, Yalcin O. The effects of posterior tibial nerve stimulation on refractory overactive bladder syndrome and bladder circulation. Arch Gynecol Obstet 2012;286(6):1453-7.

Submitted: December 14, 2012. *Revised:* January 15, 2013. *Accepted:* February 10, 2013.

In: Pain Management Yearbook 2013
Editor: Joav Merrick

ISBN: 978-1-63117-944-0
© 2014 Nova Science Publishers, Inc.

Chapter 14

Relationship of chronic low back pain and erectile dysfunction

Courtney Jacobs and Neil Baum, MD*

Louisiana State University School of Medicine and Department of Urology,
Tulane Medical School, New Orleans, Louisiana, United States of America

Abstract

Chronic low back pain is one of the most common maladies of modern man. Many of these men have accompanying erectile dysfunction (ED). The cause(s) of erectile dysfunction in men with chronic low back pain is multifactorial. This article will review the causes of erectile dysfunction in men with chronic low back pain. We will also review the noninvasive evaluation that can easily be accomplished by most physicians caring for men with chronic low back pain and erectile dysfunction. Finally, we will review the treatment options that are effective in men with chronic low back pain who are affected with erectile dysfunction. The causes of ED in these men include the side effects of medication used to treat back pain, hormone deficiency, depression and other psychological causes, and neurologic causes. Treatment of ED for men with chronic back pain can be very successful.

Keywords: Pain, low back pain, urology, erectile function, ED, opioid use, SSRI, selective serotonin reuptake inhibitors, obesity, cigarette smoking, stress, depression, testosterone, hormone deficiency

---

* Correspondence: Clinical Associate Professor Neil Baum, MD, Department of Urology, Tulane Medical School, 3525 Prytania, New Orleans, LA, United States. E-mail: doctorwhiz@gmail.com

Introduction

Back pain is a common problem affecting 80% American men over their lifetime. In the vast majority of cases, low-back pain has no identifiable cause and is termed "non-specific." In most cases, low-back pain is often benign, self-limiting and resolves in six weeks, with or without treatment. However, around 30% of individuals with low-back pain have recurrent or persistent symptoms. As a result, low-back pain is one of the most common reasons for medical visits. Many of these men with chronic low back pain also suffer from erectile dysfunction. Erectile dysfunction (ED) consists of the inability to maintain an erection suitable for sexual intercourse. Men may suffer minimal to severe ED. According to the Massachusetts Male Aging Study, 52% of men between the ages of 40 to 70 experience some degree of ED (1). The incidence of suffering with ED correlates with increasing age and health problems (2). Health problems such as hypertension, diabetes, heart disease, and high cholesterol are all associated with ED (3). The ED associated with back pain is multifactorial. Just 50 years ago the medical textbooks considered ED to be of psychogenic origin in 90% of the men. Later studies demonstrated that in men after age 50, most of the men had physical causes for their ED and younger men had mostly psychogenic causes of ED. However, even in younger men, who also have low back pain, there are often physical causes of ED.

Neurological causes of back pain and ED

Biomechanical, medication related, psychogenic and/or hormonal conditions may be to blame for chronic lower back pain and ED. Additionally, many men have neurological conditions that cause chronic lower back pain and may contribute to their ED. Bulging discs, sciatica, spondylolisthesis, spinal degeneration, and stenosis affect the spinal cord and predispose people to chronic lower back pain. Peripheral neuropathies, pelvic and pudendal nerve lesions, and spinal cord trauma may also contribute to chronic lower back pain and ED (4). Central nervous system disorders, including multiple sclerosis, may also be associated with chronic lower back pain and ED.

To evaluate the association between lower back problems and erectile dysfunction, one study found that 34% of men under 50 that underwent a surgical procedure for lumbar spine disease suffered erectile dysfunction post-surgery (5).

Those patients did not have any risk factors, except chronic lower back pain, before surgery (6). Moreover, another study found that the medical profession is underestimating neurological causes of erectile dysfunction. The study attributed neurological factors to the cause of erectile dysfunction in 69% of the patients, and concluded that physicians should perform a neurological evaluation when patients present with ED (7). Spinal cord injuries/diseases, nerve damage, and central nervous system diseases are all associated with both chronic lower back pain and ED; patients presenting with both problems should be evaluate further to explore neurological causes of organic impotence.

Opioid treatment and ED

Doctors often prescribe long-acting opioid medication to relieve the pain experienced by patients with a neurological cause for their back pain. Sexual dysfunction is a common problem among men with chronic back pain. Yet, many of these men suffer in silence. It is very common for doctors to rarely ask about patients' sexual concerns, and educational literature on the subject of ED associated with chronic opioid treatment is relatively scarce. Ironically, in many of these cases the long-acting opioid medications prescribed to relieve patients' pains may be causing or contributing to their sexual problems (8).

Since the 1990s, prescriptions written for opioid medications have significantly and steadily increased (9). Deleterious opioid effects on endocrine function and sexual health were first noticed decades ago in sexual dysfunction associated with intravenous heroin use (10). Decreased libido is common among addicts in general, but ED in men is especially common in those with opioid dependence. Recent studies show that addiction or aberrant opioid taking behaviors occur in 24% of all patients prescribed opioids for chronic back pain treatment (11).

Another problem with opioid treatment for chronic lower back pain includes concerns about the adverse consequences of opioid treatment. For example, a common side effect to narcotic medications is opioid-induced endocrine deficiency which may lead to sexual dysfunction. Considerable evidence through the years has suggested that long-acting opioids used on a daily basis for more than a month can have a number of adverse effects on the endocrine function. The most common and clinically significant effects are androgen deficiencies (12).

Opioid medications can exert a number of effects that alter the normal functioning of sex hormones found in hypothalamic-pituitary-gonadal (HPG) pathways. HPG controls the production of sex hormones and begins with secretion by the hypothalamus of gonadotropin-releasing hormone (GnRH). The GnRH stimulates the pituitary gland to secrete the gonadotropins, LH and FSH. LH and FSH stimulate the production of testosterone in the testes. Unfortunately, opioids exert an inhibitory effect on GnRH, thus decreasing LH (13). The decreased levels of LH cause the testes to decrease the production of testosterone resulting in a deficiency. Testosterone deficiency in men with and without back pain results in adverse effects such as weight gain, fatigue, depression, and sexual dysfunction including ED. Therefore, endocrine deficiencies should be considered in all men with chronic back pain who are taking daily opioids. However, opioid-induced sexual dysfunction can be successfully treated.

Opioids also exert a negative influence on adrenal androgen production. The adrenal hormones dehydroepiandrosterone (DHEA), DHEA sulfate (DHEAS), and androstenedione are weakly androgenic and they are precursors of testosterone. Serum DHEAS levels are used to determine adrenal function in general and, more specifically, adrenal androgen production. Daily use of opioids decreases adrenal androgen production as measured by DHEAS levels. Daniell et al. assessed DHEAS levels in patients treated with sustained-action oxycodone, sustained-action morphine, continuous transdermal fentanyl, or methadone and found decreased DHEAS levels in over half of those studied.

The exact mechanism by which opioids reduce DHEAS and, consequently, interfere with adrenal androgen production is not known; however, the resultant deficiency may be of clinical importance (14). It appears that all opioids cause endocrine deficiencies at least to some degree, which may influence result in sexual dysfunction. A significant proportion of men treated with sustained action opioids, estimated at 5 million in the US and Canada, are testosterone deficient (15).

Stress related back pain and ED

Back pain of stress related etiology, recently termed tension myositis syndrome (16), often frustrates both the physician and patient. Back pain due to tension myositis syndrome is caused by emotional and psychological issues. Physicians make the diagnosis after ruling out organic causes of back pain. Stress may decrease the blood flow to patients' muscles making the muscles more susceptible to strains and injuries. As well as decreasing blood flow to back muscles, stress reduces the blood flow to the penis, making it difficult for a man to achieve an erection. Psychogenic causes of ED affected 5% of men under 40 and 15% of men 65 years of age or older (17). Treatment for both stress-related back pain and ED of psychogenic origin include identifying the cause of the anxiety and stress, cognitive-behavioral therapy, pharmacological therapy to reduce the stress and anxiety, and/or relationship counseling (18). Recently, psychotherapy proved the best method of improving ED in men suffering ED of psychogenic origin (19).

Obesity and ED

Obesity is a contributing factor to back pain. Being overweight or obese (BMI >30) can significantly contribute to symptoms associated with osteoporosis, osteoarthritis (OA), rheumatoid arthritis (RA), degenerative disc disease (DDD), spinal stenosis, and spondylolisthesis.

Findings indicate that overweight and obesity increase the risk of low back pain. Being overweight and obesity have the strongest association with seeking care for low back pain and chronic low back pain (20). Obesity alone has a significant impact on male sexual health. A study, published in The Journal of Sexual Medicine, focused on 2,435 Italian male patients who sought outpatient treatment for sexual dysfunction between 2001 and 2007. Among participants, 41.5% were normal weight, 42.4% were overweight, 12.1% were obese, and 4% were severely obese.

The mean age was 52. Patients had lab blood tests and a penile Doppler ultrasound to measure penile blood flow. They also were interviewed about their ED and completed a mental health questionnaire. The study found that the degree of obesity directly correlated with a decrease in testosterone levels. Among study participants, the men who had more severe obesity had a lower level of testosterone compared to those men who were not significantly obese (21). Of course, adverse effects of low testosterone included sexual dysfunction and ED.

Smoking and ED

Patients with chronic back pain often have comorbidities, including social habits such as tobacco use (22). It has been well known that cigarette smoking has a deleterious impact on the ability to have an erection. Cigarette smoking may be related to a down regulation of the nitric oxide/cyclic guanosine monophosphate pathway in penile tissue, probably related to increased oxidative stress (23). Both smoking and ED have often been associated with endothelial dysfunction throughout the circulation including the sinusoids in the corporal bodies of the penis. It is hypothesized that acute endothelial dysfunction caused by smoking could be attributed to increased oxidative stress (24).

Human studies have demonstrated that nicotine administration via nasal spray or transdermal patch reduces pain sensitivity in both smokers and nonsmokers (25). However, patients with chronic nicotine exposure fail to show the same beneficial analgesic effect. In a group of chronic smokers who underwent general surgery requiring postoperative patient-controlled analgesia and an overnight hospital admission and who were in the immediate post-operative period reported no decrease in postoperative pain with nicotine patches. Thus is appears that chronic nicotine exposure may induce changes in receptor concentrations and be responsible for mediating or modulating nociceptive responses to stimuli, subsequently resulting in tolerance and mitigating the analgesic properties of acute use of nicotine. A study demonstrated that there is a dose response relationship between the number of cigarettes smoked per day and the prevalence of chronic low back pain. This study also found that current smokers had the strongest association with debilitating back pain (26). There are many psychological, socioeconomic, biological, and medical factors which play a role in the complex relationship between chronic back pain, smoking, and ED. But the study from the Ochsner Clinic pointed out that a dedicated physician reinforcing a smoking cessation program could have a significant positive effect on both smoking cessation and patient well-being (27). Although the study did not specifically test for ED, other studies have demonstrated that smoking cessation does have a positive impact on a man's ability to have an erection (28,29).

Depression and anti-depressants and ED

Many men with chronic back pain suffer from depression. Men who were once gainfully employed are often unable to return to work and are spending more time at home or in bed because of their pain, and, as a result, are unable to participate in life's daily activities. These men are often prescribed anti-depressants, such as SSRIs, which are frequently associated with sexual dysfunctions. Also men with chronic back pain are at risk for divorce, separation or a failed relationship all of which can contribute to or exacerbate depression. It is also of importance to note that depression even without back pain is often a major cause of ED (ED) due to both its psychological and physiological symptoms. It is well accepted that moderate or severe depression may cause ED, and ED per se may cause or exacerbate depressive mood (30). Not only can depression affect the ability to achieve an erection, it also often negatively affects libido, or sex drive. *Journal of Clinical Psychiatry* used a validated questionnaire to survey 6,297 patients taking a range of antidepressants. Overall, 37% of people taking antidepressants experienced sexual dysfunction (31). Occasional reports of sexual dysfunction associated with use of monoamine oxidase inhibitors and tricyclic antidepressants began to appear during the 1960s and 1970s. However, with the arrival of newer antidepressants in the late 1980s and 1990s, reports of sexual side effects increased, notably with regard to use of selective serotonin reuptake inhibitors (SSRIs). SSRIs may have a negative impact on any or all phases of the sexual cycle, causing decreased or complete absence of libido, impaired arousal, ED, and absent or delayed orgasm, but they are most commonly associated with delayed ejaculation and absent or delayed orgasm. The exact mechanism of sexual dysfunction is unknown. One possible mechanism is by inhibition of dopaminergic neurotransmission, resulting in described persistent sexual dysfunction (32). Estimates of sexual dysfunction associated with SSRIs vary, ranging from small percentages to more than 80% (33). The precise frequency is not known, and the issue is somewhat confounded by the fact that some studies report incidence (the number of new cases in a given population during a specified period) and some report prevalence (the number of existing cases in a given population during a specified period or at one time point).

Occasional reports of sexual dysfunction associated with use of monoamine oxidase inhibitors and tricyclic antidepressants began to appear during the 1960s and 1970s. Tricyclic antidepressants are a class of medications approved by the FDA for treating depression. While not approved by the FDA for treating pain, they may play a role in chronic back pain management. They are prescribed off-label for nerve pain, and in this role are called adjuvants. By interacting with chemicals in the nervous system, tricyclic antidepressants adjust the way the pain signals are transmitted. One pill can yield both antidepressant and pain-relieving effects, but the way in which these effects are brought about are not related to one another. Also, if a man is taking a tricyclic antidepressant for pain, the dose will likely be lower than if the man is taking it for depression. Tricyclic antidepressants are one of a few types of antidepressants used to manage chronic back pain. Others, often known as novel antidepressants, includes bupropion, venlafaxine, and duloxetine (brand name Cymbalta). Like tricyclics, some of the novel antidepressants are effective for managing neuropathic back pain. The good news is that they also incur fewer side effects than tricyclic antidepressants. But a number of novel antidepressants are so targeted to chemical interactions relating to depression that unless an underlying psychological problem is responsible for your pain, they may not be effective at relieving it. Tricyclic antidepressants, especially amitriptyline, are the most cost-effective of all off-label medications prescribed for back pain.

Clinicians caring for men with low back pain should be aware that delayed ejaculation and orgasm, symptoms most frequently associated with SSRIs, are not usually associated with depression itself, whereas decreased sexual desire is. Also important to bear in mind is that sexual functioning fluctuates in ordinary life and that sexual desire and expectations evolve over a man's life cycle. Sexual desire is also influenced by various psychological factors, such as joy, sorrow, mutual affection, disagreement, and so on (34). One of the great ironies of depression treatment is that while depression can rob you of your desire for sex, the drugs that treat it can be much worse, causing not only low libido, but also ED and difficulties with orgasm.

Post-SSRI sexual dysfunction (PSSD) is a name given to a reported iatrogenic sexual dysfunction caused by the previous use of selective serotonin reuptake inhibitor (SSRI) antidepressants. While apparently uncommon, it can last for months, years, or sometimes indefinitely after the discontinuation of SSRIs (35). It may represent a specific subtype of

SSRI discontinuation syndrome. It appears as though the majority of men regain their sexual function after discontinuing the use of SSRIs (36). But, some do not, and are faced with the persistent symptoms of post-SSRI sexual dysfunction (PSSD). In one study in which patients with SSRI-induced sexual dysfunction were switched to the dopaminergic antidepressant amineptine, 55% still had at least some type of sexual dysfunction after six months compared to 4% in the control group treated with amineptine alone. In recent placebo controlled double-blind studies testing the efficacy of SSRIs for treating premature ejaculation, it has been noted that the ejaculation-delaying effect of the medications may last for months after discontinuation in a percentage of the trial participants.

Hormonal disorders and ED

Although hormonal disorders are an uncommon cause of ED, men with lower back pain may also be suffering from hypogonadism, or other endocrine disorders, that may contribute to their ED. Around 5% of all men that suffer with ED concurrently have hypogonadism, or low testosterone levels (37). Men, especially with severe hypogonadism, found improvement in their ED after initiating testosterone therapy (38). Other endocrine disorders associated with ED include thyroid and pituitary disorders. Hyperthyroidism, or overproduction of thyroid hormones, has been associated with ED (39). Hypothyroidism, or low thyroid hormone, also plays a role in erectile and sexual dysfunction (40). Additionally, hyperprolactinemia, which usually occurs as the result of a pituitary tumor, impairs both testosterone levels and may play a role in ED (41). While low testosterone, pituitary, and thyroid disorders may coincide with ED in men with chronic lower back pain, the exact role that hormones play in ED still remains uncertain.

Adequate testosterone levels are needed for satisfactory pain control as this hormone is intricately involved in endogenous opioid activity (42). Testosterone is also necessary for opioid receptor binding, maintenance of blood-brain barrier transport, and activation of dopamine and norepinephrine activity (43). Consequently, a lack of testosterone activity in the CNS may result in poor pain control, depression, sleep disturbances, and lack of energy and motivation.

In the periphery, testosterone functions as a primary androgenic compound for tissue healing (44). A deficiency of testosterone, therefore, impairs healing and control of inflammation at pain sites. There may be two reasons for testosterone depletion in a chronic pain patient. One is pituitary insufficiency caused by severe pain, per se. Constant, persistent, uncontrolled pain will, over time, exert enough stress on the hypothalamus and pituitary (GnRH, LH, FSH) to cause the inadequate secretion of testosterone from the adrenal and gonads. When the cause of hypotestosteronemia is hypothalamic-pituitary insufficiency, other hormones such as cortisol, pregnenolone, or thyroid may likely show serum deficiencies. The second and most common cause of testosterone deficiency is opioid administration (45). Low testosterone levels have been observed with essentially all oral and intrathecal opioids (46). Low testosterone serum levels are primarily caused by opioid suppression of GnRH in the hypothalamus. Opioids may also directly impair testosterone production in the adrenal or gonads. Both causes of hypotestosteronemia may simultaneously exist. Both causes require testosterone replacement. It is unknown if testosterone suppression by opioids is opioid-specific, dose-related, or related to opioid serum levels.

Testosterone positively controls both the enzymatic steps necessary for initiation and termination of the erectile process, its net effect on erection ends up as modest. The main physiological action of testosterone is therefore to timely adjust the erectile process as a function of sexual desire, therefore finalizing erections with sex. According, sexual thoughts and motivations are universally accepted as the most testosterone dependent aspects of male sexual behavior. For these reasons, treating hypogonadism restores impaired penile erections in animal models as well as in a clinical setting (47).

Excessive alcohol use and back pain

Alcohol is widely used by patients with chronic back pain however it actually creates more problems than it solves as alcohol is a major depressant and will exacerbate any pre-existing depression. Studies have documented that there are higher levels of alcohol abuse, alcohol consumption, and alcohol blood levels in men with chronic low back pain than reported in the general population (48).

Intercourse and low back pain

Chronic pain infuses every aspect of a person's life. For some people, intercourse itself can cause pain. It is not uncommon for men with chronic back pain to state that they can obtain an erection but upon assuming the male superior position and supporting themselves on their elbows and knees, that movement of the pelvis and the lumbosaacral spine results in the loss of an erection.

Evaluating men with low back pain for ED

Causes and symptoms associated with hormonal deficiencies are summarized in the Table 1. Interview instruments have been proposed to screen men for hypogonadism. These questionnaires, however, have clinical limitations. The Androgen Deficiency in Aging Men (ADAM) questionnaire was validated for men over the age of 40 (49). Another one – the Androtest© – is a 12-item structured interview designed to screen for male hypogonadism (50).

Laboratory assessments of male testosterone levels were used to determine the predictive values of both ADAM and the Androtest. These levels are mandatory for confirming the diagnosis of hypogonadism and as a clinical basis for deciding whether or not to initiate testosterone replacement therapy. A diagnosis of endocrine deficiency should be considered in all patients receiving daily opioid treatment in an amount equivalent to or greater than 100 mg morphine (51). Patients should routinely be asked about symptoms suggestive of sex-hormone deficiency prior to treatment for their low back pain and at regularly scheduled follow-up medical visits.

Table 1. Opioid induced deficiencies

Hypogonadism
  Decreased GNRH Decreases LH Decreased testosterone

Adrenal androgen deficiency
  Decreased DHEA Decreased DHEAS Decreased androstenedione

Symptoms
  Anemia
  Decreased libido decreased muscle mass depression
  Erectile dysfunction fatigue
  Hot flashes
  Menstrual irregularities osteoporosis
  Sweating
  Weight gain

Clinical laboratories report a wide range of normal serum testosterone concentrations (e.g., 275-800 ng/dL) without specifying age-range-specific values. The normal range for free testosterone – that is testosterone not bound to protein – is also very wide (e.g., 5-21 ng/dL). Typically, young men have much higher levels of total or free testosterone than older men, so young men with clinical hypogonadism may still have testosterone levels within the normal range established by the clinical laboratory. Whenever testosterone levels are low, men also should be screened via serum prolactin levels for pituitary tumors. As a further test, decreased LH levels in men support a diagnosis of opioid-induced hypogonadism, but LH may be within the normal range. Also, testosterone maintains red blood cell production, so men with reduced testosterone associated with hypogonadism may exhibit mild anemia due to decreases in those cells.

Treating ED and chronic back pain

The mainstay of treatment of men with chronic back pain and ED should follow the three lines of therapy outline by Dr. Tom Lue (52). First line treatment consists of counseling, pharmacologic therapy, hormone replacement therapy and vacuum erection devices. Second line treatment is pharmacologic injection therapy and transurethral medication followed by third line treatment consisting of surgery.

Although organically induced ED is more common than psychogenic ED, almost all patients have a psychological component to their problem. Psychosexual counseling may therefore be helpful in many cases, especially where there are relationship difficulties, which compound the problem. Psychosexual counseling generally involves obtaining a detailed history not only from the patient but also, if possible, from the partner. Psychosexual counseling is most effective when the problem is due to technique or there are unrealistic expectations on one or both sides of the relationship. Sometimes it is simple suggestions that can help men with chronic low back pain. First, the treatment might be changed to help improve sexual functioning.

Additionally, one could consider changing the man's medication. For example decreasing the use of opiates and use more other medications that are effective for treating chronic pain with less effect on sexuality. Examples of these medications include Cymbalta (duloxetine) and Lyrica (pregabalin). For men with low testosterone levels, a prescription for testosterone may help with sexual desire. Drug treatments such as sildenafil, vardenafil, and tadalafil should be used early in the management of men with back pain and ED.

A doctor caring for men with chronic back pain needs to encourage the man and his partner to become creative about sexual intimacy. These couples should not think of sex in the same way as they always did. The positions that worked before the man struggled with chronic pain may not work with the presence of chronic back pain. The couple may need to think of new ways to initiate intimacy and different ways to be intimate. For example the couple can change sexual positions. Especially if the man has severe back pain being on top during intercourse can be painful. These men might try a male in the inferior position or on the bottom or even side-to-side position to alleviate back pain. Men might also find that placing a small pillow under the back for support may be helpful.

Another suggestion may be for men with back pain and ED is to find out the time of day, usually in the morning before they get out of bed, that they have less back pain and encourage them to engage in intercourse at those times. Also, if the man knows that sexual intimacy may exacerbate his back pain, he can be advised to take his pain medication before he plans to have intercourse. Physicians caring from men with chronic back pain can give them permission to try alternatives to intercourse. The couple can try using vibrators, manual stimulation, and other intimate acts besides just intercourse itself.

It is not uncommon for a man suffering from chronic back pain to just write off the sexual part of his life. But that puts the relationship at risk. The men should be encouraged to explore intimacy with his partner and find out about the partner's needs and wants or the man risks losing the relationship. A physician caring for a man with chronic back pain can take the time to speak to the couple and let them know that the man may not be able to engage in sexual intimacy the way they did before and that modifications and changes are going to need to be made. The man with chronic back pain also has to understand that sex is important to his partner and he will perhaps need to find alternative methods of pleasuring his partner even if it is not possible to engage in intercourse.

Of course, life style changes which include smoking cessation, starting a weight loss program, decreasing alcohol consumption, and avoiding substance abuse. If there is evidence of depression, then referral to an appropriate mental health expert is in order.

Treatment of ED in men with chronic back pain

In men, the primary treatment for opioid-induced endocrine deficiency resulting in hypogonadism is testosterone supplementation (53). Testosterone is available in gel, cream, buccal tablet, transdermal patch, intramuscular injectable formulations and subcutaneous injection of testosterone pellets that last for 4-6 months. Topical medications are preferred over injections because they provide a more physiologic testosterone concentrations not easily attainable with intramuscular injections. Also, these medications are supplied in "unit doses"; e.g., the contents of one gel pack or from a dispenser that provides a daily dose are applied once a day at approximately the same time each morning to clean dry skin of the shoulders, the abdomen, the axilla and/or upper arms. Testosterone supplementation should be administered in amounts needed to manage symptoms of hypogonadism. Amounts higher than needed may increase the risk of prostatic hypertrophy, polycythemia and prostate cancer only if prostate cancer is present but has not been diagnosed. Symptoms of hypogonadism would be expected to improve with testosterone replacement therapy, but ED may persist to some degree because of psychological factors or co-morbid medical conditions. In such cases, prescribing FDA-approved ED medications could be appropriate (e.g., sildenafil, tadalafil, vardenafil). Treatment with PDE5 inhibitors demonstrated an improvement of depressive symptoms and ED in depressed men using sildenafil, tadalafil or vardenafil (54,55).

Anecdotally, it has been observed that patients experiencing weight gain with long-term methadone treatment may lose weight when rotated to fentanyl or oxycodone. Therefore, opioid-induced endocrine deficiency syndrome also may respond to opioid rotation. This is based on an assumption that some opioids at equianalgesic doses will cause less endocrine dysfunction than others because of differential binding to opioid receptors (e.g., mu-1, mu-2, mu-3, delta, kappa) (56). Several recommendations for addressing sexual dysfunction in men with chronic back pain who are managed with opioids include:

Prior to the initiation of daily opioid treatment, physicians should inform men (e.g., with an opioid-treatment "contract") that endocrine disturbances are common with higher dose, and with long-term opioid treatment. After treatment is initiated, men should be routinely evaluated for signs and symptoms of endocrine deficiency, including sexual dysfunction. When endocrine deficiency is suspected, appropriate laboratory testing including testosterone, LH, and prolactin should be ordered.

The primary treatment of hypogonadism in men with chronic back pain is testosterone supplementation. Topical or transdermal formulations are preferred over intramuscular injections as these provide a more physiologic level than injections which provide a supraphysiologic level followed by a progressively decreasing level that may be below the normal range and result in recurrence of symptoms of hypogonadism. Also, testosterone pellets, TestopelTM, are available and provide a physiologic level that lasts from 4-6 months. Anecdotally, rotation from one opioid medication to another may also be effective. Opioid treatment is intended to reduce chronic pain, and to improve physical and social functioning. The opioid-induced endocrine syndrome with its associated sexual dysfunction – which is a common and often overlooked consequence of opioid treatment – may negate the potential benefits of this analgesic therapy. Doctors caring from men with chronic back pain, who prescribe sustained-release opioids, should inform men of potential adverse consequence, screen the men for this syndrome, and initiate treatment when clinically indicated.

Sexual dysfunction resulting from treatment with an SSRI requires a careful and sophisticated management approach. The diagnosis of SSRI-associated sexual dysfunction is difficult to make without a thorough baseline assessment and periodic clinical monitoring of sexual functioning. Adding a PDE-5 inhibitor (after a careful medical and medication history) in cases of ED and adding bupropion in cases of decreased libido seem to be the best-supported strategies, along with switching to certain non-SSRI antidepressants. Other management strategies, such as lowering the dose and drug holidays may be used. The following are some tips that can help reduce sexual side effects and restore normal sexual functioning (57):

- ***Reduce the dose***. It may be possible to lower the dose enough to reduce sexual side effects while still obtaining depression relief. For example, it has been shown that for some men 5-10 mg of Prozac may be just as effective as the standard 20 mg dose.
- ***Schedule Dosing Right After Sexual Activity***. With certain drugs, such as sertraline and clomipramine, it may be possible to schedule the daily dose right after the time a man would normally expect to engage in sexual activity, when the drug's blood level would be at its lowest.
- ***Take a Drug Holiday***. With the drugs sertraline and paroxetine it may be possible to schedule a two day drug holiday each week in order to restore sexual function without losing the efficacy of the antidepressant.
- ***Switch to an Antidepressant That Causes Fewer Sexual Side-Effects.*** Nefazodone and bupropion have been shown in double-blind studies to have less effect on sexual function than SSRIs.

Treatment of post SSRI sexual dysfunction (PSSD)

There is no known cure for PSSD, mostly because its etiology is still poorly understood. According to a survey of psychiatrists bupropion is the drug of choice for the treatment of SSRI-induced sexual dysfunction, although this is not an FDA-approved indication. Thirty-six percent of psychiatrists preferred switching patients with SSRI-induced sexual dysfunction to bupropion, and 43 percent favored the augmentation of the current medication with bupropion. A higher dose of bupropion (300 mg) may be necessary: a randomized study employing a lower dose (150 mg) failed to find a significant difference between bupropion, sexual therapy or combined treatment.

Conclusion

Chronic back pain is a common malady affecting millions of men. Many of these men also suffer from ED in addition to their back pain. The causes of ED in these men include the side effects of medication used to treat back pain, hormone deficiency, depression and other psychological causes, and neurologic causes. Treatment of ED for men with chronic back pain can be very successful.

References

[1] Feldman HA, Goldstein I, Hatzichristou DG, Krane RJ, McKinlay JB. Impotence and its medical and psychosocial correlates: results of the Massachusetts Male Aging Study. J Urol 1994;151(1):54–61.

[2] Teles AG, Carreira M, Alarcão V, Sociol D, Aragüés JM, Lopes L, et al. Prevalence, severity, and risk factors for erectile dysfunction in a representative sample of 3,548 Portuguese men aged 40 to 69 years attending primary healthcare centers: results of the Portuguese erectile dysfunction study. J Sex Med 2008;5(6):1317-24.

[3] Feldman HA, Goldstein I, Hatzichristou DG, Krane RJ, McKinlay JB. Impotence and its medical and psychosocial correlates: results of the Massachusetts Male Aging Study. J Urol. 1994;151(1):54–61.

[4] Bors E, Comarr AE. Neurological urology. Basel, Switzerland: S Karger, 1971:144-145.

[5] Siddiqui MA, Peng B, Shanmugam N, Yeo W, Fook-Chong S, Li Tat JC, et al. Erectile dysfunction in young surgically treated patients with lumbar spine disease: A prospective follow-up study. Spine 2012;37(9):797-801.

[6] Siddiqui MA, Peng B, Shanmugam N, Yeo W, Fook-Chong S, Li Tat JC, Guo CM, Tan SB, Yue WM. Erectile dysfunction in young surgically treated patients with lumbar spine disease: a prospective follow-up study. Spine. 2012;20(9):797-801.

[7] Valles-Antuña C, Fernandez-Gomez J, Fernandez-Gonzalez F. Peripheral neuropathy: an underdiagnosed cause of erectile dysfunction. BJU Int 2011;108(11):1855-9.

[8] Colameco S, Opioid-induced sexual dysfunction: causes, diagnosis, and treatment. Pain Treat Topics, August 2011.

[9] Olsen Y, Daumit GL, Ford DE. Opioid prescriptions by US primary care physicians from 1992 to 2001. J Pain 2006;7:225-35.

[10] Azizi F, Vagenakis AG, Longcope C, Ingbar SH, et al. Decreased serum testosterone concentration in male heroin and methadone addicts. Steroids 1973;22:467–72.

[11] Martell BA, O'Connor PG, Kerns RD, Becker WC, Morales KH, Kosten TR, Fiellin DA. Systematic review: opioid treatment for chronic back pain: prevalence, efficacy, and association with addiction. Ann Intern Med 2007;146(2):116-27.

[12] Kalyani RR, Gaviine S, Dobs AS. Male hypogonadism in systemic disease. Endocrinol Metab Clin North Am. 2007;36(2):333-48.

[13] Mendelson JH, Meyer RE, Ellingboe J, et al. Effects of heroin and methadone on plasma cortisol and testosterone. J Pharmacol Exp Ther 1975;195:296-302.

[14] Daniell HW, Lentz R, Mazer NA. Open-label pilot study of testosterone patch therapy in men with opioid-induced androgen deficiency. J Pain 2006;7(3):200-10.

[15] Mazer N, Chapman C, Daniell H, et al. Opioid-induced androgen deficiency in men (OPIAD): an estimate of the potential patient population in the U.S. and Canada. J Pain. 2004;5(Suppl 1):S73.

[16] 16 Schechter D, Smith AP, Beck J, Roach J, Karim R, Azen S. Outcomes of a mind-body treatment program for chronic back pain with no distinct structural pathology--a case series of patients diagnosed and treated as tension myositis syndrome. Altern Ther Health Med 2007;13 (5):26-35.

[17] Rosen RC. Psychogenic erectile dysfunction. Classification and management. Urol Clin North Am 2001;28(2):269-78.

[18] Rosen RC. Psychogenic erectile dysfunction. Classification and management. Urol Clin North Am 2001;28(2):269-78.

[19] Melnik T, Soares BG, Nasselo AG. Psychosocial interventions for erectile dysfunction. Cochrane Database Syst Rev 2007;18(3): CD004825.

[20] Rahman Shiri, Jaro Karppinen, Päivi Leino-Arjas, Svetlana Solovieva and Eira Viikari-Juntura The Association Between Obesity and Low Back Pain: A Meta-Analysis. Am J Epidemiol 2010;171(2):135-54.

[21] Corona G, Mannucci E, Fisher A, Lotti F, Petrone L, Balercia G, et al. Low levels of androgens in men with erectile dysfunction and obesity. J Sex Med 2008;5(10):2454-63.

[22] Kaye AD, Prabhakar AP, Fitzmaurice ME, Kaye RJ. Smoking cessation in pain patients. Ochsner J 2012;12(1):17-20.

[23] Imamura M, Waseda Y, Marinova GV, Ishibashi T, Obayashi S, Sasaki A, Nagai A, Azuma H. Alterations of NOS arginase and DDAH protein expression in rabbit cavernosa tissue after administration of cigarette smoke extract. Am J Physiol Regul Integr Comp Physiol 2007;293: R2081-9.

[24] Karatzi K, Papamichael C, Karatzis E, Papaioannou T, et al. Acute smoking induces endothelial dysfunction in healthy smokers. Is this reversible by red wine's antioxidant constituents? J Am Coll Nutr 2007;26 (1):10-15.

[25] Shi Y, Weingarten TN, Mantilla CB, Hooten WM, Warner DO. Smoking and pain: pathophysiology and clinical implications. Anesthesiology 2010;113(4):977-92.

[26] Shiri R, Karppinen J, Leino-Arjas P, Solovieva S, Vilkari-Juntura E. The association between smoking and low back pain: a meta-analysis. Am J Med 2010;123(1):87.

[27] Kaye AD, Prabhakar AP, Fitzmaurice ME, Kaye RJ. Smoking cessation in pain patients. Ochsner J 2012;12:(1):17-20.

[28] Guay AT, Perez JB, Heatley GJ. Cessation of smoking rapidly decreases erectile dysfunction. Endocr Pract 1998;4(1):23-6.

[29] Pourmand G, Alidaee MR, Rasuli S, Maleki A, Mehrsai A. Do cigarette smokers with erectile dysfunction benefit from stopping? A prospective study. BJU Int 2004;94:1310-3.

[30] Shiri R, Koskimaki J, Tammela TL, Hakkinen J, Auvinen A, Hakama M. Bidirectional relationship between depression and erectile dysfunction. J Urol 2007;177:669-73.

[31] James M. Ferguson, Ram K. Shrivastava, Stephen M. Stahl, James T. Hartford, Frances Borian, John Ieni, Robert D. McQuade, and Darlene Jody. Reemergence of sexual dysfunction in patients with major depressive disorder. J Clin Psychiatry 2001;62:24-9.

[32] Damsa C, Bumb A, Bianchi-Demicheli F, et al. Dopamine-dependent" side effects of selective serotonin reuptake inhibitors: a clinical review. J Clin Psychiatr 2004;65(8):1064-8.

[33] Rosen RC, Lane RM, Menza M: Effects of SSRIs on sexual function: a critical review. J Clin Psychopharmacol 1999;19:67-85.

[34] Levine SB: The nature of sexual desire: a clinician's perspective. Arch Sex Behav 2003;32:279-85.

[35] Bahrick AS. Post SSRI sexual dysfunction. Am Soc Adv Pharmacother 2006;7(3):2–10.

[36] Balon R. SSRI-associated sexual dysfunction. Am J Psychiat 2006;163: 1504-9.

[37] Mikhail N. Does testosterone have a role in erectile function? Am J Med 2006;119(5):373-82.

[38] Mikhail N. Does testosterone have a role in erectile function? Am J Med 2006;119(5):373-82.

[39] Maggi M, Buvat J, Corona G, Guay A, Torres LO. Hormonal causes of male sexual dysfunctions and their management (hyperprolactinemia, thyroid disorders, GH disorders, and DHEA). J Sex Med 2012.DOI: 10.1111/j.1743-6109.2012.02735.x).

[40] Carani C, Isidori AM, Granata A, Carosa E, Maggi M, Lenzi A, Jannini EA. Multicenter study on the prevalence of sexual symptoms in male hypo- and hyperthyroid patients. J Clin Endocrinol Metab 2005;90(12):6472-9.

[41] Zeitlin S, Rajfer J. Hyperprolactinemi and erectile dysfunction. Rev Urol 2000; 2(1): 39–42.

[42] Fednekar N and Mulgainer V. Role of testosterone on pain threshold in rats. Indian J Physiol Pharmacol 1995;39:423-4.

[43] Long JB and Holaday JW. Blood-brain barrier: Endogenous modulation by adrenal cortical function. Science 1985;227:1580-3.

[44] Dolon S, Wilke S, Aliabodi N, et al. Effects of testosterone administration in human immunodeficiency virus-infected women with low-weight. Arch Intern Med 2004;164:897-904.

[45] Daniel HW. The association of endogenous hormone levels and exogenously administered opiates in males. Am J Pain Manage 2001; 11:8-10.

[46] Ambler N, Williams AC, Hill P, et al. Sexual difficulties of chronic pan patients. Clin J Pain 2001;17:138-45.

[47] Corona G, Mondaini N, Ungar A, Razzoli E, Rossi A, Fusco F. Phosphodiesterase type 5 (PDE5) inhibitors in erectile dysfunction: The proper drug for the proper patient. J Sex Med 2011;8(12):3418-32.

[48] Gorman DM, Potamianos G, Williams KA, Frank AO, Duffy SW, Peters TJ. Relationship between alcohol abuse and low back pain. Alcohol Alcoholism 1987;22(1):61-3.

[49]   Morley J E, Carlton E, Patrick P, et al. Validation of a screening questionnaire for androgen deficiency in aging men. Metabolism 2000;49 (9):1239-42.

[50]   Corona G, M Annucci E, Petrone L. et al. Androtest: a structured interview for the screening of hypogonadism in patients with sexual dysfunction. J Sex Med 2003;3:706-15.

[51]   Daniell HW. Hypogonadism in men consuming sustained-action oral opioids. J Pain 2002;3:377-84.

[52]   Lue T. Contemporary diagnosis and management of male erectile dysfunction. Newtown, PA: Assoc Medical Marketing, 2005.

[53]   Daniell HW. Opioid-induced androgen deficiency. Discussion in opioid contracts. Am J Med 2006;120(9):e21.

[54]   Seidman SN, Roose SP, Menza MA, Shabsigh R, Rosen RC. Treatment of erectile dysfunction in men with depressive symptoms: results of a placebo-controlled trial with sildenafil citrate. Am J Psychiatr 2001;158:1623-30.

[55]   Rosen R, Shabsigh R, Berber M, Assalian P, Menz M, Rodriguez-Vela L, et al. Vardenafil study site investigators. Efficacy and tolerability of vardenafil in men with mild depression and erectile dysfunction: the depression-related improvement with vardenafil for erectile response study. Am J Psyciatr 2006;163:79-87.

[56]   Vallejo,R,, Barkin RL, Wang VC. Pharmacology of opioids in the treatment of chronic pain syndromes. Pain Physician 2011;14:E343-60.

[57]   Labbate LA et al: Sexual dysfunction induced by serotonin reuptake antidepressants. J Sex Marital Ther 24:3:1998-58.

Submitted: December 18, 2012. *Revised:* January 20, 2013. *Accepted:* February 12, 2013.

In: Pain Management Yearbook 2013
Editor: Joav Merrick

ISBN: 978-1-63117-944-0
© 2014 Nova Science Publishers, Inc.

Chapter 15

The effect of Stanford-type self-management programmes on pain and function in older people with persistent pain: A systematic review of randomised controlled trials

Denis Martin, BSc (Hons), DPhil, MSc[*1],
*Patricia Schofield, RGN, PhD, PGDipEd, DipN[2],
*Derek Jones, BA(Hons), Dip COT, PhD[3],
*Paul McNamee, PhD, CTLHE, MSc, MA[4],
*Amanda Clarke, BA(Hons), MA, PhD, RGN, PgDip[3],
Geraldine Anthony[5]
and Blair Smith, MD, MEd, FRCGP, FHEA, FRCP Edin[6]
[1]Health and Social Care Institute, Teesside University, Middlesbrough, UK
[2]School of Health and Social Care, University of Greenwich,
Avery Hill Campus, Eltham, UK
[3]School of Community and Education Studies, Northumbria University,
Coach Lane Campus, Newcastle Upon Tyne, UK
[4]Institute of Applied Health Sciences, Aberdeen University, Aberdeen, UK
[5]Centre of Academic Primary Care, Aberdeen University, Aberdeen, UK
[6]School of Medicine, Dundee University, UK

* Correspondence: Denis Martin, BSc (Hons), DPhil, Msc, Professor of Rehabilitation, School of Health and Social Care Teesside University, Centuria Building, University of Teesside, Middlesbrough, Tees Valley TS1 3BA, United Kingdom. E-mail: d.martin@tees.ac.uk

Abstract

Self-management is advocated for older people with persistent pain. Self-management can be used to describe a range of approaches. Of these, the model developed at Stanford University is one of the most well-known. To examine claims of the effectiveness of this approach for pain and function in older people we carried out a systematic review of randomised controlled trials. Trials were included in which participants were aged at least 65 years old and living in the community with persistent pain; the intervention arm was the Stanford model or a close derivative; and measures were taken of pain severity, and/or physical function and/or psychological function at a follow up of at least 6 months. Studies were excluded if the sample also contained people younger than 65 years old or if they were in a language other than English. Three RCTs were identified, each rated as moderate quality. Analysis showed a lack of convincing evidence in support of the Stanford model of self-management or close derivatives, as delivered in the trials, for reducing pain severity or improving function in people over 65 years old with persistent pain.

Keywords: Pain, persistent pain, self-management, randomised trails

Introduction

Persistent pain is defined as pain that "persists beyond the expected healing time, serves no useful purpose and often has no identifiable cause" (1). Persistent pain is more common with increasing age with figures from the UK showing that a figure of 32% of adults aged 25-34 years reporting persistent pain rising steadily to 62% in people over 75 years (2).The impact of persistent pain is more marked in older people affecting physical and mental health, independence and social function (3,4). Physiological, psychological and social changes associated with aging have been suggested as reasons why older people are especially affected by persistent pain (5,6). Therefore, in pain management particular consideration should be given to older adults, although it should also be recognised that chronological age is a crude categorisation (7).

An important aspect of pain management is self-management and it has been argued that the principle of self-management may be particularly relevant for older people (8). It has also been shown that older people can be receptive to self-management ideas (9).

Self-management is a wide term that is used to describe a range of approaches and philosophies. However, the model of self-management developed by Lorig and colleagues at Stanford University in the USA (10) has become almost synonymous with self-management in general. This model is centred around the importance of improving self-efficacy based on Bandura's theories of self-efficacy and social learning (11). The Stanford model is delivered in a formal structured way to groups by way of the Arthritis Self-Management Programme or the Chronic Disease Self-Management Programme and has strongly influenced related programmes such as the Expert Patient Programme in England and Wales.

While some investigations have shown positive effects of programmes based on the Stanford model on self-efficacy and positive behaviours in adults of working age, claims of effectiveness for pain and function in adults have been challenged as being small at best and of questionable value clinically (12). Less is known about the value of these types of programmes for older people, specifically those over 65 years of age.

The aim of this investigation, therefore, was to evaluate the evidence from randomised controlled trials of the effectiveness of self-management programmes based on the Stanford model on pain, physical function, psychological function and social function in people over 65 with persistent pain.

Methods

We undertook a systematic review of RCTs published in English from the earliest date available in the databases to 2010.

Inclusion/exclusion criteria: Studies were included if they were randomised controlled trials, in which participants were people aged at least 65 years old with persistent pain, living in the community. The intervention arm was required to comprise, either exclusively or in part, the Stanford model or a close derivative. Studies were required to report measures of pain severity, and/or physical function and/or psychological function at a follow up of at least 6 months. Studies were excluded where the sample contained people less than 65 years old. (This was determined from the actual sample recruited and analysed rather than the specific inclusion criteria. Where the minimum age was not specified we adopted an arbitrary criterion whereby the mean age minus one standard deviation had to be greater than or equal to 65 years.) Studies were excluded if they were in a language other than English.

Search strategy

MEDLINE, CINAHL plus with full text, AMED - The Allied and Complementary Medicine Database, PsycINFO; PsycARTICLES, and Psychology and Behavioral Sciences Collection were searched. The following four search terms and their associated terms were used: SELF-MANAGEMENT, PAIN, ELDERLY and RANDOMISED CONTROLLED TRIAL COMBINED using Boolean operators. Hand searching of the reference lists of relevant papers was used to identify further papers. Titles were screened and unless they were obviously inappropriate we read the abstract. Full papers were obtained when the abstract was deemed appropriate. At this point any inappropriate papers were discarded and those remaining constituted the literature for review.

Data abstraction and analysis

Two of the authors (DM & PS) independently reviewed papers. (There was no need to include a third member for arbitration as agreement was reached for each paper.)

We assessed the methodological quality of included studies (13, 14): a total of 12 criteria are judged to be met or not, yielding grades defined as high quality (10-12 criteria met), moderate quality (6-9 criteria met) or low quality (fewer than 6 criteria met). Studies with a score of 6 or more are considered to have a low risk of bias.

For each of the outcomes at 6 months and 12 months we rated the quality of evidence (13, 14). For each outcome the system yields six grades based on consideration of five domains: risk of bias; consistency of findings across studies; ability to generalise findings; sufficiency of data; and publication bias across all studies that measure that particular outcome. The evidence is defined as high quality when there are findings in at least 75% of RCTs with low risk of bias that are consistent, generalisable, based on sufficient data and not subject to publication bias. For every one domain that is not met the quality of evidence drops by one level from high quality to moderate quality, low quality and very low quality. When there are no RCTs that measure the outcome this constitutes no evidence from trials. The evidence is classified as conflicting when there is inconsistency among the findings.

Data were analysed qualitatively as pooling was not appropriate, because of heterogeneity of outcome measures and samples.

Results

Description of studies: 97 papers were identified from the search, of which two met the criteria for review. The most common reasons for exclusion were because the self-management approach was not the Stanford model or a close derivative, or the sample included participants under 65 years. A further appropriate paper was identified from hand-searching. In total therefore, three RCTs were included in the analysis, with a total sample size of 580, all conducted in the USA.

Following a pilot study, which showed no significant effects on pain and function at three months follow-up (15,16) compared a pain self-management programme with a control group receiving education only. The programme comprised 7 group sessions, one per week with each session lasting 90 minutes. The groups were facilitated by a nurse or clinical psychologist. Up to 30 weeks after the last group session participants received 4 supportive phone calls from the facilitators asking about their condition and self-management activities and offering problem solving advice. Participants in the control group received written material on self-management for persistent pain. They also received follow up phone calls though without the problem solving advice. 256 participants with a mean (1SD) age of 81.8 (6.5) years were recruited from retirement communities.

Haas et al. (17) compared their self-management intervention with a waiting list control. The intervention was the Chronic Disease Self-Management Programme. It was delivered in a group format comprising one 2.5 hour session per week for 6 weeks. The sessions were facilitated by 2 lay leaders who, like the participants, had persistent low back pain. The sample consisted of 109 community dwelling participants with a mean (1SD) age of 77.2 (7.7) years.

Hughes et al. (18) compared their programme with an education-only control. The intervention, called Fit and Strong!, was delivered to groups in three 90 minute sessions per week for 8 weeks. The groups were facilitated by a physical therapist. After completing the programme participants were encouraged to maintain physical activity. This was reinforced by a member of the research team speaking to them in person or by phone every quarter for 10 months. The control group participants were given written materials on self -management for pain. The sample was 215 community dwelling participants with a mean age of 73.3 years.

The methodological quality of each of the three studies was rated as moderate.

Pain

At 6 months Hughes et al. (18) found statistically significant differences in their two measures of pain severity in favour of the intervention. In contrast both Ersek et al. (16) and Haas et al. (17) found no statistically significant differences in pain severity between their respective interventions and controls. Only Hughes et al. (18) and Ersek et al. (16) measured pain severity at 12 months and in both studies there were no statistically significant differences between the intervention and control groups.

For people over 65 years old with persistent pain, there is *conflicting evidence* (3 trials; n=580) that the Stanford model of self-management (or a close derivative) is more effective than a comparison group for reducing pain severity at a short-term follow up.

For people over 65 years old with persistent pain, there is *moderate* evidence (2 trials; n=471) that the Stanford model of self-management (or a close derivative) is no more effective than a comparison group for reducing pain severity at a long-term follow up.

Physical function

At 6 months none of the three studies showed statistically significant benefits of intervention compared to their respective controls. At 12 months neither Hughes et al. (18) nor Ersek et al. (16) reported statistically significant differences between intervention and control. Haas et al. (17) did not take measures at 12 months. For people over 65 years old with persistent pain, there is *moderate* evidence that the Stanford model of self-management (or a close derivative) is no more effective than a comparison group for increasing self-reported physical function at a short-term (3 trials; n=580) or a long-term follow up (2 trials; n=471).

Psychological function

Only Haas et al. (17) assessed psychological function at 6 months. They reported a statistically significant benefit in the SF36 emotional well-being domain in favour of the intervention. Only Ersek et al. (16) measured psychological function at 12 months. With their measure of depression they found no statistically significant differences between intervention and control. For people over 65 years old with persistent pain, there is *limited* evidence (1 trial; n=109) that the Stanford model of self-management (or a close derivative) is more effective than a comparison group for increasing SF36 emotional well-being at a short-term follow-up. For people over 65 years old with persistent pain, there is *limited* evidence (1 trial; n=256) that the Stanford model of self-management (or a close derivative) is not more effective than a comparison group for self-reported depression at a long-term follow-up.

Social function

None of the studies reported social function. For people over 65 years old with persistent pain, there is *no* evidence from RCTs to judge the effectiveness or otherwise of the Stanford model of self-management (or a close derivative) in increasing social function at a short or long-term follow-up.

Discussion

Without making judgment on the underlying concept, the results show that from the three RCTs included in the analysis there is currently no strong evidence in support of the Stanford model of self-management or close derivatives for reducing pain severity or improving function in people over 65 years old with persistent pain.

Our findings are consistent with other reviews, which reported statistically significant but clinically trivial effects on pain and function in adults described as older though not exclusively over 65 years (12,19). One meta-analysis reported, for example, a decrease in pain of 2mm on a 100mm VAS scale as an example of a clinically trivial change that was statistically significant (12).

The lack of evidence for a reduction in pain severity in this population may not be too surprising as it is extremely resistant to any intervention. However, such claims are made and should, therefore, be tested. Functional improvements are more feasible and it is on these outcomes that the results are more disappointing.

Nunez et al. (20) argue that such self-management programmes should be judged primarily on their effects on self-efficacy. The basis of this argument is that self-efficacy is the defining philosophy underpinning the Stanford model and its close derivatives. If so, then arguably their value could be optimised by their inclusion alongside other approaches to optimise the benefits of any improvements in self-efficacy. This highlights a weakness in the current evidence base on the Stanford model and its close derivatives in that the programmes are evaluated in relative isolation, without consideration of any other simultaneous approaches to managing the participants' pain.

The review excluded studies that clearly included people under 65 years old. Focusing specifically on those over 65 limited the number of studies that met the criteria for being acceptable for review. The small number of studies identified itself points to an important gap in the literature. Ideally more data could have been obtained by extracting results for over 65s from studies that incorporated a wide age range in their samples. This level of data was not available in any of the papers identified in the review process and we did not have the resources to go beyond that.

The strict age criterion excluded studies in which the sample partially comprised people under 65. These studies could have provided further information but it was beyond the scope of the review to attempt to extract data specific to over 65s from those studies.

The review was limited to investigating the Stanford model or close derivatives. This is only one form of self-management, albeit a popular and potentially important one. To an extent this form has become synonymous with self-management. However, the varying definitions that apply to self-management make it clear that there are more approaches in use.

The review only contained randomised controlled trials on the basis that this design will provide the most robust evidence of effectiveness. Given the lack of RCTs it would be appropriate to carry out a review of non-RCT studies, to bolster current evidence, and to inform the development of broader self-management approaches and their evaluation in RCTs.

Conclusion

There is insufficient high-quality evidence to support claims that the Stanford model or close derivatives are effective for reducing pain severity or improving function in people over 65 years with persistent pain. That does not dismiss the potential value for these programmes in conjunction with other services. Structured self-management approaches in other forms of delivery remain good in principle and warrant rigorous investigation. The same applies for more ad-hoc, bespoke approaches to self-management, though these may be more difficult to investigate because of their diversity.

Acknowledgments

This review was undertaken as part of the project Engaging with Older People and their caretakers to develop Interventions for the self-management of Chronic pain (EOPIC), funded by the UK joint research councils' Lifelong Healthy Living initiative.

References

[1]   Merskey H, Bogduk N. Classification of chronic pain. Definitions of chronic pain syndromes and definition of pain terms, 2nd ed. Seattle, WA: International Association for the Study of Pain, 1994.

[2]   Elliott AM, Smith BH, Penny KI, Smith CW, Chambers WA. The epidemiology of chronic pain in the community. Lancet 1999;354:1248–52.

[3]   Thomas E, Peat G, Harris L, Wilkie R, Croft PR. The prevalence of pain and pain interference in a general population of older adults: cross-sectional findings from the North Staffordshire Osteoarthritis Project (NorStOP). Pain 2004;110:361–8.

[4]   Peat G, Thomas E, Handy J, Croft P. Social networks and pain interference with daily activities in middle and old age. Pain 2004;112:397-405.

[5]   Pickering G. Frail elderly, nutritional status and drugs. Arch Gerontol Geriatrics 2004;38:174-80.

[6]   Gibson SJ. Age differences in psychosocial aspects of pain. In: Gibson SJ, Weiner DK, eds. Pain in older persons. Progress in pain research and management. Seattle, WA: IASP Press, 2005:87-107.

[7]   Schofield P, Clarke A, Jones D, Martin D, McNamee, Smith B. Chronic pain in later life: A review of current issues and challenges. Aging Health 2011;7:551-6.

[8]   Reid MC, Papaleontiou M, Ong A, Breckman R, Wethington E, Pillemer K. Self-management strategies to reduce pain and improve function among older adults in community settings: a review of the evidence. Pain Med 2008;9:409-24.

[9]   Lansbury G. Chronic pain management: A qualitative study of elderly people's preferred coping strategies and barriers to management. Disabil Rehabil 2000;22:2-14.

[10]   Lorig KR, Holman HR. Self-management education: history, definition, outcomes, and mechanisms. Ann Behav Med 2003;26:1-7.

[11]   Bandura A. Self-efficacy: Toward a unifying theory of behavioral change. Psychol Rev 1977;84:191-215.

[12]   Chodosh J, Morton SC, Mojica W, Maglione M, Suttorp MJ, Hilton L, Rhodes S, Shekelle P. Meta-analysis: Chronic disease self-management programs for older adults. Ann Intern Med 2004;143: 427-38.

[13]   van Tulder M, Furlan AD, Bombardier C, Bouter L. Updated method guidelines for systematic reviews in the Cochrane Collaboration Back Review Group. Spine 2003;28:1290-9.

[14]   Clarke CL, Ryan CG, Martin D. Pain neurophysiology education for the management of individuals with chronic low back pain: A systematic review and meta-analysis. Manual Ther 2011;16:544-9.

[15]   Ersek M, Turner JA, McCurry SM, Gibbons L, Kraybill BM. Efficacy of a self-management group intervention for elderly persons with chronic pain. Clin J Pain 2003;19:156–67.

[16]   Ersek M, Turner JA, Cain KC, Kemp CA. Results of a randomised controlled trial to examine the efficacy of a chronic pain self-management group for older adults. Pain 2008;138:29–40.

[17]   Haas M, Groupp E, Muench J, Kraemer D, Brummel-Smith K, Sharma R, et al.. Chronic disease self-management program for low back pain in the elderly. J Manipulat Physiol Ther 2005;28:228–37.

[18]   Hughes SL, Seymour RB, Campbell RT, Huber G, Pollak, N, Sharma L, Desai P. Long-term impact of Fit and Strong! on older adults with osteoarthritis. Gerontologist 2006;46:801-14.

[19]   Warsi A, LaValley MP, Wang PS, Avorn J, Solomon DH. Arthritis self-management education programs. Arthritis Rheum 2003;48:2207-13.

[20]   Nunez D, Keller C, Ananian CD. A review of the efficacy of the self-management model on health outcomes in community-residing older adults with arthritis. Worldviews Evid Based Nurs 2009;6: 130-48.

Submitted: January 08, 2013. *Revised:* February 16, 2013. *Accepted:* February 21, 2013.

In: Pain Management Yearbook 2013　　　　　ISBN: 978-1-63117-944-0
Editor: Joav Merrick　　　　　　　　　　© 2014 Nova Science Publishers, Inc.

Chapter 16

Review of brain metastases research in the Rapid Response Radiotherapy Program (RRRP)

Natalie Pulenzas, BSc(C), Breanne Lechner, BSc(C),
*Nemica Thavarajah, BSc(C) and Edward Chow, MBBS**
Rapid Response Radiotherapy Program, Department of Radiation Oncology,
Odette Cancer Centre, Sunnybrook Health Sciences Centre, University of Toronto,
Toronto, Ontario, Canada

Abstract

Brain metastases develop in approximately 20-40% of patients, and are frequently treated with whole brain radiation therapy (WBRT) for patients ineligible for aggressive treatment. The Rapid Response Radiotherapy Program (RRRP) provides timely radiotherapy for palliative cancer patients, focusing on quality of life (QOL) as an important endpoint. This paper reviewed the past research conducted in the RRRP on brain metastases patients. QOL studies have used a wide variety of assessment tools and determined that the effect of WBRT on QOL is widely variable, ranging from decreased QOL to improvement. There is not a current standardized QOL questionnaire which has been created and validated in the brain metastases population. Research in the RRRP is lacking in other treatment options for brain metastases such as stereotactic radiosurgery (SRS), likely due to the palliative nature of our patients. Future research should focus on creating a standard QOL instrument, measuring QOL following SRS, and better determining prognostic factors of brain metastases patients before treatment.

Keywords: Brain metastases, quality of life, radiotherapy

---

* Correspondence: Professor Edward Chow MBBS, MSc, PhD, FRCPC, Department of Radiation Oncology, Odette Cancer Centre, Sunnybrook Health Sciences Centre, 2075 Bayview Avenue, Toronto, ON Canada. E-mail: Edward.Chow@Sunnybrook.ca

Introduction

Brain metastases develop in approximately 20-40% of cancer patients and are frequently treated by whole brain radiotherapy (WBRT), and more aggressively stereotactic radiosurgery (SRS), or neurosurgical resection. Candidates for more aggressive treatments such as SRS or resection, typically have a solitary brain metastasis, controlled disease elsewhere and good performance status (1). Median survival is typically one month with no intervention, and in some cases up to 3-6 months with the addition of WBRT (2). Patients may experience a reduction in symptoms while receiving corticosteroids as these medications can reduce cerebral edema. The primary objective of WBRT is to achieve some magnitude of symptom relief, allow for tapering off of corticosteroids, so as to avoid potentially debilitating long term side effects, and to possibly increase survival (1,3). Brain metastases most commonly develop from primary lung and breast cancers (1-4). The standard practice of WBRT is 2000cGy in 5 fractions in the Rapid Response Radiotherapy Program (RRRP) (2,4,5).

There have been many studies focusing on brain metastases patients in the RRRP at the Sunnybrook Odette Cancer Centre, which is a specialized clinic developed in 1996 to provide timely palliative radiotherapy with the purpose to improve or maintain quality of life (QOL) (6). This paper reviews the past research in the RRRP investigating brain metastases. A significant limitation of many brain metastases studies is a low compliance and high attrition rate due to progression of disease and neurological deficits. Questionnaires conducted in brain metastases patients can create a large patient burden, especially when these lengthy questionnaires may contain up to 50 items (3,7).

The efficacy of WBRT for treating patients with active extracranial disease and limited survival has been questioned (8). Physician expectations of the results from treatment to brain metastases are important as these physicians refer patients to the RRRP, which may lead to inappropriate treatment (5). The main focus of the past research in the RRRP is the measurement of QOL and improvement of patient-rated symptoms (2).

Methods

A retrospective review was conducted of research involving brain metastases from 2004 – present. Any research including brain metastases from the RRRP focused on QOL, prognostic factors, and use of corticosteroids was included.

Results

Doyle et al. (7) examined QOL in patients after receiving WBRT. Patient evaluations used the Functional Assessment of Cancer Therapy-Brain (FACT-BR) questionnaire at baseline, one month, and two months following completion of treatment. This assessment was originally developed in patients with primary brain cancer, and includes the general questionnaire (FACT-G) (7,9). In 2012 the FACT-BR content was successfully validated for patients with brain metastases by health care professionals (HCPs) and patients. Generally, the content was considered relevant, and patients did not report items being difficult, upsetting, or irrelevant (10). An endpoint of the study by Doyle et al. (7) was to assess the discrepancy between patient or proxy reported QOL, which was only analyzed at baseline due to small sample size at follow-ups. Sixty patients and their caregivers were enrolled. At one month post treatment only 45% of patients completed the one month follow-up, and 25% completed the two month follow up, which occurs frequently in long term studies involving this population (7). Low completion rate occurred due to various reasons such as death and deterioration in health. There was no significant difference seen in any comparisons of the Eastern Cooperative Oncology Group (ECOG) performance status between baseline, one month and two month follow-ups. Agreeability between patient and proxy rated scales was deemed to be poor, suggesting a factor to take into account in future studies using proxy questionnaires. Patient's QOL showed a non-significant trend of deterioration over time. This trend was likely clinically significant however, as the high attrition was majorly due to deterioration or death (7).

Caissie et al. (9) examined the effect of radiation to brain metastases on QOL using the 20-item European Organisation for Research and Treatment of Cancer Quality of Life Questionnaire-Brain Neoplasm (EORTC QLQ-BN20) and the EORTC Quality of Life Questionnaire - Core 15 Palliative (QLQ-C15-PAL) (9). A limitation of QOL studies in brain metastases patients is the patient burden that arises from the use of lengthy questionnaires such as the combination of the EORTC Quality of Life Questionnaire (QLQ-C30) and QLQ-BN20, which contains 50 items in total. Studies observing the combination of these two questionnaires have concluded that poor compliance and high attrition rates limit the effectiveness of these questionnaires (7,11,12). The assessment tool used by Doyle et al., FACT-BR, has also been reported to have high patient burden leading to low compliance and difficulty with data collection (7,12). Therefore the QLQ-C15-PAL was developed to help decrease patient burden, and two additional items assessing cognitive function (concentration and memory) were added to create the QLQ-BN20+2 since this was absent from shortening the QLQ-C30 (3,9). Nguyen et al. (13) successfully conducted content validation of the BN20+2 by interviewing brain metastases patients receiving radiation treatment and consulting HCPs about the relevance of each item. Majority of patients and HCPs reported all items were relevant to brain metastases patients except seizures, hair loss, and incontinence (>50% patients); itchy skin (15% HCPs); and future uncertainty (12% HCPs) were rated as irrelevant (13).

Caissie et al. (9) conducted field testing of the combination of the 37 item BN20+2 and C15-PAL, and reported 65% of the cohort completed the one month follow up (9). When compared with a previous study which conducted follow-ups using the BN20 and C-30, there was a 67% compliance rate at one month, therefore the use of the C15-PAL was shown to be successful in this population, though did not show an increase in compliance rate (14). Post treatment of WBRT, maintenance of QOL occurred in this study, which may be explained due to the wide range of KPS (median 80, range 40-100), as this included poor prognosis and good performance status patients alike (9). Wong et al. (2) conducted a study from 2005-2007 which utilized the validated Spitzer Quality of Life Index in 129 patients to assess QOL, symptom severity, and neurological function for up to three months following WBRT (2). As examined previously, benefit from WBRT would have been evident if QOL and neurological function improved, and symptom severity decreased. However, approximately half of the study cohort experienced symptom relief, as 43% had stable or improved fatigue, and 47%

improved neurological function. Similar trends were seen in improvement of daily living (29%), and health (54%). Therefore, objectives of WBRT may be appropriate to focus on the prevention of worsening or progression of symptom severity and QOL because of the general stabilization of symptoms that were found in this study (2).

A systematic review of the literature by Wong et al. (1) was conducted from 1950 to 2007 focusing on QOL outcome after WBRT. Sixty-one trials were included in the review that fit the inclusion criteria. Twenty-four QOL assessments were used including the Edmonton Symptom Assessment Scale (ESAS), QLQ-C30, BN20, FACT-G and FACT-BR. The authors concluded there is no standardized QOL instrument used consistently with brain metastases patients as stated in multiple studies, which demonstrates the importance of creating a questionnaire to be validated in brain metastases patients (1,3,11). Wong and colleagues determined that in the majority of studies, there is deterioration in at least one domain of QOL after radiotherapy (1). Three important studies highlighted in the review included patients with good performance status and/or satisfactory prognosis, and observed that certain domains of QOL improved following WBRT with follow-up time points extending up to six months. Radiation Therapy Oncology Group (RTOG) Recursive Partitioning Analysis (RPA) class I and II, or KPS of 70 or greater, formed the majority of patient groups in these three studies, suggesting better prognosis patients do benefit from radiotherapy (1). Another study randomized nineteen patients to WBRT or no additional intervention following surgery or radiotherapy. Majority of this cohort had good performance status, with one patient in RPA Class III. No change in QOL was reported in either of the arms, which could promote the notion that better prognosis patients benefit from radiotherapy, as there was no decline in QOL (1).

QOL is an important outcome to maintain or improve in patients receiving palliative radiation for brain metastases (7). All of the studies reported in this review thus far have focused on WBRT as the treatment for brain metastases.

Prognostic factors

A prospective study by Lock et al. (15) in 2004 investigated prognostic variables in brain metastases patients to determine if a certain subgroup, particularly poor prognostic status, would not benefit from WBRT. There were 275 patients with brain metastases assessed over a two year period from two cancer centers, and the median overall survival was 5.3 months (15). The rationale for this study was that patients with a poor expected survival may not achieve any symptom relief from WBRT, and their symptoms may be managed effectively by corticosteroids alone. It is demonstrated in the literature that the purpose of WBRT is generally for symptom control and it does not significantly increase survival (2,15). The patient population that would not benefit from WBRT, as defined by this study, was those with a life expectancy of less than 8 weeks. RTOG RPA is a method of determining performance status through division into three classes. RPA Class I includes patients with KPS ≥70, age <65 years, no extracranial metastases, and primary tumor controlled. RPA Class III are patients with KPS <70, and Class II encompasses the remaining patients (2). Number of metastatic sites, other than brain, and performance status, as measured by RTOG RPA, were determined to be significant predictors of survival. The study was unsuccessful in creating a model to accurately predict which patients would not benefit from WBRT (15).

Wong et al. (1) conducted a study between 2005 and 2007 and found that when compared with their opposite counterparts, patients; age <60 years, KPS≥70, and RPA Class I or II, were all significantly associated with a longer survival. Two domains of QOL (activity and daily living), vomiting, and neurological function were all associated with survival, as worse scores corresponded with poor survival (2). Chow et al. (8) also concluded that KPS≥70 was associated with longer survival. A literature review of brain metastases research was conducted by Wong and colleagues (1) in 2008, which reviewed studies that reported the Spitzer Index was superior in survival prediction when compared to KPS (1). Chow et al. determined that KPS was the most significant predictor of survival in their study; however the questionnaire used was ESAS (8).

Though there are factors which assist in determining patient prognosis, there is no consensus on how to determine which patients would not be suitable for WBRT (15). Barnes et al. (5) reported referring physicians overestimate the benefit of WBRT, therefore may be more likely to improperly refer patients for treatment (5). Further analysis into factors contributing to prognosis can contribute to reducing unnecessary treatment for poor prognosis patients, and aid in guiding physician expectations of survival and treatment.

Corticosteroids

A common limitation of many brain metastases studies is the inability to determine if the effects are due to WBRT, corticosteroids, or a combination of both. This was experienced in a QOL study by Wong et al. (2) conducted from 2005-2007 in which 35% of patients at one month, and 29% at two months following WBRT, could not be tapered off of corticosteroids (2). Corticosteroids are commonly used to first treat brain metastases, and are usually associated with the presence of symptom response. However, they can cause adverse side effects after long term use. This can be prevented in some patients through intervention with WBRT, which can improve symptoms and allow patients to tolerate tapering of steroids (16). Nguyen et al. (16) administered the dexamethasone symptom questionnaire (DSQ) to assess for steroid toxicity following WBRT (16). The study captured data for 68 patients, and at 1 month post radiation, 20% of patients were unable to be tapered off. Insomnia at week 2 post-WBRT was significantly related to a dose of ≥16mg/day, and decreased appetite loss was significantly related to longer use of steroids at baseline, but no consistent correlation between dose and QOL was determined (16).

Discussion

Factors to determine patient groups, prior to treatment, that would not benefit from WBRT is still generally inconclusive (1,8,15). It is important to continue examination into symptom outcomes and overall QOL following treatment to assess for benefit in specific patient groups. The benefit of WBRT may be diminished as patients referred to the RRRP typically have other factors disposing them to poor prognosis, such as multiple brain metastases, poor performance status, and active extracranial disease. This also contributes to the majority of our research being focused on WBRT, as more aggressive treatments in these palliative patients are rare (5). Referring physicians expectations of treatment, which are communicated to patients, may contribute to a lack of benefit seen from WBRT, as certain patients with limited survival may have been given false hope, leading to refusal of supportive care alone (5).

There is not a standardized QOL questionnaire used in brain metastases that allows for comparison across trials, decreases patient burden, and assesses symptoms related to brain metastases (1,3,11). A limitation of most of the questionnaires used in this patient population is they have been developed in a primary brain tumour population (FACT-Br, BN-20), or are general symptom assessments (ESAS). It is unknown if assessments created for brain primary correlate correctly in brain metastases as these patients may have different experiences due to active extracranial disease (9). High attrition rate is another limitation of research studies in this population due to short life span, resulting in small sample sizes at follow-up. In our centre, we developed and are currently testing a brain metastases specific questionnaire for content and psychometric validity. This may decrease patient burden as it comprises 20 items, when compared to questionnaires used previously (FACT-Br, 53 items total). Psychometric validation is also being conducted for the FACT-Br. Our questionnaire will possibly improve data collection, and appropriately assess symptoms applicable to brain metastases patients. Additional investigation into other treatment options for brain metastases, such as SRS, should be employed at our centre to examine the symptom outcomes and QOL resulting from an emerging alternative treatment for certain subsets of patients.

Conclusion

There is a wide breadth of research done in the RRRP on brain metastases patients, and especially QOL following treatment. This has resulted in the evolution of patient assessment questionnaires to be more applicable, both in content and length, for brain metastases patients. Further upcoming research in the RRRP will focus on further validation and development of appropriate assessment tools designed specifically for this patient population. Additional investigation into alternative treatment for these advanced cancer patients is also an area of future research.

Acknowledgments

We thank the generous support of Bratty Family Fund, Michael and Karyn Goldstein Cancer Research Fund, Joseph and Silvana Melara Cancer Research Fund, and Ofelia Cancer Research Fund.

References

[1]   Wong J, Hird A, Kirou-Mauro A, Napolskikh J, Chow E. Quality of life in brain metastases radiation trials: a literature review. Curr Oncol 2008;15(5):25-45.

[2]   Wong J, Hird A, Zhang L, Tsao M, Sinclair E, Barnes E, et al. Symptoms and quality of life in cancer patients with brain metastases following palliative radiotherapy. Int J Radiat Oncol Biol Phys 2009;75(4):1125-31.

[3]   Nguyen J, Sahgal A, Chow E, Danielson B. Brain metastases and quality of life. J Altern Med 2010;2(3):257-72.

[4]   Hird A, Wong J, Zhang L, Tsao M, Barnes E, Danjoux C, et al. Exploration of symptoms clusters within cancer patients with brain metastases using the Spitzer Quality of Life Index. Support Care Cancer 2010;18(3):335-42.

[5]   Barnes EA, Chow E, Tsao MN, Bradley NM, Doyle M, Li K, et al. Physician expectations of treatment outcomes for patients with brain metastases referred for whole brain radiotherapy. Int J Radiat Oncol Biol Phys 2010;76(1):187-92.

[6]   Chow E, Fan G, Hadi S, Wong J, Kirou-Mauro A, Filipczak L. Symptom clusters in cancer patients with brain metastases. Clin Oncol (R Coll Radiol) 2008;20(1):76-82.

[7]   Doyle M, Bradley NM, Li K, Sinclair E, Lam K, Chan G, et al. Quality of life in patients with brain metastases treated with a palliative course of whole-brain radiotherapy. J Palliat Med 2007;10(2):367-74.

[8]   Chow E, Davis L, Holden L, Tsao M, Danjoux C. Prospective assessment of patient-rated symptoms following whole brain radiotherapy for brain metastases. J Pain Symptom Manage 2005;30(1):18-23.

[9]   Caissie A, Nguyen J, Chen E, Zhang L, Sahgal A, Clemons M, et al. Quality of life in patients with brain metastases using the EORTC QLQ-BN20+2 and QLQ-C15-PAL. Int J Radiat Oncol Biol Phys 2012;83(4):1238-45.

[10]   Chen E, Cella D, Zeng L, Thavarajah N, Zhang L, Chang E, et al. Content validation of the FACT-Br with patients and health-care professionals to assess quality of life in patients with brain metastases. J Radiat Oncol 2012.

[11]   Leung A, Lien K, Zeng L, Nguyen J, Caissie A, Culleton S, et al. The EORTC QLQ-BN20 for assessment of quality of life in patients receiving treatment or prophylaxis for brain metastases: a literature review. Expert Rev Pharmacoecon Outcomes Res 2011;11(6):693-700.

[12]   Lien K, Zeng L, Nguyen J, Cramarossa G, Cella D, Chang E, et al. FACT-Br for assessment of quality of life in patients receiving treatment for brain metastases: a literature review. Expert Rev Pharmacoecon Outcomes Res 2011;11(6):701-8.

[13]   Nguyen J, Zhang L, Clemons M, Vassiliou V, Danielson B, Fairchild A, et al. Content validation of the EORTC QLQ-BN20+2 with patients and health care professionals to assess quality of life in brain metastases. J Radiat Oncol 2012;1:397-409.

[14]   Chen E, Nguyen J, Zhang L, Zeng L, Holden L, Lauzon N, et al. Quality of life in patients with brain metastases using the EORTC QLQ-BN20 and QLQ-C30. J Radiat Oncol 2012;1:179-86.

[15]   Lock M, Chow E, Pond GR, Do V, Danjoux C, Dinniwell R, et al. Prognostic factors in brain metastases: can we determine patients who do not benefit from whole-brain radiotherapy?. Clin Oncol (R Coll Radiol) 2004;16(5):332-8.

[16]   Nguyen J, Caissie A, Zhang L, Zeng L, Dennis K, Holden L, et al. Dexamethasone toxicity and quality of life in patients with brain metastases following palliative whole-brain radiotherapy. J Radiat Oncol 2012.

[17]   Cramarossa G, Chow E, Zhang L, Bedard G, Zeng L, Sahgal A, et al. Predictive factors for overall quality of life in patients with advanced cancer. Support Care Cancer 2013 Jan 22.

[18]   Koo K, Zeng L, Chen E, Zhang L, Culleton S, Dennis K, et al. Do elderly patients with metastatic cancer have worse quality of life scores? Support Care Cancer 2012;20(9):2121-7.

[19]   Lien K, Zeng L, Zhang L, Nguyen J, Di Giovanni J, Popovic M, et al. Predictive factors for well-being in advanced cancer patients referred for palliative radiotherapy. Clin Oncol (R Coll Radiol) 2012;24(6):443-51.

Submitted: February 01, 2013. *Revised:* March 03, 2013. *Accepted:* March 10, 2013.

In: Pain Management Yearbook 2013
Editor: Joav Merrick

ISBN: 978-1-63117-944-0
© 2014 Nova Science Publishers, Inc.

Chapter 17

Barriers to prescription of sublingual fentanyl tablets for breakthrough cancer pain in an outpatient cancer center

Marissa Slaven, MD[*1], *Frederick A Spencer, MD*[2]
and Edward Chow, MBBS[3]

[1]Division of Palliative Care, Department of Family Medicine,
McMaster University, Hamilton, Canada
[2]Department of Medicine, McMaster University, Hamilton, Canada
[3]Department of Radiation Oncology, Sunnybrook Health Sciences Centre,
Toronto, Ontario, Canada

Abstract

Breakthrough cancer pain (BTcP) is a significant source of distress for patients with cancer. Sublingual fentanyl tablets are the first rapid onset opioid targeted to treat BTcP available in Canada. Objectives: In this study we sought to review the use of this product in consecutive patients for efficacy and safety. Methods: A retrospective chart review was conducted of patients attending an outpatient palliative care clinic who received prescriptions for fentanyl tablets over six months. Data extracted included age, gender, palliative performance status (PPS), primary and secondary disease sites, concurrent cancer therapy, concurrent analgesics, and efficacy of sublingual fentanyl. Efficacy was defined as titration of sublingual fentanyl to achieve satisfactory control of pain as per patient report. Results: Twenty charts were reviewed. The mean age of patients was 58 years and the mean PPS score was 77%. The dose range of sublingual fentanyl was 100 micrograms (mcg) up to 800 mcg. The drug was documented to be effective and was

---

* Correspondence: Marissa Slaven, MD, 699 Concession St, Hamilton, Ontario L9H 1Z8, Canada. E-mail: Marissa.slaven@jcc.hhsc.ca

continued through the follow-up period in nine patients. It was ineffective by ten patients. Only one patient experienced side effects. Conclusion: Successful titration of sublingual fentanyl for BTcP occurred in 50% of patients managed in our clinic. The safety profile in our case review was excellent with only one patient experiencing side effects requiring discontinuation of the medication. Coordinated efforts to improve outpatient titration (e.g., written instructions) as well as research into initiation of drug at higher doses (thereby requiring fewer titration steps) may improve the utility of this agent.

Keywords: Pain, cancer, fentanyl, palliative care

Introduction

Breakthrough cancer pain (BTcP) is a common problem distinct from persistent background pain, which is defined as a constant or continuous pain that is experienced by the patient for more than 12 hours per day. In contrast, breakthrough pain is defined as an exacerbation of pain that occurs on a background of otherwise stable pain in patients receiving chronic opioid therapy (1). Breakthrough cancer pain is characterized by rapid onset, short duration and severe intensity (1).

Breakthrough cancer pain represents a significant burden. A review of the literature demonstrates a prevalence of 51-89% of patients with controlled levels of background pain (1-6).

Research shows that cancer patients with chronic pain are less satisfied with their pain control if they have breakthrough pain (9).

Cancer patients with breakthrough pain also report higher levels of peak pain, higher levels of depression and anxiety, and greater functional impairment (7-10). Rapid onset opioids are particularly well suited to address the problem of breakthrough cancer pain. Sublingual fentanyl products are delivered through the oral mucosa rapidly (within a few minutes), avoid first pass metabolism, and are very potent. They are generally well tolerated with side effect profiles similar to other narcotics (11-13).

The fentanyl sublingual tablet was approved for use by Health Canada in 2011 for the treatment of breakthrough pain in opioid-tolerant adult patients who are already receiving around the clock opioid therapy for their underlying persistent cancer pain. Current guidelines suggest patients should be on a minimum of sixty milligrams oral morphine equivalent (MME) in twenty four hours for two weeks before starting on sublingual fentanyl.

Regardless of opioid dose prescribed to control chronic pain, sublingual fentanyl must be titrated up from a 100 mcg starting dose whenever it is started, or re-started, by increments (100, 200, 300, 400, 600 and 800mcg). Two clinical trials have shown fentanyl sublingual tablets to be an effective and well-tolerated treatment for the relief of breakthrough pain (11, 12).

This paper reviews the use of a fentanyl sublingual tablet in patients in an outpatient palliative care clinic over a six month period. The purpose of this case report is to better understand demographics of patients receiving treatment, efficacy of treatment, potential barriers to use, and side effects of treatment.

Methods

An outpatient pain and symptom management clinic was established in our regional cancer center six years ago. The interdisciplinary team is composed of a physician, an advanced practice nurse, two registered nurses and a social worker. Referrals are for patients eighteen years or above who have a cancer diagnosis and an expected prognosis of one year or less. The clinic operates eight half days each week and sees approximately three hundred and fifty new patients each year. Patients are typically given appointments at one month intervals unless they call the clinic with a request to be seen sooner. All medications are reviewed with patients at each visit for compliance, safety and effectiveness.

Patients with breakthrough pain (BTP) were prescribed a starting dose of 100 mcg of sublingual fentanyl tablet and were instructed that if there was insufficient pain relief after 30 minutes to take rescue medication as allowed. The fentanyl sublingual dosage was then increased by the patient by 100 mcg for subsequent BTP episodes. Patients were instructed to wait two hours before treating subsequent BTP episodes. Patients were asked to call the clinic if they reached a dose of 300 mcg and did not have relief of their breakthrough pain. If there were no adverse effects they were then prescribed tablet strengths of 400, 600 and 800 mcg and dosing continued in this manner until an effective dose was reached or until a maximum dose of 800 mcg is reached. Patients were told they could take up to four doses in a twenty four hour period.

We conducted a retrospective chart review for twenty consecutive patients newly prescribed Abstral, a sublingual rapid onset fentanyl tablet beginning May 1st 2011 through October 31st 2011. Data extracted included age, gender, palliative performance status (PPS), primary and secondary disease sites, concurrent cancer therapy, concurrent analgesics, and use and efficacy of sublingual fentanyl. For the purpose of this study efficacy was defined as patient successful titration of sublingual fentanyl to achieve satisfactory control of breakthrough pain as per patient report. Pain control was deemed inadequate in patients who stopped sublingual fentanyl and/or failed to call for further dose titration despite continued pain. Charts were reviewed through to April 30th 2012. Institutional ethics approval for this retrospective study was obtained.

Results

Twenty patients were prescribed sublingual fentanyl tablets over a six month period. One chart had insufficient documentation regarding the dosing and efficacy of the fentanyl and was excluded. Of the remaining nineteen patients, ten were male and nine female. The age range was 29-78 years old with a mean age of 58 years. The palliative performance scale (PPS) at the time that sublingual fentanyl was started ranged from 60 to 100% with a mean PPS score of 77%. Primary cancer sites included: sarcoma [3], lung [3], breast [3], renal [2], melanoma, lymphoma, prostate, penile, rectal, mesothelioma, ovarian, and hepatocellular cancer. Eighty percent of patients had metastatic disease with the most common sites being bone [11], lung [4] and liver [4]. Many patients were receiving disease modifying therapy with 11 receiving chemotherapy, 11 received radiation and four received no therapy.

Patients also received co-analgesics including: steroids [6], neurontin [5], NSAIDs [5], pregabalin [1], cannabinoid [1] and tylenol [1]. Patients in this review had a MME range of 60-2250 milligrams with a mean dose of 508 milligrams and a median dose of 200 milligrams prior to starting fentanyl.

The dose range of sublingual fentanyl used ranged from 100 micrograms (mcg) up to the maximum dose of 800 mcg with the median dose being 300 mcg. The drug was documented to be effective and was continued through the follow-up period in nine of the nineteen patients. It was deemed ineffective by ten patients and discontinued by them without consultation with the physician.

The median dose in those for whom it was effective was 300 mcg (range 200to 800 mcg) compared to a medium dose of 100 mcg (range 100 to 800) in those for whom it was deemed ineffective. Six patients for whom the drug was discontinued were not titrated up to maximum dose before discontinuing the drug. The vast majority (90%) of patients for whom it was deemed ineffective were on it for less than one month (median of <1 month, range<1 month to 2 months). For those for whom it was effective half were treated for longer than four months and one was treated for more than one year (median of 18 weeks, range<1 month to 1 year). One of 19 patients had a side effect, delirium, related to the administration of sublingual fentanyl which led to its discontinuation. Three patients for whom it was effective were subsequently transferred to institutions where it was not available and so were forced to discontinue it.

Discussion

Although sublingual fentanyl products have been studied in clinical trial settings it is important to understand what barriers exist to prevent their effective use in real clinical settings.

In our clinic we were successful in managing breakthrough cancer pain in half of the patients for whom the drug was prescribed. The mean effective dose was 300 mcg, well below the maximum recommended dosage of 800 mcg. It is noteworthy that 8 of the 10 patients in whom sublingual fentanyl was deemed "ineffective" in the management of breakthrough pain were not titrated to maximum dose. These patients opted to discontinue the drug without further titration beyond 300 mcg as they lost confidence in sublingual fentanyl products after two to three failures in titration.

It is possible that the overall efficacy would have been higher if more patients had been titrated up to maximum dose before deciding the treatment was ineffective and ceased. Titrating narcotics in an outpatient clinical setting can be challenging. Although patients are given teaching during their clinic visit and are asked to contact the clinic should they have any questions or concerns not all patients remember the teaching on titration or take advantage of the opportunity to receive help. Subsequent to this review we have been providing written instructions to patients for titration in addition to the teaching done in clinic. In clinical trials the mean effective dose of fentanyl sublingual tablet was greater than or equal to 300 mcg (13,14). It would be helpful to identify those patients in whom 100 mcg would not be effective so that a higher initial dose could be used and patients could achieve pain relief with a minimum number of titrations. One study has suggested that it is safe to start titration at higher doses in patients on higher daily MME doses (15). Again; more research is called for in this area.

A limitation of our study is its retrospective design. Other factors that may have impacted successful titration may not have been adequately captured by chart review. Prospective studies evaluating titration strategies and utilizing response to treatment pain scales should be performed. It is noteworthy, that the safety profile in our case review was excellent with only one patient experiencing side effects requiring discontinuation of the medication

In conclusion, successful titration of sublingual fentanyl tablets for management of breakthrough pain occurred in 50% of patients managed in our outpatient clinic. In the majority of patients for whom it was ineffective it was not titrated to maximal dose before stopping - this was not due to development of side effects. Coordinated efforts to improve outpatient titration (e.g., written instructions) as well as research into initiation of drug at higher doses (thereby requiring fewer titration steps) may improve the utility of this agent.

References

[1]   Portnoy RK, Hagen NA. Breakthrough pain: definition, prevalence and characteristics. Pain 1990;41:273-81.

[2]   Fine PG, Busch MA. Characterization of breakthrough pain by hospice patients and their caregivers. J Pain Symptom Manage 1998;16(3):179-83.

[3]   Mercadante S, Radbruch L, Caraceni A, Cherny N, Kaasa S, Nauck F, et al. Episodic (breakthrough) pain: consensus conference of an expert working group of the European Association for Palliative Care. Cancer 2002;94(3):832-9.

[4]   Breivik H, Vherny N, Collett B, Collett B, de Conno F, Filbet M, et al. Cancer-related pain: a pan-European survey of prevalence, treatment and patient attitudes. Ann Oncol 2009;20(8):1420-33.

[5]   Zeppetella G, Riberiero M. Pharmacotherapy of cancer-related episodic pain . Expert Opin Pharmacother 2003;4(4):493-502.

[6]   Gomez-Batiste X, Madrid F, Moreno F, Gracia A, Trelis J, Fontanals et al. Breakthrough cancer pain: prevalence and characteristics in patients in Catalonia, Spain. J Pain Symptom Manage 2002;24(1):45-52.

[7]   Caraceni A, Martini C, Zecca E, Portenoy RK, Ashby MA, Hawson G, et al. Breakthrough pain characteristics and syndromes in patients with cancer pain. An international survey. Palliat Med 2004;18:177-83.

[8]   Portenoy RK, Payne D, Jacobsen P. Breakthrough pain: characteristics and impact in patients with cancer pain. Pain 1999;81:129-34.

[9]   Zeppetella G, O'Doherty CA, Collins S. Prevalence and characteristics of breakthrough pain in cancer patients admitted to a hospice. J Pain Symptom Manage 2000;20(2):87-92.

[10]   Skinner C, Thompson E, Davies A. Clinical features. In: Davies A. Cancer related breakthrough pain. Oxford: Oxford University Press, 2006:13-22.

[11]   Rauck RL, Tark M, Reyes E, Hayes TG, Bartkowiak AJ, Hassman D, et al. Efficacy and long-term tolerability of sublingual fentanyl orally disintegrating tablet in the treatment of breakthrough cancer pain. Curr Med Res Opin 2009;25:2877-85.

[12]   Nalamachu S, Hassman D, Wallace M, Dumble S, Derrick R, Howell J. Long-term effectiveness and tolerability of sublingual fentanyl citrate orally disintegrating tablet for the treatment of breakthrough cancer pain. Curr Med Res Opin 2011;27:519-30.

[13]   Nalamachu SR, Rauck RL, Wallace MS, Hassman D, Howell J. Successful dose finding with sublingual fentanyl tablet: combined results from 2 open-label titration studies. Pain Pract 2012;12(6):449-56.

[14] Ward J, Laird B, Fallon M; BTcP Registry Group. The UK breakthrough cancer pain registry: Origin, methods and preliminary data. Presented at The Compass Collaboration Annual Scientific Meeting, Edinburgh 2011 Apr 14-15.

[15] Mercadante S, Gatti A, Porizio G, Lo Presti C, Aielli F, Adile C, et al. Dosing fentanyl buccal tablet for breakthrough cancer pain: dose titration versus proportional doses. Curr Med Res Opin 2012;28(6); 963-8.

Submitted: December 15, 2012. *Revised:* January 15, 2013. *Accepted:* January 26, 2013.

In: Pain Management Yearbook 2013
Editor: Joav Merrick

ISBN: 978-1-63117-944-0
© 2014 Nova Science Publishers, Inc.

Chapter 18

Mother-child concordance for pain location in a pediatric chronic pain sample

Lindsay F Schwartz, BS[1], Laura C Seidman, BS[2],
Lonnie K Zeltzer, MD[2] and Jennie CI Tsao, PhD[2]

[1]University of Illinois at Chicago, Chicago, Il USA
[2]Pediatric Pain Program, Department of Pediatrics,
David Geffen School of Medicine at UCLA, Los Angeles, Ca, USA

Abstract

Body maps have long been used to assess pain location in adult and pediatric chronic pain patients. Assessing agreement between parent and child reports of pain location using such maps may help establish a unified picture of children's pain experience. However, few studies have examined the extent of agreement between mothers and children on the location of the child's pain. Using kappa coefficients and other determinants of the magnitude of kappa we assessed mother-child concordance in pain location using body maps with 21 standardized areas in 41 children with chronic pain (65.9% female, mean age = 14.60) and their mothers. The highest level of agreement was found for the abdominal region; agreement for the head region was moderate and not superior to the other body areas. Approximately half of the body map areas yielded poor to fair mother-child agreement, while the other half yielded moderate or better agreement. There was more agreement between mothers and sons than between mothers and daughters on the total number of body areas considered painful, but there were no effects of pubertal status, race, and ethnicity on agreement. Our results are consistent with previous studies indicating that parent assessments of children's pain do not necessarily

*Correspondence: Jennie C. I. Tsao, PhD, Pediatric Pain Program, Department of Pediatrics, David Geffen School of Medicine at UCLA, Box 951752, #22-464 MDCC, Los Angeles, California 90095-1752, USA, Telephone: (310) 825-0731, Fax: (310) 794-2104, E-mail: jtsao@mednet.ucla.edu.

mimic their child's report. Future research should test additional psychosocial factors that may contribute to parent-child discordance regarding the location of the child's pain.

Keywords: Children, adolescents, parents, pediatric pain, chronic pain

Introduction

Pain perception in children is complex and often difficult to assess. Although parents are often seen as the "experts" regarding their child's pain (1), it is now recognized that children themselves can provide accurate reports of their own pain (2-4). In accord, the majority of recent studies have examined the child's own account of his/her pain in addition to reports from the child's parents. A key question posed by researchers and clinicians alike is the extent to which parents and children agree regarding the child's pain. Extant work in this area has focused primarily on indicators such as pain intensity or pain frequency with few studies examining parent-child agreement on the location of the child's pain. Despite the usual focus on the chief presenting complaint during clinical encounters, children often experience pain in more than one location (5). Therefore, understanding parent-child agreement on the location(s) of the child's pain may enhance the accuracy of pain assessment and treatment in pediatric chronic pain.

Body maps (i.e., pain charts, manikins) have long been used as part of the multidimensional assessment of pain in pediatric samples, and such maps can be completed without assistance by children as young as 8 years of age (5). Only three prior studies have utilized body maps to assess parent-child agreement regarding the child's pain. Using a body map with 17 different locations in pediatric spina bifida patients, one such investigation found that children who reported more intense pain also reported more pain locations; there was higher parent-child concordance for pain intensity in locations where pain of severe intensity was reported (6). However, parent-child agreement regarding specific pain locations was not examined. Another investigation in Duchene (DMD) and Becker (BMD) muscular dystrophy patients found poor parent-child concordance for pain duration and frequency using a body map with nine distinct areas, but agreement on pain location was not assessed (7). Graumlich et al. (8) in their study of pediatric patients with sickle cell disease (SCD), reported parent-child concordance rates using a body map with 14 body locations. The percent agreement between parents and children regarding pain location ranged from 58.3-95.8% across all body sites, but agreement for individual areas was not reported.

Recently, von Baeyer, et al. (5) proposed the use of a body map developed by the SUPER-KIDZ research group (9) containing 21 standardized and demarcated areas. Use of a standardized body map facilitates comparisons across studies, and pain locations may be more accurately assessed using a body map than by interview (5). The aim of the current study was to examine agreement between mothers and children regarding the location of the child's pain using the SUPER-KIDZ body map in a sample of pediatric chronic pain patients. Because prior studies have not done so, we tested mother-child agreement for each of the body regions. As noted by Chambers et al. (10), previous reports showing high parent-child concordance have mostly relied on correlational analyses which may over-estimate parent-child agreement. Thus, following Chambers, we calculated kappa coefficients to assess mother-child agreement as well as additional statistics, i.e., prevalence index, bias index, and the maximum obtainable kappa, to aid in the interpretation of kappa. Since headaches and abdominal pain are the most common pain complaints in children (11), we hypothesized that agreement for these areas would be greater than that of the other body regions. Based on the findings of Chambers (10) and others (6-9) we expected the overall extent of agreement to be moderate. We also conducted exploratory analyses to examine sex and racial/ethnic differences in overall mother-child agreement regarding the number of painful locations.

Methods

All recruitment and study procedures were approved by the University of California, Los Angeles Institutional Review Board (IRB). Subjects were part of a larger study on sex and pubertal differences in laboratory pain responses. The study sample consisted of children and adolescents with chronic pain aged 8-17 years (*n* = 46), as well as their mothers (*n* = 46). All fathers were also invited to participate; however, only a small number of fathers did so (*n* = 5). Therefore, only data on mothers and children will be presented. The sample was primarily recruited through a multidisciplinary tertiary clinic specializing in pediatric chronic pain. Prior to the patient's initial consultation with the clinic physicians, the patient and his/her parents met with a trained research associate who gave an initial overview of the study. If the patient and his/her family were interested in participating, the research associate then asked a series of questions to ascertain study eligibility. Inclusion and exclusion criteria are further discussed below.

Seven participating families were originally recruited as well-child control participants for the larger laboratory pain study but were found to meet criteria for chronic pain (15.2% of the sample). These participants were recruited through advertisements, community events, and via referrals from previous participants (who earned an additional $25 for each referred family that completed the study). Study advertisements were posted on online forums (e.g., Craigslist) and at physical locations (e.g., libraries, pediatricians' offices, etc.). Participants were also recruited by study staff at community events (festivals/fairs, etc.). The study PI (LKZ) reviewed each of these cases and re-assigned them to the chronic pain group. Seven additional participating families (15.2% of the sample) were recruited from other local clinics and by physicians at private practices and university-based clinics. Physicians and clinic staff provided patients with the study flyer to enable interested families to contact the study coordinator regarding participation. Each of these cases was reviewed by the study PI to determine eligibility.

Inclusion criteria followed the commonly accepted definition of chronic/recurrent pain as pain that has persisted for three months or longer (12). Subjects were excluded from the study if they presented with a developmental delay, autism, or significant anatomic impairment that could preclude understanding of or participation in study procedures. Siblings of the child/adolescent participants were also excluded. Mothers could be biological or adoptive parents of the child; however, the child had to reside at least half of the time in the household with their mother for her to be eligible to participate. Each participating family member was compensated with $50 for their participation.

Of the original 46 mother-child pairs enrolled in the study, five pairs (10.9%) were excluded because participants did not complete a body map (i.e., they reported that the child did not experience pain in the last month). Therefore, data from 41 children (65.9% female, 75.6% late puberty, mean age = 14.60, age range = 9.33) and 41 mothers were analyzed in this study. See Table 1 for additional demographic information. Table 1 also displays the presenting pain complaints for girls, boys, and the total sample. As shown in Table 1, over 60% of the patient sample presented with more than one pain complaint.

Procedure

Mothers provided written informed consent and children provided written assent. Mothers and children each independently completed a body map assessing the location of the child's pain in separate rooms; each participant was also interviewed separately by a trained research assistant about the child's pain. The procedure for completing the body maps conformed to that recommended by von Baeyer et al. (5). Participants were first asked by a trained research assistant whether the child had experienced pain in the past month. Those who answered affirmatively were given a body map (described below; see *Measures* section) and asked to shade all areas where the child had experienced pain in the past month. Markings were completed using a dark colored pen.

Completed body maps were independently scored by two trained research assistants. Any mark in an area was recorded as positive for pain in that area. Any area that was not marked was recorded as negative for pain in that area. Laterality was ignored (i.e., a mark on the left foot, right foot, or both feet all scored as positive for pain in the feet). For the 1,722 body map areas scored (i.e., 21 body map areas for 82 subjects – 41 mothers and 41 children), there were a total of 28 discrepancies between the two scorers (1.6% error rate). These discrepancies were addressed and resolved by two additional independent researchers through collaborative conferencing on each discrepancy.

Measures

Demographics: A questionnaire designed for the larger laboratory pain study was used to assess the child's/parent's ethnicity and race, child's/parent's age, and child's biological sex.
Pain interview: A series of open-ended questions about the child's pain were administered using an interview developed for the laboratory pain study. The interview included questions about pain intensity, pain duration, and which pain bothered them the most.

Stage of puberty: Children completed a self-report measure based on diagrams representing different stages of pubertal development (13). This instrument consisted of schematic drawings with written descriptions of five stages of secondary sexual characteristics on two separate dimensions based on the Tanner's Sexual Maturity Scale (14). Such self-assessment ratings correlate with ratings based on physical examination by physicians (13,15). Subjects were given sex-appropriate measures and asked to rate her/himself on each of two dimensions by selecting the drawing closest to his/her stage of development. A single score, ranging from I (prepubertal) to V (adult) level of development, was computed by averaging the two ratings.

Body map: The body map used in this study is the pain chart recommended by the Childhood Arthritis and Rheumatology Research Alliance (CARRA; CA, USA) for studies of recurrent and chronic pain and first adopted as part of the SUPER-KIDZ pain assessment project (9). There are 21 distinct body areas identifiable on the map, and both front and back views are represented. As noted above, participants were asked to shade all areas in which the child had experienced pain in the past month.

Table 1. Demographic characteristics and presenting pain complaints for girls, boys, and the total sample

	Boys (*N* = 14)	Girls (*N* = 27)	Total Sample (*N* = 41)
Child mean age in years (SD)	13.5 (2.5)	15.3 (2.3)	14.6 (2.5)
Child pubertal state [Late Puberty – n (%)]	8 (57.1)	23 (85.2)	31 (75.6)
Child race [Caucasian – n (%)]	8 (57.1)	18 (66.7)	26 (63.4)
Child ethnicity [Hispanic – n (%)]	3 (21.4)	6 (22.2)	9 (22.0)
Mother mean age in years (SD)	45.2 (5.0)	45.47 (7.8)	45.38 (6.9)
Mother race [Caucasian – n (%)]	9 (64.3)	19 (70.4)	28 (68.3)
Mother ethnicity [Hispanic – n (%)]	3 (21.4)	3 (11.1)	6 (14.6)
Pain Diagnosis			
Headaches	9 (64.3)	15 (55.6)	24 (58.5)
Abdominal Pain	4 (28.6)	16 (59.3)	20 (48.8)
CRPS	1 (7.1)	2 (7.4)	3 (7.3)
Fibromyalgia	2 (14.3)	9 (33.3)	11 (26.8)
Joint Pain	1 (7.1)	2 (7.4)	3 (7.3)
Neck Pain	1 (7.1)	1 (3.7)	2 (4.9)
Shoulder Pain	0 (0.0)	1 (3.7)	1 (2.4)
Back Pain	3 (21.4)	6 (22.2)	9 (22.0)
Leg Pain	1 (7.1)	1 (3.7)	2 (4.9)
Chest Pain	0 (0.0)	1 (3.7)	1 (2.4)
Hand Pain	0 (0.0)	1 (3.7)	1 (2.4)
Foot Pain	1 (7.1)	1 (3.7)	2 (4.9)
Multiple Pain Diagnoses	7 (50.0)	19 (70.4)	25 (61.0)

Note: Frequencies for pain diagnoses sum to more than 100% due to multiple pain diagnoses. CRPS = complex regional pain syndrome, type 1 or type 2.

Statistical analyses

Kappa coefficients were calculated for each of the 21 body map areas. Kappa statistics are typically used to indicate the amount of agreement between two raters (e.g., clinicians) regarding the presence or absence of a disease state or diagnosis. In the current study, we calculated kappa coefficients to assess the extent of concordance between mothers and children. Kappa (κ) is defined as a measure of "true" agreement. It indicates the proportion of agreement beyond that expected by chance (that is, the *achieved* agreement beyond chance as a proportion of the *possible* agreement beyond chance). Kappa values range from -1 to 1, with 1 signifying perfect agreement between raters, 0 signifying agreement no better than that expected by chance, and negative numbers signifying agreement worse than that expected by chance. The latter only rarely occurs in smaller samples as a result of sampling variation (16,17).

Kappa values were categorized using the scale Landis and Koch (18) proposed as standards for strength of agreement: <0.000 = poor, $0.001–0.200$ = slight, $0.201–0.400$ = fair, $0.401–0.600$ = moderate, $0.601–0.800$ = substantial, and $0.801–1.000$ = almost perfect agreement. Although these standards are controversial, they provide a simple heuristic by which the magnitude of kappa may be evaluated. To reduce the possibility of Type 1 error in evaluating the statistical significance of the kappa values, a Bonferroni correction for 21 tests was performed; $p < 0.002$ was considered significant (i.e., agreement was significantly better than would be expected by chance alone).

As suggested by Sim and Wright (19), the following statistics were also calculated to assist in interpreting the magnitude of kappa. As noted by these authors, the interpretation of the value of kappa on its own is problematic without taking into account key factors such the prevalence of an attribute (base rates) and inter-rater bias (19).

Prevalence index (PI): This statistic measures the proportions of positive and negative responses from each observer and determines if they are equally probable or if their probabilities vary (20). If the PI is high (i.e., the prevalence of a positive rating is either very high or very low), chance agreement is also high, and kappa is reduced (21). Thus, when PI is large, kappa is lower than when PI is low or zero; the effect of PI on kappa is greater for large values of kappa than for small values (22).

Bias index (BI): The extent to which two observers differ in their assessment of the occurrence of a condition is referred to as bias (22). BI measures the extent to which the raters disagree on the proportion of positive (or negative) cases. As BI increases, the proportion of agreement expected by chance decreases, and the value of kappa increases (19,22). Therefore, a large BI has the effect of inflating kappa (19,22).

Kappa max (κ_{Max}): This statistic refers to the maximum attainable kappa for each body map area. To calculate κ_{Max}, the proportions of positive and negative judgments by each rater are taken as fixed, and the distribution of paired ratings is then adjusted to represent the greatest possible agreement. κ_{Max} serves to gauge the strength of agreement while preserving the proportions of positive ratings given by each rater. In effect, it provides a reference value for kappa that preserves the individual's overall propensity for a positive endorsement (19). Greater the discrepancy between kappa and κ_{Max} indicates poorer agreement than kappa alone would suggest.

Additional exploratory analyses used independent *t*-tests to test for differences based on the sex of the child, the child's pubertal status (early vs. late puberty), and the race/ethnicity of the child (Caucasian vs. non-Caucasian and Hispanic vs. non-Hispanic, respectively). The following dependent variables were evaluated: 1) the total number of body areas endorsed by the child; 2) the total number of body areas endorsed by the mother; 3) the total number of mother-child body areas endorsed by both mother and child (the number of mother-child agreements); 4) the total number of mother "positive" and child "negative" occurrences (i.e., the mother indicated that the child experienced pain in a body area(s), but the child did not); 5) the total number of mother "negative" and child "positive" occurrences (i.e., the mother indicated that the child did not experience pain in a body area(s), but the child did). For these exploratory tests, a standard probability level of $p < 0.05$ (two-tailed) was used to evaluate the results.

Results

Table 2 displays the descriptive data for the 21 body map areas for mothers and children. Table 3 shows the kappa, PI, BI, and κ_{Max} statistics, indicating the extent of agreement between mothers and children for the 21 body map areas. The mean number of painful areas endorsed by children was 5.51 (SD: 3.802; Range: 1-17) and 4.42 for mothers (SD: 2.585; Range: 1-12). Only 6 children (14.6%) and 2 mothers (4.9%) reported a single body area as being painful.

Table 2. Descriptive statistics for mother-child pairs

	Mother-Child Disagreement	Mother-Child Both "Positive"	Mother-Child Both "Negative"	Mother "Positive", Child "Negative"	Child "Positive", Mother "Negative"
Upper Arm	4 (9.8%)	0 (0.0%)	37 (90.2%)	1 (2.4%)	3 (7.3%)
Forearm	5 (12.2%)	0 (0.0%)	36 (87.8%)	1 (2.4%)	4 (9.8%)
Face	6 (14.6%)	0 (0.0%)	35 (85.4%)	2 (4.9%)	4 (9.8%)
Groin	1 (2.4%)	1 (2.4%)	39 (95.1%)	0 (0.0%)	1 (2.4%)
Wrist	9 (22.0%)	1 (2.4%)	31 (75.6%)	5 (12.2%)	4 (9.8%)
Elbow	4 (9.8%)	2 (4.9%)	35 (85.4%)	2 (4.9%)	2 (4.9%)
Thigh	5 (12.2%)	2 (4.9%)	34 (82.9%)	1 (2.4%)	4 (9.8%)
Calf	9 (22.0%)	2 (4.9%)	30 (73.2%)	4 (9.8%)	5 (12.2%)
Chest	10 (24.4%)	2 (4.9%)	29 (70.7%)	3 (7.3%)	7 (17.1%)
Hand	4 (9.8%)	3 (7.3%)	34 (82.9%)	1 (2.4%)	3 (7.3%)
Hip	6 (14.6%)	4 (9.8%)	31 (75.6%)	1 (2.4%)	5 (12.2%)
Ankle	10 (24.4%)	4 (9.8%)	27 (65.9%)	4 (9.8%)	6 (14.6%)
Upper Back	14 (34.1%)	4 (9.8%)	23 (56.1%)	3 (7.3%)	11 (26.8%)
Foot	9 (22.0%)	6 (14.6%)	26 (63.4%)	2 (4.9%)	7 (17.1%)
Neck	9 (22.0%)	6 (14.6%)	26 (63.4%)	1 (2.4%)	8 (19.5%)
Shoulder	15 (36.6%)	7 (17.1%)	19 (46.3%)	6 (14.6%)	9 (22.0%)
Mid-Back	9 (22.0%)	11 (26.8%)	21 (51.2%)	1 (2.4%)	8 (19.5%)
Knee	11 (26.8%)	11 (26.8%)	19 (46.3%)	3 (7.3%)	8 (19.5%)
Lower Back	8 (19.5%)	12 (29.3%)	21 (51.2%)	2 (4.9%)	6 (14.6%)
Abdomen	6 (14.6%)	16 (39.0%)	19 (46.3%)	5 (12.2%)	1 (2.4%)
Head	11 (26.8%)	20 (48.8%)	10 (24.4%)	7 (17.1%)	4 (9.8%)

Poor mother-child agreement (κ < 0.000): Upper arm, forearm, wrist

κ values for the upper arm, forearm, and wrist were extremely low or negative, indicating poor agreement by the Landis and Koch scale. Moreover, the large discrepancies between κ and κ_{Max} support the categorization of poor mother-child agreement. Although high PI values have the effect of lowering κ, this effect is greater for large values of κ than for small values. Given the very low values for kappa, the effect of high PI values on agreement for these regions is likely to be minimal. BI values were very low suggesting little impact on κ values. None of the kappa values in this group were statistically significant.

Slight mother-child agreement (0.001 < κ < 0.200):
Calf, chest, upper back

κ values for calf, chest, and upper back were low, suggesting slight agreement by the Landis and Koch scale. Very large discrepancies between κ and $κ_{Max}$ support the classification of only slight agreement. Since κ values were low, the likely effects of PI values on κ are small. BI values were low indicating minimal impact on κ. None of the kappa values for these areas were statistically significant.

Fair mother-child agreement (0.201 < κ < 0.400):
Shoulder, ankle, face, thigh

Moderately low κ values were found for the shoulder, ankle, face, and thigh, suggesting fair agreement by the Landis and Koch scale. Similar to the results for the poor and slight categories above, there were large discrepancies between κ and $κ_{Max}$ as well as very low BI values across all areas.

Table 3. κ $κ_{Max}$, prevalence index, and bias index for the 21 body map areas

	κ	$κ_{Max}$	Prevalence Index (PI)	Bias Index (BI)	κ Significance Level (p)
Forearm	-0.041	0.376	0.878	0.063	0.739
Upper Arm	-0.038	0.788	0.902	0.049	0.776
Wrist	0.056	0.895	0.732	0.024	0.717
Chest	0.153	0.661	0.659	0.098	0.298
Upper Back	0.171	0.526	0.463	0.195	0.215
Calf	0.178	0.909	0.683	0.024	0.252
Shoulder	0.204	0.841	0.293	0.073	0.185
Ankle	0.291	0.858	0.561	0.049	0.060
Face	0.32	0.774	0.756	0.049	0.035
Thigh	0.384	0.631	0.78	0.073	0.008
Head	0.433	0.845	0.244	0.073	0.005
Foot	0.435	0.686	0.488	0.122	0.003
Elbow	0.446	1.00	0.805	0.00	0.004
Knee	0.451	0.75	0.195	0.122	0.003
Neck	0.445*	0.568	0.488	0.171	0.002*
Hip	0.492*	0.661	0.659	0.098	0.001*
Hand	0.547*	0.774	0.756	0.049	<0.001*
Mid-Back	0.547*	0.648	0.244	0.171	<0.001*
Lower Back	0.594*	0.797	0.22	0.098	<0.001*
Groin	0.655*	0.655	0.927	0.024	<0.001*
Abdomen	0.709*	0.806	0.073	0.098	<0.001*

Note: * = p < .002.

High PI values for the face and thigh suggest that chance agreement was also high and the kappa values for these regions were somewhat reduced. None of the kappa values in this group were statistically significant.

Moderate mother-child agreement (0.401 < κ < 0.600): Head, foot, neck, elbow, knee, hip, hand, mid-back, low-back

Although the κ values for head, foot, neck, elbow, knee, hip, hand, mid-back, and low-back all suggested moderate agreement, examination of the other agreement statistics indicates that the extent of agreement for these regions may be further categorized into two distinct subgroups.

The subgroup with the poorer agreement statistics included the elbow, head, knee, and foot regions. κ values for this group ranged from 0.43 to 0.45, and all the regions in this subgroup had low BIs (ranging from 0 to 0.12). The difference between κ and $κ_{Max}$ for the regions in this subgroup ranged from 0.55 to 0.25, indicating a substantial divergence between the obtained agreement and the maximum possible agreement. Although the elbow region had a high PI, this is offset by the fact that it also had the greatest difference between its κ and $κ_{Max}$ value. None of the kappa values for the areas in this subgroup were statistically significant.

The subgroup with better agreement statistics included the neck, hand, hip, mid-, and low-back regions. The κ values for these five areas were similar ranging from 0.45 to 0.59, and the discrepancies between their κ and $κ_{Max}$ values were lower than that of the above subgroup (ranging from 0.10 to 0.22), indicating better agreement. High PI values for the hip and hand suggested that chance agreement was high and that kappa values for these regions are somewhat reduced. Low BI values across all areas suggest little impact on κ values. All of the κ values for these areas were statistically significant.

Substantial mother-child agreement (0.601 < κ < 0.800): Groin, abdomen

The groin and abdomen both had high κ values that were statistically significant and reflected substantial agreement according to Landis and Koch's scale. The discrepancy between the κ and $κ_{Max}$ values was very small for the abdomen (0.1) and zero for the groin region.

The abdomen region had a low PI, indicating low chance agreement resulting in a higher kappa. The groin region had a high PI suggesting that chance agreement was high and that kappa was therefore reduced. Even though there was substantial agreement for the groin region, it should be noted that there were very few cases of groin pain—one case in which both mother and child agreed the pain was present and one case in which the child endorsed pain in this region but the mother denied that the child experienced pain in this region (see table 2). Low BI values again indicated minimal effects on kappa values.

Overall mother-child agreement: Effects of gender, puberty, and race/ethnicity

Results of the *t*-tests indicated that there was a trend for girls to endorse more total body areas than boys ($p = 0.054$), but there was no difference in the total number of body areas endorsed by mothers of sons versus mothers of daughters. There was significantly more agreement on the total number of body areas between mothers and sons (M = 18.5; SD = 2.0) than between mothers and daughters (M = 16.2; SD = 3.0) (t(39) = 2.62, p < 0.02), but there were no other significant differences based on child sex. There were no significant differences on any of the variables based on pubertal status, race, or ethnicity.

Discussion

We hypothesized that mother-child agreement regarding the location of the child's pain would be greater for the head and abdominal regions compared to other body regions when assessed using a standardized body map with 21 demarcated areas (5). Our hypothesis was partially supported in that agreement was greatest for the abdominal region. Although agreement was also high for the groin region, there were only two cases endorsing this area as painful. Contrary to our hypothesis, agreement for the head region was not superior to the other body areas. We also hypothesized that the overall magnitude of mother-child agreement would be moderate. This hypothesis was also partly supported in that roughly half of the body map areas showed moderate or better agreement (head, foot, neck, elbow, knee, hip, hand, mid-back, low-back, groin, abdomen), whereas the other half showed poor to fair agreement (forearm, upper arm, wrist, chest, upper back, calf, shoulder, ankle, face, thigh). Our exploratory analyses found that agreement regarding the total number of painful body areas was higher between mothers and sons than between mothers and daughters. However, there were no differences in mother-child agreement based on child race/ethnicity or pubertal status.

The current methodology allowed for a more nuanced examination of mother-child agreement and represents a significant advance over prior work. Since reliance on kappa values alone to assess agreement between observers is controversial (19), we calculated prevalence index (PI), bias index (BI), and maximum obtainable kappa (κ_{Max}) to aid the interpretation of kappa. High PI values indicate that the prevalence of a positive rating is either very high or very low, chance agreement is also high and therefore kappa is reduced; the effects of PI on kappa are greater for larger values of kappa (19,22). Thus, the high PI values for the groin, hip and hand regions suggest that the obtained kappas for these areas were attenuated. Smaller differences between κ and κ_{max} indicate better agreement and thus, the large discrepancies between κ and κ_{Max} values for the head, foot, elbow and knee regions indicated poorer agreement than that suggested by kappa alone. Even though these areas met criteria for moderate agreement, their kappa coefficients were not statistically significant, indicating that agreement was no better than that expected by chance alone. Within the same moderate agreement category, the discrepancy between κ and κ_{Max} values was much smaller for the neck, hip, hand, mid- and low-back, indicating that these regions evidenced relatively better agreement; in accord, the kappas for these regions were statistically significant. Low BI values across all body regions indicated little bias in the sample (i.e., disagreement on the proportion of positive or negative cases).

Only one prior study by Graumlich et al. (8) in pediatric SCD patients has utilized a body map to examine parent-child agreement regarding pain location. (Two other studies using body maps focused on other indices such as pain intensity (6,7)). It is difficult to draw comparisons between the Graumlich study and current one for several reasons. Although Graumlich reported parent-child percent agreement for pain location ranged from 58.3% to 95.8%, they did not report parent-child agreement for each individual body area. Moreover, these authors did not detail the method used to assess agreement other than to indicate that parent-child concordance rates were examined by calculating "percent agreement ratios" for all pain sites. As discussed by Chambers et al. (1), the use of correlational analysis does not take into account error variance between parents and children and may result in overestimates of these associations. Moreover, the Graumlich sample included patients who presented with a single disease (SCD) whereas our sample consisted of patients with various chronic pain complaints, which likely yielded more heterogeneity in the body locations endorsed as painful and, consequently, a lower likelihood of mother-child agreement for specific body areas. Nevertheless, our findings regarding the overall magnitude of agreement are at least partially consistent with previous research showing moderate mother-child agreement for pain indices such as pain severity and frequency (1,6-9).

Epidemiological research indicates that headaches and abdominal pain are the first and second most common pain complaints among children (11). In line with these findings, the most common presenting pain complaints in the current sample were head pain (58.5%) and abdominal pain (48.8%). Notably, mothers were more likely than children to endorse each of these areas as painful (see table 2). It is unclear why mother-child agreement was much better for the abdomen than for the head region. During pain interviews conducted after completion of the body maps, we asked mother and children separately which pain bothered the child the most (if more than one location was considered painful). Whereas the number of children ($n = 8$) and mothers ($n = 9$) who indicated the abdomen was most bothersome was similar, there was a somewhat greater discrepancy between the number of children ($n = 9$) and mothers ($n = 12$) indicating that head pain was the most bothersome. The interviews also ascertained the duration of the most bothersome pain by both child and mother report. The duration of pain was much longer for the abdomen (mean = 6.6 years by child report and 5.3 years by mother report), than for head pain (mean = 2.9 years by child report and 3.0 years by mother report). Thus, it is possible that the longer duration of abdominal pain relative to head pain may explain the better agreement for the former compared to the latter body region.

Our finding of greater agreement between mothers and sons than between mothers and daughters on the total number of painful body areas is new and somewhat unexpected. We previously found stronger associations between mother's fear of anxiety symptoms and girls' acute laboratory pain responses compared to boys' (23). Others have similarly reported that the impact of mothers' pain-related behavior on children's laboratory pain responses is more pronounced among girls than boys (24,25). Prior work on mother-child concordance for pain using body maps has not examined sex differences in agreement. Our findings of sex-based differences in mother-child agreement cannot be explained by variations in the prevalence of pain as there were no sex differences in the total number of body sites considered painful by either child or parent report. However, girls were substantially older than boys (mean age boys = 13.4 vs. girls = 15.3), and a possible explanation is that mother-child agreement may be generally higher among younger compared to older children.

The current findings have clear implications for the assessment and treatment of chronic pain in children. In clinical practice, the use of interviews to assess pain is a common approach with emphasis typically being placed on the chief presenting complaint (5). The utility of body maps to assess pain location is underscored by our findings that nearly all of the patients in our sample reported more than one pain location. Only two mothers (4.9%) and 6 children (14.6%) endorsed a single area as being painful. Our results support the current recognition that the optimal route to acquiring an accurate portrayal of a child's pain experience is to obtain both parent and child report. However, given the observed discrepancy between mother and child reports even for common pain locations such as the head, additional work is needed to develop better methods to integrate child and parent information.

Limitations of this study should be mentioned. First, we only included participants who indicated that the child had experienced pain in the past month, and thus 5 of the 46 enrolled families did not complete body maps.

Given the fluctuating and cyclical nature of chronic/recurrent pain, asking about usual pain location(s) may have yielded different findings. However, the one month time frame was used to temper the possible effects of memory bias over an extended time period. Second, we were not able to assess father-child agreement due to the small number of enrolled fathers. Further work may examine father-child agreement as well as the extent of agreement between mothers and fathers regarding their child's pain. Third, our results may not generalize to other pediatric samples. As noted previously, the extent of mother-child agreement may have been diluted by the large number of different pain complaints represented. It is possible that higher levels of agreement may be obtained in patient populations with more focal pain problems or specific disease states.

In sum, in this sample of pediatric chronic pain patients, agreement between mothers and children regarding the location of the child's pain was greatest for the abdomen, with moderate or better agreement for approximately half of the 21 areas assessed using a standardized body map. Future research may assess whether factors such as mother and/or child psychological characteristics (e.g., anxiety) may contribute to differences in mother-child agreement, as well as further examining the potential impact of pain duration, child development and sex-based effects. Additional work may test whether the current results are applicable to other patient populations as well as healthy populations. Such studies may enhance efforts to understand the underlying reasons for parent-child disagreement regarding the child's pain.

Acknowledgments

This study was supported by R01DE012754, awarded by the National Institute of Dental and Craniofacial Research (PI: Lonnie K. Zeltzer), and by UCLA Clinical & Translational Research Center CTSI Grant UL1TR000124 (PI: Lonnie K. Zeltzer). There are no conflicts of interest in this article.

References

[1]   Chambers CT, McGrath PJ. Pain measurement in children. In: MA Ashburn LR, ed. The management of pain. New York: Churchill Livingstone, 1998:625-34.

[2]   McGrath P. Pain in children: Nature, assessment, and treatment. New York: Guilford, 1990.

[3]   Ross D, Ross S. Childhood pain: Current issues, research, and management Baltimore: Urban Schwarzenberg, 1988:75-100.

[4]   Ross DM, Ross SA. Assessment of pediatric pain: an overview. Issues Compr Pediatr Nurs 1988;11(2-3):73-91.

[5]   von Baeyer CL, Lin V, Seidman LC, Tsao JC, Zeltzer LK. Pain charts (body maps or manikins) in assessment of the location of pediatric pain. Pain Manage 2011;1(1):61-8.

[6]   Clancy CA, McGrath PJ, Oddson BE. Pain in children and adolescents with spina bifida. Dev Med Child Neurol 2005;47(1):27-34.

[7]   Zebracki K, Drotar D. Pain and activity limitations in children with Duchenne or Becker muscular dystrophy. Dev Med Child Neurol 2008;50(7):546-52.

[8]   Graumlich SE, Powers SW, Byars KC, Schwarber LA, Mitchell MJ, Kalinyak KA. Multidimensional assessment of pain in pediatric sickle cell disease. J Pediatr Psychol 2001;26(4):203-14.

[9]   Stinson JN, Connelly M, Jibb LA, Schanberg LE, Walco G, Spiegel LR, et al.. Developing a standardized approach to the assessment of pain in children and youth presenting to pediatric rheumatology providers: a Delphi survey and consensus conference process followed by feasibility testing. Pediatr Rheumatol Online J 2012;10(1):7.

[10] Chambers CT, Reid GJ, Craig KD, McGrath PJ, Finley GA. Agreement between child and parent reports of pain. Clin J Pain 1998;14:336-42.

[11] Croft F, Blyth F, van der Windt D. Chronic pain epidemiology: From aetiology to public health. New York: Oxford University Press, 2010.

[12] McGrath PJ, Walco GA, Turk DC, Dworkin RH, Brown MT, Davidson K, et al. Core outcome domains and measures for pediatric acute and chronic/recurrent pain clinical trials: PedIMMPACT recommendations. J Pain 2008;9(9):771-83.

[13] Morris NM, Udry JR. Validation of a self-administered instrument to assess stage of adolescent development. J Youth Adolesc 1980;9(3):271-80.

[14] Tanner JM. Growth at adolescence: with a general consideration of the effects of hereditary and environmental factors upon growth and maturation from birth to maturity. Oxford: Blackwell Scientific, 1962.

[15] Schlossberger NM, Turner RA, Irwin CE, Jr. Validity of self-report of pubertal maturation in early adolescents. J Adolesc Health 1992;13(2):109-13.

[16] Bartko JJ, Carpenter WT, Jr. On the methods and theory of reliability. J Nerv Ment Dis 1976;163(5):307-17.

[17] Fleiss J, Nee J, Landis J. Large sample variance of kappa in the case of different sets of raters. Psychol Bull 1979(86):974 -7.

[18] Landis JR, Koch GG. The measurement of observer agreement for categorical data. Biometrics 1977;33(1):159-74.

[19] Sim J, Wright CC. The kappa statistic in reliability studies: use, interpretation, and sample size requirements. Phys Ther 2005;85(3):257-68.

[20] Kilpikoski S, Airaksinen O, Kankaanpaa M, Leminen P, Videman T, Alen M. Interexaminer reliability of low back pain assessment using the McKenzie method. Spine (Phila Pa 1976) 2002;27(8):E207-14.

[21] Fleiss J. Measuring nominal scale agreement among many raters. Psychol Bull 1971;76:378-82.

[22] Byrt T, Bishop J, Carlin JB. Bias, prevalence and kappa. J Clin Epidemiol 1993;46(5):423-9.

[23] Tsao JCI, Lu Q, Myers CD, Kim SC, Turk N, Zeltzer LK. Parent and child anxiety sensitivity: Relationship to children's experimental pain responsivity. J Pain 2006;7(5):319-26.

[24] Chambers CT, Craig KD, Bennett SM. The impact of maternal behavior on children's pain experiences: an experimental analysis. J Pediatr Psychol 2002;27(3):293-301.

[25] Walker L, Williams S, Smith C, Garber J, Van Slyke D, Lipani T. Parent attention versus distraction: impact on symptom complaints by children with and without chronic functional abdominal pain. Pain 2006;122(1-2):43-52.

Submitted: November 01, 2012. *Revised:* January 10, 2013. *Accepted:* January 26, 2013

In: Pain Management Yearbook 2013
Editor: Joav Merrick

ISBN: 978-1-63117-944-0
© 2014 Nova Science Publishers, Inc.

Chapter 19

The influence of music on temporal perception and pain in a dental clinic

Nicolas Guéguen, PhD and Céline Jacob, PhD*
Université de Bretagne Sud, Vannes, France

Abstract

Several experiments have shown that music has a relaxation effect, reduces anxiety and influences time perception. The purpose of the study was to assess whether music influenced dental patients' perception of time spent in the waiting room and the feeling of pain. Soft music was either present or absent in a dental clinic. After the treatment, the patients were asked to estimate the time they had spent in the waiting room and their level of pain felt during the dental care. Results showed that music reduced the subjective perception of time spent in the waiting room and decreased the level of pain felt during the dental care. The interest in using audio distraction as an effective means of reducing pain during dental care is discussed.

Keywords: Pain, perception, music, dental treatment

Introduction

Dental treatment and the surrounding dental environment may elicit some negative emotions among people. These negative emotions include anxiety, fear and discomfort. Dental anxiety and/or fear act as barriers to receiving dental care by reducing initial treatment (1,2). Experiencing pain during dental care increases anxiety and fear, which in return establishes a vicious cycle where invasive treatment is required for a problem that has deteriorated over time which then increases pain and discomfort and leads to a reinforcement of fear, further

---

* Correspondence: Nicolas Guéguen, PhD, Université de Bretagne Sud, Campus de Tohanic 56000 Vannes, France.
E-mail: nicolas.gueguen@univ-ubs.fr

avoidance of dental treatment and as a result, continued disease (3). Thus it becomes important to be able to find techniques and methods that could help the practitioner reduce negative feelings and the level of pain experienced by patients. Some studies have found that atmospherics could have a positive impact on a patient's feelings. Research found reduced patient anxiety in dentist waiting rooms when they exposed patients to the odor of orange essential oil (4,5). Our objective was to test the effect of music on patients' cognition and level of subjective pain experienced during dental care.

Background music is known to influence people's behavior, and in particular the time for which they are prepared to wait (6-10). For instance, when people had to wait in a room, background music resulted in fewer people leaving the room and/or doing so only after a longer period (11). Similarly, instrumental music used as a waiting tune for an answering machine made people stay on the telephone longer before hanging up (7). For these authors, the pleasure induced by background music could lead the participants to estimate that less time has passed than in reality. Since patients commonly experience the time spent waiting for dental treatment as particularly anxiety provoking because it provides them time to think about what will (or could) happen and to ruminate on worst-case outcomes (12), it could be hypothesized that patients in the waiting room of a dental clinic with background music probably would estimate having spent less time waiting than those not exposed to background music.

Research on background music also found that it could be used as a pain management technique. A study found that during childbirth women reported that music distracted them from labor pain (13). Further research also reported a reduction in pain evaluation in postoperative surgery (14) and reduced chronic pain (15). For these authors, the limbic system would be involved with emotional output for music and pain, and because perception of both music and pain travel along similar neural pathways, each would affect the other. Thus, it could be hypothesized that patients exposed to music during dental care would experience less pain than those not exposed to it.

Methods

The participants were 80 adult patients (46 women and 34 men between the ages of 19 and 64 years), divided into two groups while in the waiting room. Forty patients were exposed to music in the waiting room and in the treatment room while the other 40 were not.

Procedure

This experiment was approved by the ethical committee of the laboratory (CRPCC-LESTIC EA 1285). The experiment took place on an individual basis. According to random distribution, when a patient entered the dental clinic, music was either present or absent with the help of a high fidelity sound system using stereo speakers. The music was played both in the waiting and in the dental care room. The music used was that selected and evaluated in a previous study (16), which evaluated thousands of musical pieces in order to select those considered soft and relaxing by listeners. When the patient left the dental clinic he/she was asked by an interviewer to respond to two survey questions (all agreed). The interviewer asked the participant to estimate the time he/she had waited in the waiting room before entering the dental care room. After that, the participant was asked orally to evaluate his/her level of pain felt during the dental care. The evaluation was made on a semantic scale with six steps. The participants were informed that they had participated in a study that evaluated the relation between music and pain, and were given details of the procedure used. They were asked if they would consent to the use of data collected. They were carefully informed that all the data would remain anonymous. All of them consented.

Results

On all measures employed in this study, no differences were found between male and female scores. Hence, the data were pooled and are presented in table 1.

Table 1. Means and standard deviations

	Music	No music
Estimation of time passed (in minutes)	M = 10.3 SD = 0.89	M = 13.5 SD = 0.90
Pain level experienced (6 max level)	M = 3.1 SD = 0.78	M = 3.8 SD = 0.84

An independent means test comparison was performed and demonstrated a significant difference on estimations of time spent between the two groups ($t(78) = 15.98$, $p < .001$, $d = 3.61$) revealing that the time spent waiting was judged as being longer in the control condition than in the music condition. With the level of pain felt during the care period, a significant difference was found ($t(78) = 3.86$, $p < .001$, $d = 0.87$) revealing that patients exposed to music experienced less pain that those not exposed to music.

In order to study the link between these two dependent measures, we calculated Bravais-Pearson correlation coefficients for each group. We found a positive correlation between the two measures for both the with-music ($r = .48$, $p = .002$) and the with-out-music control groups ($r = .51$, $p = .001$). Thus, the longer the estimation of time-passed, the higher the pain experienced was.

Discussion

The results of the present study confirm the positive effect of music on time perception. Indeed, music decreases estimates of time passed compared with a control situation where no music was played. These results confirm those obtained in a previous study (17) that showed the same difference when music was played in a waiting room. It was also found that music reduced the level of pain experienced by the patients during dental care. These results are in accordance with those found in a study (14), which found that music reduced pain evaluation in postoperative surgery. Our results confirmed that soft music also appeared to be a good way to reduce the level of pain evaluated during dental treatment. Perception of both music and pain probably travel along similar neural pathways, and each would affect one another (13).

Of course, we can imagine the practical interests of such a study. Music seems to be a useful tool in making dental treatment less painful for the patient which in return would lead him/her to increase the rate of regular dental visits which would then likely prevent the deterioration of oral health.

References

[1]   Klingberg G. Dental fear and behavior management problems in children: A study of measurement, prevalence, concomitant factors, and clinical effects. Swed Dent J 1995; 103:1–78.

[2]   Milgrom P, Weinstein P. Dental fears in general practice: New guidelines for assessment and treatment. Int Dent J 1993;43:288–93.

[3]   Armfield JM, Stewart JF, Spencer AJ. The vicious cycle of dental fear: Exploring the interplay between oral health, service utilization and dental fear. BMC Oral Health 2007;7:1186-92.

[4]   Lehrner J, Eckersberger C, Walla P, Pötsch G, Deecke L Ambient odor of orange in a dental office reduces anxiety and improves mood in female patients. Phys Behav 2000;71:83–5.

[5]   Lehrner J, Marwinski G, Lehr S, Johren P, Deecke L Ambient odors of orange and lavender reduce anxiety and improve mood in a dental office. Phys Behav 2005;86: 92–5.

[6]   Areni C, Kim D. The influence of background music on shopping behavior : classical versus top-forty music in a winestore. Adv Con Res 1993 20: 336-346.

[7]   North A, Hargreaves D, McKendrick J. Music and on-hold waiting time. Br J Psychol 1999;90:161-4.

[8]   Milliman R. Using Ancienne music to affect the behavior of supermarket shoppers. J Mark 1982;46:86-91.

[9]   Milliman, R. The influence of Ancienne music on the behavior of restaurant patrons. J Con Res 1986;13:286-9.

[10]   Yalch R, Spangenberg E. Using store music for retail zone : a field experiment. Ad Cons Res 1993;20:632-6.

[11]   North A, Hargreaves D, McKendrick J. The influence of in-store music on wine selections. J Appl Psychol 1999;84:271-6.

[12]   Cohen SM, Fiske J, Newton JT The impact of dental anxiety on daily living. Br Dent J 2000;189:385–90.

[13]   Browning C A. Using music during childbirth. Birth 2000;27:272-6.

[14]   Locsin, R. The effect of music on the pain of selected post-operative patients. J Adv Nurs 1981;6:19-25.

[15]   Zimmerman L, Pozehl B, Duncan K, Schmitz R. Effects of music in patients who had chronic cancer pain. West J Nurs Res 1989;11:296-307.

[16]   Guéguen N, Jacob C. Music congruency and consumer behaviour: An experimental field study. Int Bull Business Adm 2010;9:56-63.

[17]   Stratton V. Influence of music and socializing on perceived stress while waiting. Per Mot Skills 1992;75:334.

Submitted: November 15, 2012. *Revised:* January 15, 2013. *Accepted:* February 10, 2013.

In: Pain Management Yearbook 2013
Editor: Joav Merrick

ISBN: 978-1-63117-944-0
© 2014 Nova Science Publishers, Inc.

Chapter 20

Comparison of baseline quality of life scores in patients with bone and brain metastases as assessed using the EORTC QLQ-C15-PAL

Julia Di Giovanni, BSc(C)[1], Liang Zeng, MD(C)[1],
Liying Zhang, PhD[1], Vassilios Vassiliou, MD[2],
Takefumi Satoh, MD[3], Palmira Foro, MD[4], Brigette B.Y. Ma, MD[5],
Wei-Chu Chie, MD[6], Arjun Sahgal, MD[1], Michael Poon, BSc(C)[1]
and Edward Chow, MBBS[1]*

[1]Rapid Response Radiotherapy Program, Department of Radiation Oncology,
Odette Cancer Centre, Sunnybrook Health Sciences Centre, University of Toronto,
Toronto, Ontario, Canada
[2]Department of Radiation Oncology, Bank of Cyprus Oncology Centre, Nicosia, Cyprus
[3]Department of Urology, Kitasato University School of Medicine, Kanagawa, Japan
[4]Hospital de l'Esperança, Sant Josep de la Muntanya, Barcelona, Spain
[5]Department of Clinical Oncology, Prince of Wales Hospital, Shatin,
New Territories, Hong Kong, SAR
[6]Department of Public Health and Institute of Epidemiology and Preventative Medicine,
National Taiwan University, Taipei, Taiwan

* Correspondence: Professor Edward Chow MBBS, MSc, PhD, FRCPC, Department of Radiation Oncology, Odette Cancer Centre, Sunnybrook Health Sciences Centre, 2075 Bayview Avenue, Toronto, ON, Canada M4N 3M5. E-mail: Edward.Chow@sunnybrook.ca.

Abstract

From February 2009 to May 2010, patients receiving treatment for bone or brain metastases from five cancer centers across the world completed the EORTC QLQ-C15-PAL. Demographic information as well as various disease characteristics were recorded. To compare baseline QLQ-C15-PAL scores between patients with bone and brain metastases, univariate linear regression analysis was performed with or without confounders. A Bonferroni adjusted p-value < 0.003 (0.05/15 items) was considered statistically significant. A total of 109 patients with brain metastases and 233 patients with bone metastases completed the QLQ-C15-PAL. As expected, primary cancer site and previous systemic treatments were different between groups: there was a significantly greater number of patients with prostate and renal cell cancers and fewer patients with lung or gastrointestinal cancers with bone metastases, compared to patients with brain metastases (p<0.005). Prior to accounting for these two confounding factors, there were two QLQ-C15-PAL symptom scales significantly different between patients with bone metastases and patients with brain metastases. Patients with bone metastases had greater severity in pain (baseline mean score: 53.7 vs. 22.8; p<0.001) and fatigue (47.8 vs. 40.4; p=0.0029), compared to those with brain metastases. After accounting for confounders, only pain was significantly different (p<0.0001). Patients with bone metastases experience more pain at baseline compared to those with brain metastases. Patients with either bone or brain metastases otherwise experienced similar QOL profiles as assessed by the QLQ-C15-PAL. Supplementing of QLQ-C15-PAL by disease-specific instruments such as the QLQ-BM22 or QLQ-BN20 is therefore recommended in future trials depending on patient population included.

Keywords: QLQ-C15-PAL, EORTC, quality of life, bone metastases, brain metastases, radiotherapy

Introduction

Advanced cancer patients often have significant symptom burden and poor performance status. It has previously been shown that symptoms increase in severity with reduced survival (1). As patients have shorter life expectancies, traditional clinical trial endpoints such as survival are no longer appropriate in this population and therefore, clinicians tend to focus more on quality of life (QOL) (2).

QOL is commonly assessed using validated self-administered questionnaires. The European Organization for Research and Treatment of Cancer (EORTC) offers a core module (QLQ-C30) along with more disease specific modules, such as the QLQ-BM22 for patients with bone metastases (5). However, these questionnaires can be cumbersome, especially if multiple assessments are required. Shorter questionnaires may therefore be beneficial as they can reduce patient burden (3). For this reason, a shorter, palliative version of the core module was developed, the QLQ-C15-PAL (4).

The QLQ-C15-PAL contains 15-items originally from the QLQ-C30 that was identified to be most representative of subscales within the core module itself (8). A previous study conducted by Steinman et al. which used the QLQ-C15-PAL for patients with brain metastases found this instrument reduced the burden of repeated questionnaire completion for patients with advanced disease. Patients themselves even favored this instrument over the longer QLQ-C30 (7).

Bone metastases are a common cause of intractable pain in the advanced cancer population, and cause skeletal related events (SREs) including pathological fractures, bone pain requiring radiotherapy, surgery to bone, spinal cord compression and hypercalcaemia (7). Brain metastases constitute the most common intracranial neoplasm in adults, occurring in 10-15% of patients with advanced cancer (6, 9). Depending on the location of the brain metastases, patients may exhibit a range of neurological symptoms such as headaches, focal weakness, mental disturbance, behavioral changes, seizures, speech difficulty, and ataxia (10).

Although the QLQ-C15-PAL has been successfully shortened through rigorous statistical means, its adoption has been relatively slow in the palliative setting. Few prospective studies have detailed its use in the population. To date, comparisons among broad patient subgroups within the palliative cancer patient setting have not been made. The purpose of the present study was to compare QLQ-C15-PAL scores in patients with brain metastases to those with bone metastases.

Methods

From February 2009 to May 2010, patients receiving treatment for bone or brain metastases from cancer centers in Canada (three sites in total: Odette Cancer Centre, Toronto; Cross Cancer Institute, Edmonton; Tom Baker Cancer Centre, Calgary; Japan, Hong Kong, Cyprus and Taiwan completed the QLQ-C15-PAL at baseline. Demographic information along with various disease characteristics was recorded. All research was conducted after approval from all local research ethics boards.

QLQ-C15-PAL

All items of the QLQ-C15-PAL are rated on a 4 point Likert scale from 1-4. The items are then scored as single or multi-item scales in the following domains: physical functioning, emotional functioning, fatigue, nausea/vomiting, pain, dyspneoa, insomnia, appetite loss, constipation and overall quality of life. For functional scales and the global QOL scale, a higher score indicates better function whereas for symptom scales, a higher score indicates a greater severity.

Statistical analyses

Demographic results were expressed as mean, standard deviation (SD), median and ranges for continuous demographics, and proportions for categorical values. To compare baseline characteristics in patients with bone and brain metastases, the Chi-square test was performed for categorical variables and the Wilcoxon rank-sum test for age and KPS. A two-sided p-value of <0.05 was considered statistically significant.

Individual items (un-scored subscales) were compared between both patient groups (brain vs. bone metastases) using the Chi-square test. A Bonferroni adjusted p-value < 0.003 (0.05/15 items) was considered statistically significant. To compare baseline QLQ-C15-PAL scores between patients with bone and brain metastases (BM and BN), univariate linear regression model (GLM) was performed. To normalize the distribution, natural log-transformation was applied for each score. A Bonferroni adjusted p-value < 0.003 was used for this step. After adjusting for confounding factors (i.e., significant demographics between groups, in this case, previous systemic treatment and primary cancer site), univariate linear regression analysis was performed to compare QLQ-C15-PAL baseline scores in patients with BM or with BN as well. In this step, the outcome was natural log scale of each QLQ-C15-PAL scale, the independent variables were the binary variable of group (1=BM, 0=BN), and 2 confounders, such as *ln (QLQ-C15-PAL scale) = a + b×Group + c×previous systemic treatment + d×Primary Cancer Site*. All analyses were conducted using Statistical Analysis Software (SAS version 9.2 for Windows).

Results

A total of 109 patients with brain metastases and 233 patients with bone metastases were enrolled for this study (Table 1). Genders were balanced (51% female). In all patients, the median age and Karnofsky Performance Status (KPS) were 62 years (range: 22-87) and 80 (range: 10-100), respectively. The most common primary cancers were of the breast (n=107, 31%), lung (n=99, 29%) and prostate (n=65; 19%).

Descriptive statistics on QLQ-C15-PAL scores for patients with bone and brain metastases at baseline are available in Table 2. For patients with bone metastases, emotional functioning was better (mean score: 71.5±27.33) than physical functioning (57.7±28.89). Pain was the most severe symptom (53.7±31.12) while nausea/vomiting was the least (15.1 ± 27.4). Fatigue was the most severe symptom (40.4 ±28.25) while nausea was the least severe symptom (9.7 +/-21.02). Overall QOL was slightly better in patients with brain metastases compared to patients with bone metastases (61.4 and 54.8 respectively).

Comparison of baseline characteristics

Primary cancer site and previous systemic treatment were significantly different between the two groups and as a result were included in additional analyses as confounding factors.

Patients with bone metastases have higher proportions with previous systemic treatment, in comparison to patients with brain metastases (83.9% vs. 63.6%).

In the patients with bone metastases, there were higher proportions of patients with breast, prostate or renal cell cancer site and lower proportions of patients with lung or GI, compared to patients with brain metastases (P<0.0001). There were no significant differences between the age of patients who completed the assessment, the KPS, the gender, married status, or patient status.

Comparison of QLQ-C15-PAL scores unadjusted for confounders

Table 3 summarizes findings of the simple univariate linear regression model. There were two QLQ-C15-PAL symptom scales significantly different between patients with bone metastases and patients with brain metastases, namely, fatigue (47.8 vs. 40.4; p=0.0029) and pain (53.7 vs. 22.8; p<0.0001). Patients with bone metastases reported greater severity in pain and fatigue, compared to those with brain metastases.

Comparison of QLQ-C15-PAL scores adjusting for confounders

After accounting for previous systemic treatment and primary cancer sites as confounders, results were similar (Table 4). Only pain symptom scale was significantly different between both groups.

Table 1. Demographics in Patients with Bone Metastases (BM) and in Patients with Brain Metastases (BN)

	Total N=342	BM N=233	BN N=109	p-value *
Age (years)				0.2467
Mean (SD)	61.3 (11.7)	61.8 (11.9)	60.2 (11.2)	
Median (range)	62 (22-87)	62.5 (28-87)	61 (22 – 83)	
KPS at baseline				0.1105
Mean (SD)	75.9 (14.8)	75.0 (14.9)	77.7 (14.4)	
Median (range)	80 (0-100)	80 (0-100)	80 (40-100)	
Gender				0.9583
Female	175 (51.17%)	119 (51.07%)	56 (51.38%)	
Male	167 (48.83%)	114 (48.93%)	53 (48.62%)	
Married status				0.3338
Married	222 (67.89%)	153 (69.86%)	69 (63.89%)	
Widowed	22 (6.73%)	17 (7.76%)	5 (4.63%)	
Single	36 (11.01%)	23 (10.50%)	13 (12.04%)	
Partner	11 (3.36%)	10 (4.57%)	1 (0.93%)	
Other	36 (11.01%)	16 (7.31%)	20 (18.52%)	
Primary cancer site				**<0.0001**
Breast	107 (31.29%)	88 (37.77%)	19 (17.43%)	
Lung	99 (28.95%)	36 (15.45%)	63 (57.80%)	
Prostate	65 (19.01%)	65 (27.90%)	0 (0.00%)	
Gastrointestinal	20 (5.85%)	13 (5.58%)	7 (6.42%)	
Renal Cell	14 (4.09%)	11 (4.72%)	3 (2.75%)	
Others	37 (10.82%)	20 (8.58%)	17 (15.60%)	
Patients status				0.6210
Outpatient	312 (91.50%)	212 (90.99%)	100 (92.59%)	
Inpatient	29 (8.50%)	21 (9.01%)	8 (7.41%)	
Previous systemic treatment				**<0.0001**
Yes	261 (77.45%)	193 (83.91%)	68 (63.55%)	
No	76 (22.55%)	37 (16.09%)	39 (36.45%)	

* P-value was obtained by Chi-squared test for categorical variables and Wilcoxon rank-sum test for age and KPS. Bold indicates statistical significance.

Table 2. Mean Symptom Scores between Bone and Brain Metastases Patients at Baseline

		N	Mean	Std	Median	Min	Max
Overall QOL	group						
	BM-PAL15	230	54.8	25.28	50.0	0	100
	BN-PAL15	107	61.4	25.04	66.7	0	100
Physical Functioning	group						
	BM-PAL15	231	57.7	28.89	60.0	0	93
	BN-PAL15	107	69.5	27.06	73.3	0	93
Emotional Functioning	group						
	BM-PAL15	229	71.5	27.33	66.7	0	100
	BN-PAL15	106	73.8	23.41	75.0	0	100
Fatigue	group						
	BM-PAL15	228	47.8	27.09	44.4	0	100
	BN-PAL15	105	40.4	28.25	33.3	0	100
Nausea / Vomiting	group						
	BM-PAL15	230	15.1	27.40	0.0	0	100
	BN-PAL15	108	9.7	21.02	0.0	0	100
Pain	group	231	53.7	31.12	50.0	0	100
	BM-PAL15						
	BN-PAL15	108	22.8	29.59	16.7	0	100
Dyspnea	group	231	19.3	27.12	0.0	0	100
	BM-PAL15						
	BN-PAL15	108	18.5	25.51	0.0	0	100
Insomnia	group	231	36.2	35.59	33.3	0	100
	BM-PAL15						
	BN-PAL15	107	34.0	35.46	33.3	0	100
Appetite loss	group	230	27.7	35.54	0.0	0	100
	BM-PAL15						
	BN-PAL15	107	20.2	31.31	0.0	0	100
Constipation	group	231	27.4	32.88	0.0	0	100
	BM-PAL15						
	BN-PAL15	107	17.8	28.34	0.0	0	100

Table 3. Comparing baseline QLQ-C15-PAL scores in patients with BM and in patients with BN by univariate linear regression analysis without accounting for confounders

At Baseline	Coefficient	SE	p-value *	MSE
Overall QOL	-0.154	0.107	0.1520	0.840
Physical Functioning	-0.284	0.107	0.0085	0.839
Emotional Functioning	-0.106	0.096	0.2721	0.671
Fatigue	0.421	0.140	0.0029	1.413
Nausea / Vomiting	0.390	0.195	0.0464	2.799
Pain	1.713	0.178	<.0001	2.321
Dyspnea	-0.013	0.219	0.9524	3.540
Insomnia	0.121	0.234	0.6044	3.994
Appetite loss	0.425	0.234	0.0696	3.988
Constipation	0.633	0.229	0.0060	3.832

A Bonferroni adjusted p-value < 0.003 was considered statistical significant.

Table 4. Comparing baseline QLQ-C15-PAL scores in patients with BM and in patients with BN by univariate linear regression analysis with accounting for confounders

At Baseline	p-value of Group (BM vs. BN)	p-value of Confounders		MSE
		Previous Systemic Treatment	Primary Cancer Site	
Overall QOL	0.2477	0.6858	0.0014	0.816
Physical Functioning	0.0047	0.5102	0.6081	0.852
Emotional Functioning	0.1614	0.8278	0.5538	0.684
Fatigue	0.0159	0.9113	0.8821	1.449
Nausea / Vomiting	0.0562	0.8881	0.8058	2.810
Pain	<0.0001	0.4863	0.7702	2.341
Dyspnea	0.3867	0.6311	0.0030	3.394
Insomnia	0.2723	0.2355	0.7733	4.021
Appetite loss	0.0636	0.5992	0.9124	4.041
Constipation	0.0106	0.1869	0.3477	3.832

A Bonferroni adjusted p-value < 0.003 was considered statistical significant.

Patients with bone metastases had more pain than those with brain metastases. The average pain scale was 53.7 for patients with bone metastases, compared to 22.8 for those with brain metastases (p<0.0001). Other scales were not significant different after adjusting for confounders. The confounders of previous systemic treatment was not significant related to any QLQ-C15-PAL score; primary cancer site was only significantly associated with overall QOL (p = 0.0014).

Discussion

Few studies have reported on the use of the QLQ-C15-PAL for patients with advanced cancer. The present study assessed whether the QLQ-C15-PAL scores were different between patients with bone and brain metastases. In the palliative setting when facing treatment decisions for patients with poor prognosis, symptom control and QOL become arguably the most important goals of care rather than the traditional endpoint of survival. There have been several editorials discussing the use of QLQ-C15-PAL along with several papers discussing the planned use of QLQ-C15-PAL in upcoming studies. Furthermore, as the QLQ-C15-PAL extracts items already included in the QLQ-C30, this instrument is available in many languages (7).

After adjusting for confounders, patients with bone metastases had significantly greater pain than those with brain metastases; as the majority of patients with bone metastases present with pain. We did not find other scores to be significantly different and this may be due to the fact that both groups of patients were experiencing these issues, albeit possibly due to different causes. For example, physical functioning deficits may be observed patients with bone metastases due to pain and whereas for those with brain metastases, due to dizziness or other neurologic symptoms.

We would however, expect other domains not assessed by the QLQ-C15-PAL, such as cognitive functioning to be different in patients with bone and brain metastases. Unfortunately, these items were removed when the QLQ-C30 was shortened. Therefore, we recommend that future trials involving patients with brain metastases elect to supplement core instruments such as the QLQ-C15-PAL in conjunction with disease specific instruments such as the QLQ-BN20 to assess these domains.

In a similar study done on QLQ-C15-PAL symptoms in advanced cancer, it was found that domains of physical and emotional functioning, pain, and appetite loss were significant predictors of overall QOL in these patients with advanced cancer (7). Both appetite loss and emotional functioning were independently predictive of overall QOL in patients with bone metastases (n = 190). In patients with brain metastases (n = 150), independent predictors of overall QOL included physical and emotional functioning as well as fatigue.

The QLQ-C15-PAL domains of physical and emotional functioning, pain and appetite loss were significant predictors of overall QOL in this cohort of patients with advanced cancer (7). Similarly to our study in which it was found that patients with bone metastases were affected primarily by pain and brain metastases by fatigue. Overall QOL on average was slightly better in patients with brain metastases, but both were affected by these symptoms.

A limitation in this study here is that patients were grouped by their reason for referral. If a patient requires palliative radiotherapy for painful bone metastases but also previously had brain metastases, they would be included in the bone metastases group only.

This therefore may confound our findings. In addition, although we divided patients by treatment for bone or brain metastases, significant heterogeneity may still exist for patients included in these subgroups. Previously it has been shown that symptoms increase in severity with reduced survival (1). However, no information as to patients' disease trajectory was collected and we are unable to comment on this potential confounding factor in our analysis (1). Overall, the QLQ-C15-PAL demonstrated the ability to detect QOL issues expected in patients with bone and brain metastases. Future studies requiring more disease-specific findings should include disease-specific tools such as the QLQ-BM22 and QLQ-BN20.

Acknowledgments

We thank the generous support of the Bratty Family Fund, Michael and Karyn Goldstein Cancer Research Fund, Joseph and Silvana Melara Cancer Research Fund, and the Ofelia Cancer Research Fund. The authors have no conflicts of interest to disclose.

References

[1]   Zeng L, Zhang L, Culleton S, Jon F, Holden L, Kwong J, Khan L, Tsao M, Danjoux C, Sahgal A, Barnes E, Chow E. Edmonton symptom assessment scale as a prognosticative indicator in patients with advanced cancer. J Palliat Med 2011;14(3):337-42.

[2]   Zeng L, Chow E, Zhang L, Tseng LM, Hou MF, Fairchild A, Vassiliou V, Jesus-Garcia R, El-Din MA, Kumar A, Forges F, Chie WC, Bedard G, Bottomley A. An international prospective study establishing minimal clinically important differences in the EORTC QLQ-BM22 and QLQ-C30 in cancer patients with bone metastases. Support Care Cancer 2012;20(12):3307-13.

[3]   Lien K, Zeng L, Bradley N, Culleton S, Popovic M, Di Giovanni J, Jamani R, Cramarossa G, Nguyen J, Koo K, Jon F, Chow E. Poor accrual in palliative research studies: An update from the Rapid Response Radiotherapy Program. World J Oncol 2011t;2(5):217-24.

[4]   Groenvold M, Petersen MA, Aaronson NK, Arraras JI, Blazeby JM, Bottomley A, Fayers PM, de Graeff A, Hammerlid E, Kaasa S, Sprangers MA, Bjorner JB. The development of the EORTC QLQ-C15-PAL: a shortened questionnaire for cancer patients in palliative care. Eur J Cancer 2006;42(1):55-64.

[5]   Chow E, Hird A, Velikova G, Johnson C, Dewolf L, Bezjak A, Wu J, Shafiq J, Sezer O, Kardamakis D, van der Linden Y, Mak B, Castrol M, Foro Arnalot P, Ahmedzai S, Clemons M, Hoskin P, Yee A, Brundage M, Bottomley A. The European Organization for Research and Treatment of Cancer Quality of Life Questionnaire for patients with bone metastases: The EORTC QLQ-BM22. Eur J Cancer 2009;45:1146-52.

[6]   Diagnostics of central nervous system metastatic disease. Arch Oncol 2006;14(1):41-3.

[7]   Caissie A, Culleton S, Nguyen J, Zhang L, Zeng L, Holden L, Dennis K, Chan E, Jon F, Tsao M, Danjoux C, Sahgal A, Barnes E, Koo K, Chow E. What QLQ-C15-PAL symptoms matter most for overall quality of life in patients with advanced cancer? World J Oncol 2011;2(4):166-74.

[8]   Lien K, Zeng L, Nguyen J, Cramarossa G, Culleton S, Caissie A, Lutz S, Chow E. Comparison of the EORTC QLQ-C15-PAL and the FACIT-Pal for assessment of quality of life in patients with advanced cancer. Expert Rev Pharmacoecon Outcomes Res 2011;11(5):541-7.

[9]   Schiff D, Kesari S, Wen PY. Cancer neurology in clinical practice. Brain 2004;127(3):714.

[10] Cheng J, Zhang X, Liu B. Health-related quality of life in patients with high-grade glioma. Neuro Oncol 2009;11(1):41–50.

Submitted: January 05, 2013. *Revised:* February 15, 2013. *Accepted:* February 21, 2013.

In: Pain Management Yearbook 2013
Editor: Joav Merrick

ISBN: 978-1-63117-944-0
© 2014 Nova Science Publishers, Inc.

Chapter 21

Pediatric pain assessment: A pragmatic analysis of dialogues in the interactions of healthcare providers, children and their parents

Marc Zabalia, PhD[*,1], *Denis Jacquet, PhD*[1], *Corinne Grasménil, RPsychol*[1] *and Chantal Wood, MD*[2]

[1]PALM EA 4649, Normandy University, Caen, France
[2]Assessment and Treatment of Pain Unit, Robert Debre Hospital, Paris, France

Abstract

In pediatric care, despite a triadic communication system, only physician and parent are involved in the definition of symptoms, diagnosis and treatment. However, children are competent participants when parents are absent. In this study, our interest is to highlight the pragmatic aspect of the adult-child dialogue comparing chronic versus acute pain and to understand the stages of construction of a common ground. Twenty-three children aged 6 to 15 years (12 girls and 13 boys, m= 9,8 years old) were recorded during a pain assessment interview. Fifteen children aged 7 to 15 years consulted for acute pain (7 girls, 8 boys, m= 10 years old) and eight children aged 6 to 15 years were seen in a chronic pain consultation (4 girls and 4 boys, m= 9,6 years old). In the interviews for pain assessment, healthcare providers can benefit of knowing their referencing process to adapt their discourse in way to promote an understanding of the patient's pain experience. Verbal self-report of pain is an important way to understand the subjectivity of pain, it also becomes necessary to highlight the dialogue cues. In a patient-centered approach, the child's role in the consultation should be as important as the parent's. In the chronic pain context, all the speakers are taking an active part in the interaction. It is now relevant to

[*] Correspondence: Marc Zabalia, Université de Caen Basse-Normandie, Esplanade de la Paix. CS 14032, 14032 CAEN cedex 5 France. E-mail: marc.zabalia@unicaen.fr.

investigate what is said and especially by who, when there are confused data about the reliability of information given by the parents.

Keywords: Pediatrics, child health, pain, assessment

Introduction

The healthcare provider-patient communication has been gaining interest within the last decade (1,2). In the patient-centered approach, the focus of the studies has been on interactions between physicians and patients (3). There is growing evidence that patient-centered approach is particularly positively associated with patient satisfaction (4-6), patient compliance (7-9) and a greater partnership in decision-making (10). The development of the patient-centered approach has also led to a more egalitarian relationship between clinician and patient (11).

In pediatric care, despite a triadic communication system, only physician and parent are involved in the definition of symptoms, diagnosis and treatment (12). However, children are competent participants when parents are absent, despite the fact that they stay inactive when a parent is talking (13). The study of children's roles in communication with their pediatricians should be included (14). Studies who paid attention to the structural aspects of clinician-parent-child communication revealed that it was mainly the parent who was responsible for excluding the child from medical conversation but they also showed an increase in the number of initiatives on the part of the child itself in the course of time (15).

In the pediatric pain management domain, studies have first paid attention to the abilities of children to self-report their pain. Most of the studies about the development of children's understanding of illnesses concluded that the cognitive developmental level had not only a significant effect (16-19) but it had a more decisive role on the child's understanding of illness and its treatment compared to gender, socio-economic or nurses' explanations (20). These data, widely reported in the medical literature, have established a theoretical background to the research on pain assessment, including self-assessment in children. Children give helpful information about their pain when special attention is given to the questions that are made, when the psychological climate is free from coercion, and particularly when the child is considered as a full partner. Ross and Ross (21) have shown that 70% of children aged 5 to 12 years (n = 994) use many adjectives to describe a single pain (stabbing, burning, crushing, puncture, pressure, dull pain, excruciating pain). In addition, a significant number of children (n = 286) produce specific sentences to describe their pain. Similarly, a majority of children respond spontaneously with a wide variety of adjectives, words and sentences describing the pain (22). The verbal communication quality of the child about the intensity of pain increases with age. Children older than 7 years are those for which data are the most consistent (23). The descriptions of pain, the causes of it, and the assessment of its intensity gradually evolve with the cognitive development of the child (19).

In the context of chronic pain in children, the diagnose process is often describe by children and families as a negative experience (24,25). This is due to the increasing number of consultations requiring the child to repeat its symptoms. In addition, it is difficult for him to identify useful information to the clinician. In the healthcare provider-patient encounter, the dialogue does not involve only the patient's ability to self-report his problem. It is even more true when the patient is a child, because children do not always speak spontaneously and do not give answers easily to questions asked in a clinical setting. Clemente and colleagues (26) have shown that non-focused questioning presents opportunities for children to format a pain account of their symptoms and concerns in their own words. The assessment of child's pain is a patient-adult interaction which involves more than the adult's medical knowledge and the child's verbal level. More recently, the Craig's social communication of pain model describes the adults decoding of the child's verbally and nonverbally encoded communication about pain, and influences back from the adult to the child (27).

In the case of a child's self-report, the dialogue involves an adult's interpretation. The aim of the interaction is to share a set of representations for a common purpose: understanding the pain. Consequently, this requires an interpretation from the adult of what the child is saying about this subjective phenomenon. The child too, must interpret the perspectives and expertise of adults. From the perspective of patient-centred care, the child's role in the consultation should be as important as the parent's (28). In this study, our interest is to highlight the pragmatic aspect of the adult-child dialogue comparing chronic versus acute pain and to understand the stages of construction of a "common ground" (29). Literature has provided a comprehensive review of the role of common ground in language processing (30). First, we expected that healthcare providers would use multiple dialogue control utterances and would favour paraphrases to ensure their understanding of child's pain. The psycholinguistic literature has shown that is the good way to integrate knowing and meaning (31). Second, we expected that dialogue control utterances would vary depending on the types of pain. Understanding chronic pain would require more summaries than understanding acute pain.

Methods

Twenty-three children aged 6 to 15 years (12 girls and 13 boys, m= 9,8 years old) were recorded during a pain assessment interview. Fifteen children aged 7 to 15 years consulted for acute pain (7 girls, 8 boys, m= 10 years old) and eight children aged 6 to 15 years were seen in a chronic pain consultation (4 girls and 4 boys, m= 9,6 years old).

The eight chronic pain interviews were conducted by pediatricians, eleven of the acute pain interviews were conducted by physicians, one by a pediatrician and one by a pain team nurse. In each case, one parent was present. All participants gave full informed consent. Approval was obtained by ethical boards of hospitals and scientific committee of funding source. The interviews were recorded with a pocket digital recorder Edirol R09® from March 2008 to June 2010 in Paris, Lisieux and Caen, France.

Interviews context : Clinicians have assessed several aspects of pain the interviews: types of pain and the location in the child's body, pain descriptors, pain duration. They have also used scales, questionnaires was used in the chronic pain assessment. All clinicians have used a more narrative approach rather than focused-questioning. The interviews include establishment of pain symptoms, history-taking in chronic pain, and physical exam.

Data coding: The dialogues were coded focusing on their pragmatic framework rather than on the linguistic meanings. For each speaker (health-provider, child and parent), we recorded eight components of the conversation: (1) the number of turn-takings, (2) the number of utterances, (3) the number of original wordings introducing a new topic, (4) the number of dialogue control utterances divided in (5) number of paraphrases (paraphrases and self-paraphrases) (6) number of repetitions, (7) number of summaries, and finally we recorded (8) the number of phatic expressions of the social components of communication.

The 6196 utterances in 4183 turn-takings were transcribed by two independent coders. The intraclass correlation was .89.

Statistical analyses: Data was analysed using Statistica® 9.0 StatsSoft® software. Alpha was set at .05. A MANOVA test examined the speaker (health-provider, child and parent), the types of pain (acute, chronic) and the interaction of both independent variables effects. One-way ANOVAs test was conducted to test the effect of speaker on dependant variables. Independent samples T test was used to test the effect of types of pain on dependant variables.

Results

The healthcare providers produced more than a half of utterances and they introduced new topics in 82.8% of cases (see table 1). The parents' role in the dialogue was less obvious. It seems that they played an active and equal part in the interaction compared to the child. But 71.8% of their utterances occurred mainly in the context of chronic pain.

Healthcare providers used more dialogue control utterances than the children and their parents $(F(2,66)=14,77$ $p<.0001)$. But they did not use the different components equally (see table 2). The paraphrases were significantly more used than others components in healthcare providers' utterances $(F(6,122)= 4,74$ $p=.0002)$. In 78.52 % of cases, healthcare providers paraphrased the child or the parent's utterances. In the other cases, it was self-paraphrases. In the children and the parents too, the paraphrases were the most used dialogue control cue (see table 2).

Like in any social interaction, healthcare professionals spent time to manage the verbal relationships between the different partners. They produced 57.3 % of the phatic expressions of the social components of communication, almost three times more than children and parents $(F(2,66)= 6,25$ $p=.003)$.

Table 1. Percentages of dialogue components in healthcare provider, child and parent

	Health-provider	Child	Parent	p
Turn-taking	47,1	26,3	26,5	.01
Utterances	56,4	20,3	20,1	.0003
Original wording introducing a new topic	82,8	5,5	11,5	.0001

Table 2. Percentages of dialogue control utterances in health-provider, child and parent

	Health-provider	Child	Parent	p
Paraphrases	36,2	14,9	14,9	.001
Repetitions	15,1	2,6	4,3	.0001
Summaries	6,3	0,2	5,1	.2

Table 3. Percentages of dialogue control components in healthcare providers in acute versus chronic pain interviews

	Acute pain	Chronic pain	p
Original wording introducing a new topic	96,4	67,7	.02
Paraphrases	68,59	54	.2
Repetitions	29,01	22,15	.19
Summaries	2,39	23,92	.0001
Number of phatic expressions of social components of communication	46,45	53,54	.14

Acute versus chronic pain interviews

The mean length of the acute pain interviews was 11.6 minutes (σ= 5,19 mn) and the chronic pain interviews lasted on average 19.18 minutes (σ= 6,4 mn). The length of the acute versus chronic pain interviews are significantly different (t(19)= 2,73 $p<.01$). However, the number of turn-takings and the number of utterances are not significantly different in health-providers when comparing the acute versus chronic pain interviews. As shown in table 3, healthcare providers used some dialogue control components differently in the two situations.

Children use significantly more paraphrases (F(3,19)= 5,25 $p=.008$) as did their parent (F(3,19)= 9,6 $p=.0004$) in the chronic pain context.

Healthcare providers were not the only ones to introduce new topics during the chronic pain interviews. Parents produced original wording in 21.11% of theses utterances (11.18% in the children). Paraphrases and repetitions were used equally in the two kinds of consultations, but summaries were more used in the chronic pain context. There was a difference in the number of utterances produced by the children in the two conditions (t(21)= 1,51 $p=.0003$). The number of wordings introducing a new topic was more higher in children presenting with chronic pain compared to children presenting with acute pain (t(21)= 5,55 $p<.0001$), but it was only 5.75% of the utterances.

Discussion

As expected in the first hypothesis, healthcare providers used different kinds of dialogue control components to lead the pain interviews. Because of the goal of pain assessment, the healthcare providers were conducting the interviews. Results show that the dialogues were directed-interviews. The psycholinguistic literature has shown that paraphrases can serve as a cohesive tie as well as a way to put ideas in our own words. Repetition was often seen as the central meaning-making strategy (32). All conversations include repetition, it occurs in all types of discourses (33). To reduce referential ambiguity, speakers continue using the same expression even it was over-informative (34).

In this study, nurses and physicians as the children and their parents used more paraphrases. The paraphrase appeared to be an important dialogue component in the acute pain context and it kept a central function in the chronic context too. In the particular condition of pain interviews, it seems to be the more relevant dialogue component to share meaning. It could be understood as a way for healthcare providers to ensure an agreement with partners and to keep ideas in mind for the process of diagnosis. It could probably be used by the children and the parent as a way to reinforce meaning and to increase the referents of the common ground.

Summaries are also a way to ensure that partners are sharing a representation, but they were little used in the chronic pain interviews contrary to our assumptions. The question is raised to know if this dialogue control cue is too complex for children during interactions on medical themes. Even if healthcare providers used some dialogue components differently in both situations, the pragmatic of the interviews was nearly the same.

To succeed in the activities of meaning-making, healthcare providers used a system of control, called "correction loops" (35). With these reformulations, they did not simply repeat, they added, they replaced or modified the syntax order. This process of referencing is a dynamic co-referencing that can lead to a convergence of the partners towards the same meaning. This kind of language-specific adaptation promotes the meaning, and makes the speaker's behaviour predictable.

Despite a same pragmatic framework, the children took a different role in the two pain conditions. We were not surprised that the children answered many questions in the chronic pain interviews, but it was unexpected that they would introduce very little topics about their pain.

In the chronic pain context, the assessment pain interview was not only a speaker-listener dyad. Parents played an active role. As they had more knowledge about their child's pain and disease, it is possible that they could easily consider their interlocutor's informational needs.

In children with severe intellectual disabilities, parents would be able to provide relevant estimates of their child's pain intensity (36). But in typical children, the literature gives contrary data about the reliability of parents' pain ratings and pain reported by the child (37-40). Future studies need to explore the relevance of information given by the parents during chronic pain interviews.

Limitations

Because the interviews was audio-recorded, it was not possible in this study to conduct triadic analyses to take into account the allocation of utterances (who the speaker is addressing), and by analysing the communication between all three interlocutors. The number of interviews does not allow us to employ a developmental perspective, when children's communication skills and their understanding of diseases may change with age.

Conclusion

In the interviews for pain assessment, healthcare providers can benefit of knowing their referencing process to adapt their discourse in way to promote an understanding of the patient's pain experience. Verbal self-report of pain is an important way to understand the subjectivity of pain, it also becomes necessary to highlight the dialogue cues.

The importance of the child in decisions about their health care is now recognized (28). In a patient-centered approach, the child's role in the consultation should be as important as the parent's.

In the chronic pain context, all the speakers are taking an active part in the interaction. It is now relevant to investigate what is said and especially by who, when there are confused data about the reliability of information given by the parents.

Acknowledgments

The authors would like to thank Laure Pupin-Guérin, registered psychologist (Centre Hospitalier Robert Bisson, Lisieux), Thierry Moreaux et Nathalie Duparc, nursing staff (Centre d'Evaluation et de Traitement de la Douleur, Hôpital Robert Debré, Paris). This study was supported by La Fondation de France (grant number 2006012445).

References

[1] Larsen H, Risor O, Putnam S. P-R-A-C-T-I-C-A-L: a step-by-step model for conducting the consultation in general practice. Fam Pract 1997;14:295-301.

[2] Marvel MK, Epstein RM, Flowers K, Beckman HB. Soliciting the patient's agenda: Have we improved? JAMA 1999;28:283-7.

[3] Drotar D. Physician behavior in the care of pediatric chronic illness: Association with health outcomes and treatment adherence. J Dev Behav Pediatr 2009;30(3):246-54.

[4] Nobile C. Drotar D. Comer D, et al. Parent-provider communication and satisfaction with children's primary health care. J Dev Behav Pediatr 2000;21(5):383-4.

[5] Roter DL, Stewart M, Putman SM, et al. Communication patterns of primary care physicians. JAMA 1997;277:350-6.

[6] Gattellari M, Buttow PN. Tattersall MH. Sharing decision in cancer care. Soc Sci Med 2001;52:1855-78.

[7] Cecil DW, Kileen I. Control, compliance and satisfaction in the family practice encounter. Fam Med 1997;29:653-7.

[8] Hall JA, Roter DL, Rand CS. (1981). Communication of affect between patient and physicians. J Health Soc Behav 1981;22:18-30.

[9] Henbest RJ, Stewart M. Patient-centeredness in the consultation 2: Does it really make a difference? Fam Pract 1990;7:28–33.

[10] Newes-Adeyi G, Helitzer DL, Roter D et al. Improving client-provider communication: evaluation of a training program for women, infants and children (WIC) professionals in New York State. Patient Educ Couns 2004;55:210-7.

[11] Borne HW. The patient from receiver of information to informed decision-maker. Patient Educ Couns 1998;34:89-102.

[12] Tates K, Elbers E, Meeuwesen L et al. Doctor-parent-child relationships: a 'pas de trois'. Patient Educ Couns 2002;48(1):5-14.

[13] Pyörälä E. The participation roles of children and adolescents in the dietary counselling of diabetics. Patient Educ Couns 2004;55(3):385.

[14] Nobile C. Drotar D. Research on the quality of parent-provider communication in pediatric care: Implications and recommendations. J Dev Behav Pediatr 2003;24(4):279-90.

[15] Meeuwesen L, Kaptein M. Changing interactions in doctor-parent-child communication. Psychol Health 1996;11:787-95.

[16]   Bibace R, Walsh ME. Development of children's concepts of illness. Pediatrics 1980;66:912-7.

[17]   Perrin EC, Gerrity PS. There's a demon in your belly: children's understanding of illness. Pediatrics 1981;67(6):841-9.

[18]   Thompson K, Varni JW. A developmental cognitive-biobehavioral approach to pediatric pain assessment. Pain 1986;25:283-96.

[19]   Harbeck C, Petersen L. Elephant dancing in my head: a developmental approach to children's concept of specific pains. Child Dev 1992;63:138-49.

[20]   Beales JG, Lennox Holt PJ, Kenn JH et al. Children with juvenile chronic arthritis: their beliefs about their illness and therapy. Ann Rheum Dis 1983;42:481-6.

[21]   Ross DM, Ross SA. The importance of type of question, psychological climate and subject set in interviewing children about pain. Pain 1984;19:71-9.

[22]   Jerrett M, Evans K. Children's pain vocabulary. J Adv Nurs1986;11:403-8.

[23]   Lehmann HP, Bendebba M, DeAngelis C. The consistency of young children's assessment of remembered painful events. J Dev Behav Pediatr 1990;11(3):128-34.

[24]   Carter B. Chronic pain in childhood and the medical encounter: professional ventriloquism and hidden voices. Qual Health Res 2002;12(1):28-41.

[25]   Kenny DT. Constructions of chronic pain in doctor-patient relationships: bridging the communication chasm. Patient Educ Couns 2004;52(3):297-305.

[26]   Clemente I. Lee S-H. Heritage J. Children in chronic pain: Promoting pediatric patients' symptom accounts in tertiary care. Soc Sci Med 2008;66:1418-28.

[27]   Craig KD. The social communication model of pain. Can Psychol 2009;50(1):22-32.

[28]   Tates K. Meeuwesen L. Doctor-parent-child communication. A (re)view of the literature. Soc Sci Med 2001;52:839-51.

[29]   Clark H, Murphy GH. Audience design in meaning and reference. In: LeNy JF, Kintsch W, eds. Language and comprehension. Amsterdam: North-Holland, 1982;287–99.

[30]   Barr DJ, Keysar B. Anchoring comprehension in linguistic precedents. J Mem Lang 2002;46:391-418.

[31]   Szmrecsanyi B. Morphosyntaxic persistence in spoken English: a corpus study at the intersection of variationist sociolinguistics, psycholinguistics and discourse analysis. Berlin: Walter de Gruyter, 2006.

[32]   Tannen D. Talking voices. Cambridge: Cambridge University Press,1989.

[33]   McCarthy M, Carter R. Language as Discourse: Perspectives for language teaching. London: Longman, 1994.

[34]   Barr DJ, Keysar B. Perspective taking and the coordination of meaning in language use. In: Traxler MJ, Gernsbacher MA, eds. Handbook of psycholinguistics. New York: Academic Press, 2007:901-38.

[35]   Vivier J. Coopération entre psychologie et intelligence artificielle dans une expérimentation sur le dialogue homme-machine, Intellectica 1996;22:145-68. [French]

[36]   Voepel-Lewis T, Malviya S, Tait AR. Validity of parent ratings as proxy measures of pain in children with cognitive impairment. Pain Manag Nurs 2005;6(4):168-74.

[37]   Rajasagaram U, Taylor DM, Braitberg G, Pearsell, JP, Capp BA. Paediatric pain assessment: differences between triage nurse, child and parent. J Paediatr Child Health 2009;45(4):199-203.

[38]   Singer AJ, Gulla J, Thode HCJr. Parents and practitioners are poor judges of young children's pain severity. Acad Emerg Med 2002;9(6):609-12.

[39]   Kelly A M, Powell CV, Williams A. Parent visual analogue scale ratings of children's pain do not reliably reflect pain reported by child. Pediatr Emerg Care 2002;18(3):159-62.

[40]   Zhou H, Roberts P, Horgan L. Association between self-report pain ratings of child and parent, child and nurse and parent and nurse dyads: meta-analysis. J Adv Nurs 2008;63(4):334-42.

In: Pain Management Yearbook 2013
Editor: Joav Merrick

ISBN: 978-1-63117-944-0
© 2014 Nova Science Publishers, Inc.

Chapter 22

Focal myositis as a presentation of paraneoplastic syndrome in pancreatic cancer

Erin Wong, BSc (C)[1], Gillian Bedard, BSc(C)[1], Linda Probyn, MD[2], Natalie Pulenzas, BSc(C)[1], Breanne Lechner, BSc(C)[1], Lori Holden, MRTT[1], Edward Chow, MBBS[1] and Natalie Lauzon, MRTT[,1]*

[1]Rapid Response Radiotherapy Program, Department of Radiation Oncology, Odette Cancer Centre, Sunnybrook Health Sciences Centre, University of Toronto, Toronto, Ontario, Canada
[2]Department of Medical Imaging, Sunnybrook Health Sciences Centre, University of Toronto, Toronto, Ontario, Canada

Abstract

Paraneoplastic syndrome is rare in the field of oncology, with approximately 8 out of 100 patients displaying some manifestation of this syndrome. In terms of dermatological and rheumatological manifestations of paraneoplastic syndromes, dermatomyositis and polymyositis are common presentations. In the same family of inflammatory muscle disease as polymyositis, focal myositis occurs infrequently and its presentation as a paraneoplastic syndrome has only been suggested in a few cases. Here we present the case of a 42-year-old female with focal myositis of the right quadriceps muscles, who also has known primary pancreatic cancer, suggesting its presentation as a paraneoplastic syndrome.

Keywords: Myositis, paraneoplastic syndrome, pancreatic cancer, external beam radiation

* Correspondence: Ms. Natalie Lauzon BSc, MRTT Department of Radiation Therapy, Odette Cancer Centre, Sunnybrook Health Sciences Centre, 2075 Bayview Avenue, Toronto, ON Canada. Email: Natalie.Lauzon@Sunnybrook.ca.

Introduction

Paraneoplastic syndrome is uncommon, correlating clinical features or symptoms that occur as a result of an underlying malignancy (1-3). What characterizes this syndrome is that it is not due to the infiltration of the primary tumor, compression caused by the primary tumor or the metastasized spread of the tumor (4,5). Conversely, paraneoplastic syndrome is hypothesized to be the result of tumor biological mediators produced by the primary tumor such as hormones, peptides, autocrine and paracrine mediators or immune-mediated response such as cytotoxic lymphocytes and antibodies (3,4). As there are a wide variety of causes, intuitively, there are multiple manifestations of paraneoplastic syndromes such as neurological (motor/autonomic neuropathy or Lambert-Eaton myaesthenic syndrome), endocrine (hypercalcemia or cushing syndrome), hematological (eosinophilia or granulocytosis), and dermatological and rheumatological (dermatomyositis and polymyositis) (5,6).

Dermatomyositis (DM) and polymyositis (PM) are a group of autoimmune inflammatory disorders. PM is characterized by proximal muscle weakness, while DM is characterized by both skin involvement as well as proximal muscle weakness (3,5,6). Focal myositis, which is similar to DM and PM, is the painful enlargement of muscle mass which is localized to one area of the body (7). However, unlike DM and PM, its association with a primary malignancy is very rare and has not been thoroughly studied with only a few reported cases in literature (8-12).

In this report, we present the case of a young female with metastatic pancreatic cancer experiencing significant right knee pain. Radiological imaging of this region demonstrated findings suggestive of focal myositis, as a presentation of the rheumatological manifestation of paraneoplastic syndrome.

Case report

A 42 year old female was diagnosed with pancreatic cancer in November 2011. Initially, lymphadenopathy was found in the retroperitoneal region which was subsequently biopsied. Pathology of the specimen was consistent with metastatic adenocarcinoma with the differential diagnosis of upper gastrointestinal or pancreaticobiliary tract primary. Later in July 2012, a CT scan of the chest, abdomen and pelvis revealed a multicystic mass in the pancreatic tail (see figure 1). Therefore a diagnosis of metastatic pancreatic cancer was made due to subsequent findings of enhancement in the bone of the pelvis and spine seen in the staging scans.

This patient was initially referred to the Rapid Response Radiotherapy Program (RRRP) for radiotherapy treatment to palliate bone pain in August 2012. At that time, she had pain in the pelvis and lumbar spine region radiating down the right leg which was treated with a single dose of 800 cGy. This patient also had bony metastases in the cervical spine, specifically C2, with soft tissue mass on the thecal sac which was radiated with 2000 cGy in five fractions.

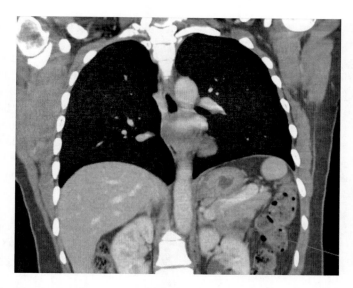

Figure 1. Coronal reformatted CT image through the upper abdomen demonstrating a cystic pancreatic lesion (arrow) compatible with the primary pancreatic carcinoma.

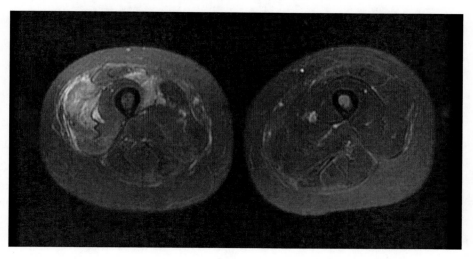

Figure 2. Axial T2 fat suppressed MR image through the bilateral femurs above the knee demonstrating increased signal compatible with edema in the right quadriceps muscle, predominately the vastus medialis and lateralis compatible with myositis.

Soon after, in October 2012, this patient was referred to the RRRP again, this time for right knee pain. An MRI of the bilateral lower extremities was ordered by her medical oncologist to diagnose the pain. In comparison to a previous MRI scan of the pelvis, this current MRI scan showed progression of the bony metastases along the right ischium, iliac crest, acetabulum to the symphysis pubis and intertrochanteric region of the right femur. In addition, multiple femoral low density endosteal lesions were seen which, in the opinion of the radiologist, was consistent with metastatic disease. However signal abnormality was also seen extending into the right vastus lateralis, abductor magnus and vastus medialis throughout the length of the muscles (see figure 2). This abnormality was thought to be focal myositis as a presentation of paraneoplastic syndrome.

This patient arrived by ambulance to the RRRP and at that time was bed-ridden. She had a Karnofsky performance status of 40. After discussion between the radiation and medical oncologist on her situation, it was decided that her knee (region of myositis) and right hemi-pelvis which had a reoccurrence of pain, would be radiated (see figure 3). The patient was informed of the possible side effects which included pain flare, gastrointestinal side effects, nausea, vomiting, and diarrhea and was then consented to a single radiation dose of 8 Gy, pre-medicated with Ondansetron. This treatment was prescribed in hopes of controlling the myositis in the knee region and to provide pain relief in the hemi-pelvis region.

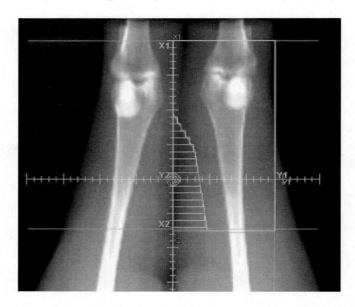

Figure 3. Anterior digitally reconstructed radiograph (DRR) depicting the radiation treatment area of the distal RT femur and knee.

Discussion

Paraneoplastic syndrome is a complex disease, with multiple manifestations and different combinations of multiple, heterogeneous clinical features, making it difficult to diagnose (1,2). It is currently estimated to be present in 8 out of 100 oncology patients; however this statistic may be under-estimated due to the difficulty in diagnosis of this syndrome (5). Conversely, the number of patients with certain symptoms manifestations which are later determined to be paraneoplastic in nature is greater. In current literature, it has been reported by Andras et al., in a small cohort of 217 patients with either DM or PM, approximately 19% of patients with DM had or were later diagnosed with malignancy (3). Similarly, in a Taiwanese cohort of 143 patients studied by Chen et al., it was found that 13% of patients with DM and PM had an associated malignancy (6). Although not significantly substantial, this percentage of patients suggests it may still be worthwhile to screen patients who have certain disorders such as DM or PM for cancer, as the disorder may later be discovered to be paraneoplastic in nature.

In the current case, focal myositis was seen in a patient with pancreatic cancer and is believed to be paraneoplastic in nature as suggested by the referring medical oncologist, radiologist and radiation oncologist.

In a case reported by Zenone et al., a 51-year-old women developed hypertrophy of her right calf prior to the diagnosis of cancer. Less than a year later, the patient presented to the same hospital with bone pain which was confirmed to be poorly differentiated adenocarcinoma of unknown primary. For this case, because of the temporal synchronicity of the two incidences, the authors believe that this focal myositis was a presentation of paraneoplastic syndrome (8).

Similar to the previous case, Naschitz et al. presented a case on a 78-year-old male who presented to his doctor with a tender mass in the left forearm that had been present for 5 months. This muscle mass was found to be normal with some inflamed fibrous tissue through a biopsy. Approximately 6 months afterwards, he was diagnosed with Hodgkin's disease (9). Terrier et al. also presented a case of a 74-year-old female that was simultaneously diagnosed with both chronic lymphocytic leukemia and focal myositis of the right deltoid muscle (10). Two older case reports originally suggested the association of focal myositis with squamous cell carcinoma of the head and neck and with phaeochromocytoma of the adrenals (11,12).

Different treatment options used for patients with focal myositis in conjunction with primary malignancy have been suggested by these case reports. In the case reported by Zenone et al., prednisone was prescribed to the patient for treatment of her focal myositis (8). Alternatively, Naschitz et al. reported on surgical excision of the focal myositis followed by subsequent chemotherapy and radiation targeting the primary malignancy once it was discovered (9). In the case by Terrier et al., chemotherapy alone was used in the treatment of the focal myositis (10). In all of these cases, treatment was successful in the management of the focal myositis, with patients experiencing significant improvement (8-10).

In most of these cases, diagnoses of focal myositis either preceded or were simultaneously discovered with the primary malignancy. This similar timeline of events also occur for paraneoplastic syndrome of other manifestations. (3,13). Though this current case does not follow this timeline, it does add to the collection of evidence towards the possible paraneoplastic nature of focal myositis. As such, the knowledge and presentation of paraneoplastic syndrome can assist health care professionals in the early detection of an underlying cancer.

Acknowledgments

We thank the generous support of Bratty Family Fund, Michael and Karyn Goldstein Cancer Research Fund, Joseph and Silvana Melara Cancer Research Fund, and Ofelia Cancer Research Fund.

References

[1] Hueber AJ, Rech J, Kallert S, Requadt C, Cavallaro A, Kalden JR, et al. Paraneoplastic syndrome, infection or arthritis: Difficulties in diagnosis. Int J Clin Pract 2006;60(10):1310-2.

[2] Ozdogu H, Boga C, Bolat F, Kilic D, Habesoglu MA, Karatas M. Paraneoplastic syndrome associated with desquamative interstitial pneumonia mimicking lung cancer: A case report. Turkish J Cancer 2008;38(2):78.

[3] Andras C, Csiki Z, Ponyi A, Illes A, Danko K. Paraneoplastic rheumatic syndromes. Rheumatol Int 2006;26(5):376-82.

[4] Wood JP, Haynes AP, Cheung KL. A paraneoplastic manifestation of metastatic breast cancer responding to endocrine therapy: a case report. World J Surg Oncol 2008;6:132.

[5] Pelosof LC, Gerber DE. Paraneoplastic syndromes: an approach to diagnosis and treatment. Mayo Clin Proc 2010;85(9):838-54.

[6] Chen YJ, Wu CY, Shen JL. Predicting factors of malignancy in dermatomyositis and polymyositis: a case-control study. Br J Dermatol 2001;144(4):825-31.

[7] Caldwell CJ, Swash M, Van der Walt JD, Geddes JF. Focal myositis: a clinicopathological study. Neuromuscul Disord 1995;5(4):317-21.

[8] Zenone T, Ghadban R, Leveque-Michaud C, Chan V. Focal myositis: a paraneoplastic syndrome? Joint Bone Spine 2011;78(4):426-7.

[9] Naschitz JE, Yeshurun D, Dreyfuss U, Best LA, Misselevich I, Boss JH. Localized nodular myositis. A paraneoplastic phenomenon. Clin Rheumatol 1992;11(3):427-31.

[10] Terrier B, Lavie F, Miceli-Richard C, Azria A, Mariette X. Focal myositis with fasciitis and vasculitis revealing chronic lymphocytic leukaemia. Rheumatology (Oxford) 2005;44(10):1324-6.

[11] Bhatnagar D, Carey P, Pollard A. Focal myositis and elevated creatine kinase levels in a patient with phaeochromocytoma. Postgrad Med J 1986;62(725):197-8.

[12] McLendon CL, Levine PA, Mills SE, Black WC. Squamous cell carcinoma masquerading as focal myositis of the tongue. Head Neck 1989;11(4):353-57.

[13] Kurzrock R, Cohen PR. Cutaneous paraneoplastic syndromes in solid tumors. Am J Med 1995;99(6):662-71.

SECTION THREE: RADIATION, PELVIC PAIN AND HEADACHE

In: Pain Management Yearbook 2013
Editor: Joav Merrick

ISBN: 978-1-63117-944-0
© 2014 Nova Science Publishers, Inc.

Chapter 23

Review of symptom cluster research in the Rapid Response Radiotherapy Program (RRRP)

Breanne Lechner, BSc(C), Natalie Pulenzas, BSc(C),
*Nemica Thavarajah, BSc(C) and Edward Chow, MBBS**
Rapid Response Radiotherapy Program, Department of Radiation Oncology,
Odette Cancer Centre, Sunnybrook Health Sciences Centre, University of Toronto,
Toronto, Ontario, Canada

Abstract

Patients with cancer often experience various concurrent symptoms which can predict changes in patient functioning, treatment outcomes and affect their quality of life. Clinical evidence of patients frequently experiencing multiple symptoms has prompted research in the identification and analysis of symptom clusters. The Rapid Response Radiotherapy Program (RRRP) provides timely radiotherapy for palliative cancer patients, focusing on quality of life (QOL) as an important endpoint. This paper reviewed the past research in the RRRP on symptom clusters in patients with advanced cancer. Research in the RRRP has addressed symptom clusters in patients with brain metastases, bone metastases and reviewed external publications concerning symptom clusters in cancer patients. Further research should aim to standardize statistical methods used for symptom cluster identification and validate symptom clusters in advanced cancer patients.

Keywords: Symptom cluster, advanced cancer, radiotherapy

* Correspondence: Professor Edward Chow MBBS, MSc, PhD, FRCPC, Department of Radiation Oncology, Odette Cancer Centre, Sunnybrook Health Sciences Centre, 2075 Bayview Avenue, Toronto, ON Canada. Email: Edward.Chow@Sunnybrook.ca.

Introduction

Patients with cancer often experience various concurrent symptoms associated with the cancer itself, its treatment, or a combination of the two (1). These symptoms frequently predict changes in patient functioning, treatment outcomes and affect their quality of life (2). Symptoms are multidimensional concepts which can involve cognitive sensations and the biophysical functioning of the patient (2). Clinical evidence of patients frequently experiencing multiple symptoms simultaneously rather than in isolation has identified the need for further research investigating symptom clusters (2). The definition of symptom clusters by Kim et al. (3) indicates that at least two or more symptoms must be related to each other, occur together, be a stable group, and be relatively independent of other clusters. Evaluating multiple symptoms can provide information regarding the relationship between symptoms, predictors of patient outcomes and identify ideal treatment to manage specific symptom clusters (2). Thus, research in this area benefits health care providers, patients and caregivers. Symptom clusters in cancer patients can be affected by various treatments, including palliative radiotherapy (RT). Therefore, it is imperative to conduct longitudinal studies to evaluate symptom clusters in patients at baseline and at follow-up points after treatment.

Research in the Rapid Response Radiotherapy Program (RRRP) has strived to derive and analyze symptom clusters and increase the knowledge base of symptom management research. The RRRP is an outpatient clinic established in 1996 to provide timely palliative RT. Located at the Odette Cancer Centre, the RRRP provides quick access to RT to relieve symptoms and improve quality of life (QOL) in advanced cancer patients. This paper reviews previous research in the RRRP on symptom clusters in advanced cancer patients receiving RT.

Methods

A literature search was conducted to identify studies investigating symptom clusters in cancer patients conducted by the RRRP from 2007 to present. Studies examining symptom clusters in patients with various primary cancer types and previous literature reviews regarding symptom clusters were included in the review.

Results

The literature review identified relevant studies published between 2007 and 2013. Extensive research has been conducted regarding symptom clusters in areas including bone metastases, brain metastases, and broader literature reviews.

Symptom clusters in bone metastases

A study by Chow et al. (4) explored symptom clusters in patients with bone metastases in the RRRP to determine whether bone pain was associated with any other symptoms using the Edmonton Symptom Assessment Scale (ESAS). A total of 518 patients with bone metastases provided analgesic intake information and completed the ESAS at baseline, one, two, four, eight, and twelve weeks following RT. Three clusters were identified and accounted for 66% of the total variance at baseline. Cronbach's alpha coefficient demonstrated high internal reliability in the clusters, with a coefficient ranging from 0.61 to 0.81. It was found that pain clustered with fatigue, drowsiness, and poor sense of well-being at baseline. It was also observed that the clusters changed post-radiation in both responders and non-responders to RT and that pain clustered with different symptoms. In non-responders, three symptom clusters were consistently present, except in week eight. RT influenced the structure of symptom clusters in both responders and non-responders. This dataset of patients was reanalyzed by Khan et al. (5) using different statistical methods to determine whether symptom clusters in patients with bone metastases vary when extracted using three different statistical methods. Clusters derived using Principal Component Analysis (PCA) in the previous study by Chow et al. (4) were compared to symptom clusters extracted using Hierarchical Cluster Analysis (HCA) and Exploratory Factor Analysis (EFA). Clusters were derived at baseline, one, two, four, eight and twelve weeks after RT. The patient sample was further divided into responders versus non-responders to RT. A complete consensus between HCA, EFA and PCA for the number and composition of symptom clusters was not reached at any time point despite the use of an identical data set. As expected, different symptom clusters were observed in the responders and non-responders with all three statistical methods. In addition, clusters varied at each time point within each subgroup. Depression and anxiety were consistently found in the same cluster. The use of a common analytical method is necessary for consistency and comparison purposes in future symptom cluster research.

A study published in 2008, conducted in the RRRP explored symptom clusters in cancer patients with pain due to bone metastases. This study by Hadi et al. (6) enrolled 348 patients with bone metastases between May 2003 and January 2007 referred for palliative RT, receiving either single or multiple fractions. The patients' worst pain at the site of treatment and seven functional interference scores were assessed using the Brief Pain Inventory (BPI) at baseline, four, eight, and twelve weeks post RT (6). PCA was performed on these items to determine interrelationships between symptoms. Principal components with an Eigenvalue higher than 0.90 and explaining more than 10% of the variance were selected. The Cronbach alpha statistic was used to estimate the internal consistency and reliability of the derived clusters. Two symptom clusters were identified. Cluster one included walking ability, general activity, normal work, enjoyment of life, and worst pain (6). Cluster two included relations with others, mood, and sleep (6). The two clusters at baseline accounted for 67% of the total variance with a Cronbach's alpha of 0.87 and 0.70 respectively (6). In patients that responded to RT, the two symptom clusters were no longer detected at four, eight, and twelve weeks post-RT. In non-responders, the same two clusters were not present at week four, re-emerged at week eight, and disappeared at week twelve (6). Hadi et al. (6) concluded that the significant correlations between worst pain score and the functional interference items demonstrate the importance of pain reduction as a goal for RT, as reducing pain can reduce functional interference and improve QOL.

This dataset was reanalyzed by Chen et al. (7) in 2012 to determine whether symptom clusters in patients with bone metastases varied when derived using three different statistical methods. The previous BPI data was reanalyzed using HCA and EFA. Little correlation was observed in the symptom cluster findings of PCA, EFA, and HCA in the total patient sample. Absolute consensus among all three statistical methods was never reached at any assessment time point. Varying patterns of symptom cluster presentation over time were observed in the responders versus non-responders subgroups regardless of the analytical method employed. A core cluster of symptoms composed of worst pain, general activity, walking ability, normal work, and enjoyment of life frequently presented in the same cluster (7).

An additional validation study was conducted in the RRRP by Hadi and colleagues (8). This study enrolled 52 patients between February and September 2007 with bone metastases receiving either a single fraction or multiple fractions of RT (8). Again, patients provided worst pain at the site of RT and functional interference scores were assessed using the BPI at baseline, four, eight, and twelve weeks post-RT. Two symptom clusters were identified. Cluster one included worst pain, interference with general activity, normal work, and walking ability. Cluster two consisted of interference with mood, sleep, enjoyment of life, and relations with others (8). These symptom clusters were not identical to those in the previous study, therefore, the authors concluded that these differences may be an indicator of the instability of the discovered symptom clusters or may be the result of a fewer number of patients in this validation study (6, 8). Thus, further research is warranted to determine if the previously discovered symptom clusters are in fact reproducible.

Another study on symptom cluster research by Chen et al. (9) was initiated to identify symptom clusters at baseline in a subgroup of bone metastases patients reporting non-zero ESAS scores. A subgroup of patients reporting severity scores greater than zero for all nine ESAS symptoms at baseline was compiled from a pre-existing database of bone metastases patients identified in the RRRP. At baseline, notably different symptom clusters were identified in the non-zero subgroup compared with the total patient population regardless of the statistical method utilized. When clusters derived using different statistical methods were compared, symptom cluster results varied depending on the method employed, with a few exceptions where analogous clusters were derived using two different statistical methods at a specific time point. A complete consensus between all three methods was never observed, which emphasizes the importance of the use of standardized statistical methods in symptom cluster research (9).

Symptom clusters in brain metastases

Chow et al. (10) explored the presence of symptom clusters in patients with brain metastases. Between January 1999 and January 2002, 170 patients with brain metastases referred to the RRRP completed the ESAS at baseline, one, two, four, eight, and twelve weeks after whole brain radiotherapy (WBRT). To determine interrelationships between symptoms a PCA with varimax rotation was carried out on the nine ESAS items. Three symptom clusters were found at baseline. Cluster one included fatigue, drowsiness, shortness of breath, and pain and accounted for 37% of the total variance. Cluster two included anxiety and depression, and accounted for 12% of the total variance. Cluster three included poor appetite, nausea, and a poor sense of well-being, and accounted for 13% of the total variance (10). The internal reliabilities of the three clusters using Cronbach's alpha coefficient ranged from 0.61 to 0.74 (10). This study concluded that symptom clusters appeared to exist in patients with brain metastases. Limiting factors of this study included high attrition rate due to profound deterioration in this patient population, as well as incomplete data on steroid usage, as certain symptoms can be affected by steroid usage (10).

A reanalysis of this data by Chow et al. (10) was published by Chen et al. (11) in 2013 to determine whether symptom clusters in patients with bone metastases varied when derived using different statistical methods. The ESAS data was reanalyzed using HCA and EFA. Symptom clusters extracted at baseline and each subsequent follow-up generally varied depending on the analytical method employed. Twelve unique clusters were found at each follow-up with each method, and only at the eight week follow up did all three methods demonstrate the same cluster of symptoms. Symptom cluster findings using PCA and HCA correlated more strongly with each other than either did with the findings of EFA. Inconsistency in symptom cluster composition was also observed at different time intervals. While the symptom clusters differed between the three analytical methods, symptoms within determined clusters such as anxiety and depression or fatigue and drowsiness consistently clustered together over time. The authors concluded that the stability of symptom pairs observed indicates a robust interrelationship existed between the symptoms involved (11).

An additional study by Hird et al. (12) involved 129 patients with brain metastases referred to the RRRP between August 2005 to October 2007 who completed the Spitzer Quality of Life Index (SQLI) and a study designed 17 item symptom questionnaire at baseline, one, two, and three months after WBRT. PCA was again used along with the Cronbach's alpha statistic. In analysis of the SQLI, the first cluster identified consisted of activity, daily living, and health (12). The second cluster consisted of support and outlook (12). Cronbach's alpha was 0.69 and 0.40 respectively, and the two clusters accounted for 64% of the variance (12). Analysis of the symptom questionnaire items revealed three clusters at baseline. Though these clusters changed slightly over time, certain symptoms remained to together despite WBRT: trouble concentrating and confusion, memory loss and decreased alertness, nausea and vomiting, dizziness and headache (12). Thus, this article concluded that symptom clusters do exist in patients with brain metastases.

A reanalysis of this compiled SQLI data was conducted by Khan et al. (13) to determine whether the use of different statistical methods influenced the composition of symptom clusters derived from patients with brain metastases. Symptom clusters extracted using PCA in the previous study were compared to clusters determined using HCA and EFA at baseline, one, two, and three months following WBRT. The number and composition of symptom clusters at each time point varied based on the statistical method employed, despite the use of an identical dataset. However, some domains consistently clustered together, such as activity and daily living from the SQLI items. Additionally, memory loss, confusion, and trouble concentrating were always present in the same cluster. Nausea and vomiting also occurred in conjunction regardless of the analytical method employed. This analysis concluded that symptom clusters vary with respect to occurrence, quantity, and composition based on the statistical method utilized to extract them (13). The use of a single analytical method is essential for consistency and comparison purposes in future symptom cluster research.

Reanalysis and literature reviews

A review by Chen et al. (14) was conducted to reanalyze data from the previous symptom cluster study by Fan et al. (15) using different statistical methods. The previous study by Fan et al. explored symptom clusters in advanced cancer patients by applying PCA on ESAS data collected at baseline, one, two, four, eight, and twelve week follow up for 1296 patients (15). The more recent reanalysis by Chen et al. (10) used this same data set and extracted symptom clusters with HCA and EFA. The symptom cluster findings of HCA and PCA correlated more frequently with each other than either did with EFA. Complete consensus of all three statistical methods was never reached (14). Thus, the authors concluded that the presence of symptom clusters in cancer patients vary depending on which statistical analysis is used (14).

A literature review published in 2011 by Chen et al. (16) examined past literature on symptom clusters in lung cancer patients. Five relevant studies were identified which investigated symptom clusters in lung cancer patients. The number of symptoms in a cluster ranged from two to eleven (16). The only cluster that was consistently identified was composed of nausea and vomiting symptoms in the two studies reviewed (16). Respiratory clusters identified in two studies were also comparable, containing both dyspnea and cough, among other symptoms (16). Chen et al. (16) concluded that differences in sample population characteristics, assessment tools and statistical analyses resulted in a lack of consensus in symptom clusters in patients with lung cancer.

Nguyen et al. (17) published a review of research reporting symptom clusters in breast cancer patients between 2005 and 2009. Five relevant studies were identified that differed from each other in statistical methodology, number of symptom clusters produced, and the symptoms comprising the clusters. The number of symptom clusters extracted between the five studies varied from one to four, while the number of symptoms in a cluster ranged from two to five. One study examining symptom clusters between different patient groups and a second study examining clusters across a time trajectory had certain reproducible clusters comprising similar symptoms. There were no clusters across different studies that contained the same symptoms, though fatigue was present in at least one cluster in all five studies and depression/psychological distress was noted in four of the studies. Nausea and appetite were the only two symptoms that associated together across three of the five studies. Although there were common symptoms assessed across the five studies, no common symptom clusters could be derived from these reports. This lack of commonality may have been the result of the disparities in subpopulations of patients, assessment tools, and methodological approaches (17).

In 2012, Thavarajah et al. (2) reviewed empirically determined symptom clusters in patients with metastatic cancer. A total of eight relevant studies published between 2005 and 2011 were identified. The number of symptom clusters extracted varied from two to eight clusters per study, comprising of two to eight symptoms per cluster. There were no clusters consistently identified within all eight studies. Notable differences in symptoms assessed, assessment tools, statistical analysis and patient demographics were observed between the studies. The lack of consensus among the inter-study symptom clusters are likely due to the differences in patient population as well as study methodology.

A further literature review by Thavarajah et al. (18) explored symptom clusters specifically in prostate cancer patients which identified two relevant studies on this topic. Both studies were longitudinal in nature and utilized cluster analysis to derive symptom clusters, though one of the studies also used three additional statistical methods. Both studies identified several symptom clusters in prostate patients, though several disparities between the two studies were determined. Differences in sample populations, assessment tools, symptoms observed and statistical methods can account for discrepancies between the two studies. Thus, the authors concluded that further research in prostate cancer symptom clusters is necessary to establish clinically relevant findings.

Discussion

Extensive research has been conducted in the RRRP regarding symptom clusters. Studies have explored symptom clusters in specific patient types with metastases to bone and brain. Symptom cluster research has also been conducted in the general population of patients with advanced cancer from various primary sites. Research identifying and analyzing symptom clusters is relevant for medical professionals in the oncology field as well as their patients. Identifying symptom clusters and their trends over time also has clinical relevance for symptom treatment and QOL improvement.

Evidently, through examination of research on symptom clusters in the RRRP, it is necessary to conduct longitudinal studies to identify symptom clusters over time. It is important for studies to determine how symptom clusters change or deteriorate over time from baseline to multiple follow up points. Longitudinal studies are also essential for examining the effect of treatment, including RT, on symptom clusters in cancer patients by assessing symptoms both at baseline and following treatment.

In addition to completing studies that are longitudinal in nature, involving large patient populations in studies is also important for symptom cluster research in order to establish findings and clusters that can be deemed significant. Conclusions from studies with smaller patient sample sizes were less definitive as discrepancies between identified symptom clusters in different studies may be the result of small patient populations (8).

For symptom cluster research, statistical analysis is also imperative. It has been identified by many of the studies conducted in the RRRP that symptom clusters can vary depending on which method of statistical analysis is used. Studies in the RRRP have used statistical methods of detecting symptom clusters including PCA, HCA, and EFA. It is important to find a standardized method of analysis for identifying symptom clusters and validate this method in the identification of symptom clusters in various patient populations (9, 14). The use of a single universal statistical method will allow various studies on symptom clusters in advanced cancer patients to be compared and analyzed together (13).

Symptom cluster investigation is a developing area of research and is promising in providing insights into symptom management for cancer patients. Symptom clusters can interfere with patients' functional status, QOL and relationships with others (3). It may be more effective to initiate interventions and assess their effects on symptom clusters rather than on single symptoms. Further research identifying underlying mechanisms of symptom clusters and impeding or manipulating these mechanisms may offer ways to treat a cluster of symptoms simultaneously (3). Research in the RRRP has shown that methodological inconsistencies between studies have resulted in a lack of consensus amongst symptom clusters for certain patient populations and have thus impeded the determination of clinically relevant findings (16).

Conclusion

Although there is still debate in the literature on what defines a symptom cluster and which statistical method should be used to identify symptom clusters, it is evident that research in the area is significant. The efforts of the RRRP have aimed to broaden the available information on symptom clusters in patients with advanced cancer and how these clusters are impacted by RT. There are still inconsistencies in research methodologies and results for patients with various primary cancers and sites of metastases. Thus, continued research in the RRRP is warranted to further determine the clinical implications of symptom clusters and validate the methods used to identify them.

Acknowledgments

We thank the generous support of Bratty Family Fund, Michael and Karyn Goldstein Cancer Research Fund, Joseph and Silvana Melara Cancer Research Fund, and Ofelia Cancer Research Fund.

References

[1]   Bedi H, Hird A, Campos S, Chow E. Symptom clusters in metastatic cancer: A critical appraisal. J Pain Manage 2010;3(1):17-29.

[2]   Thavarajah N, Chen E, Zeng L, Bedard G, Di Giovanni J, Lemke M, et al. Symptom clusters in patients with metastatic cancer: A literature review. Expert Review of Pharmacoecon Outcomes Res 2012;12(5):597-604.

[3]   Kim HJ, McGuire DB, Tulman L, Barsevick AM. Symptom clusters: Concept analysis and clinical implications for cancer nursing. Cancer Nurs 2005;28:270-82.

[4]   Chow E, Fan G, Hadi S, Filipczak L. Symptom clusters in cancer patients with bone metastases. Support Care Cancer 2007;15(9):1035-43.

[5]   Khan L, Cramarossa G, Chen E, Nguyen J, Zhang L, Tsao M, et al. Symptom clusters using the edmonton symptom assessment system in patients with bone metastases: A reanalysis comparing different statistical methods. World J Oncol 2012;3(1):23-32.

[6]   Hadi S, Fan G, Kirou-Mauro A, Hird A, Filipczak L. Symptom clusters in cancer patients with metastatic bone pain. J Palliat Med 2008;11(4):591-600.

[7]   Chen E, Khan L, Zhang L, Nguyen J, Cramarossa G, Tsao M, et al. Symptom clusters in patients with bone metastases - A reanalysis comparing different statistical methods. Supportive Care Cancer 2012;20(11):2811-20.

[8]   Hadi S, Zhang L, Hird A, de Sa E, Chow E. Validation of symptom clusters in patients with metastatic bone pain. Curr Oncol 2008;15(5):211-8.

[9]   Chen E, Nguyen J, Cramarossa G, Khan L, Zhang L, Tsao M, et al. Symptom clusters in patients with advanced cancer: Sub-analysis of patients reporting exclusively non-zero ESAS scores. J Palliat Med 2012;26(6):826-33.

[10]   Chow E, Fan G, Hadi S, Wong J, Kirou-Mauro A, Filipczak L. Symptom clusters in cancer patients with brain metastases. Clin Oncol (R Coll Radiol) 2008;20(1):76-82.

[11]   Chen E, Khan L, Zhang L, Nguyen J, Zeng L, Bedard G, et al. Symptom clusters in patients with brain metastases-a reanalysis comparing different statistical methods. J Radiat Oncol 2013;2(1):95-102.

[12]   Hird A, Wong J, Zhang L, Tsao M, Barnes E, Danjoux C, et al. Exploration of symptoms clusters within cancer patients with brain metastases using the spitzer quality of life index. Support Care Cancer 2010;18(3):335-42.

[13]   Khan L, Cramarossa G, Lemke M, Nguyen J, Zhang L, Chen E, et al. Symptom clusters using the spitzer quality of life index in patients with brain metastases--a reanalysis comparing different statistical methods. Support Care Cancer 2013;21(2):467-73.

[14]   Chen E, Nguyen J, Khan L, Zhang L, Cramarossa G, Tsao M, et al. Symptom clusters in patients with advanced cancer: A reanalysis comparing different statistical methods. J Pain Symptom Manage 2012;44(1):23-32.

[15]   Fan G, Hadi S, Chow E. Symptom clusters in patients with advanced-stage cancer referred for palliative radiation therapy in an outpatient setting. Support Cancer Ther 2007;4(3):157-62.

[16]   Chen E, Nguyen J, Cramarossa G, Khan L, Leung A, Lutz S, et al. Symptom clusters in patients with lung cancer: A literature review. Expert Rev Pharmacoecon Outcomes Res 2011;11(4):433-9.

[17]   Nguyen J, Cramarossa G, Bruner D, Chen E, Khan L, Leung A, et al. A literature review of symptom clusters in patients with breast cancer. Expert Rev Pharmacoecon Outcomes Res 2011;11(5):533-9.

[18]   Thavarajah N, Chen E, Bedard G, Lauzon N, Zhou M, Chu D, Chow E. Symptom clusters in patients with prostate cancer: a literature review. J Pain Manage 2012;5(4): 303-10.

In: Pain Management Yearbook 2013
Editor: Joav Merrick

ISBN: 978-1-63117-944-0
© 2014 Nova Science Publishers, Inc.

Chapter 24

Review of radiation-induced nausea and vomiting research in the Rapid Response Radiotherapy Program

Natalie Pulenzas, BSc(C), Breanne Lechner, BSc(C), Nemica Thavarajah, BSc(C) and Edward Chow, MBBS*

Rapid Response Radiotherapy Program, Department of Radiation Oncology, Odette Cancer Centre, Sunnybrook Health Sciences Centre, University of Toronto, Toronto, Ontario, Canada

Abstract

Research conducted by the Rapid Response Radiotherapy Program (RRRP) on radiation induced nausea and vomiting (RINV) is examined in this review. RINV develops in approximately 50-80% of patients, and severity is dependent on factors such as treatment volume, overall dose, current chemotherapy, and pre-existing nausea and vomiting (N/V). RINV has an acute phase, during and immediately after radiation, and a delayed phase in the days following treatment. The most commonly prescribed anti-emetic in practice was 5-hydroxytryptamine-3 (5-HT3) receptor antagonists (RA), which is also recommended by Multinational Association for Supportive Care in Cancer (MASCC) and the American Society of Clinical Oncology (ASCO). The international patterns of RINV management strategies for radiation oncologists and trainees were reviewed through an online survey. Awareness of guidelines and standards of practice varied across all groups. Prospective studies that used 5-HT3 RAs for the prophylaxis of RINV resulted in low control rates of N/V, most markedly in the delayed phase. A prospective study used the Functional Living Index of Emesis (FLIE), and developed a daily diary to assess N/V, however had a very low compliance rate due to no follow-up calls and complicated instructions. There

* Correspondence: Professor Edward Chow MBBS, MSc, PhD, FRCPC, Department of Radiation Oncology, Odette Cancer Centre, Sunnybrook Health Sciences Centre, 2075 Bayview Avenue, Toronto, ON Canada. Email: Edward.Chow@Sunnybrook.ca.

is no current standardized assessment for RINV that is applicable to palliative cancer patients.

Keywords: Radiation-induced nausea and vomiting, quality of life, radiotherapy

Introduction

Radiation therapy is used to obtain symptom relief for painful bone metastases and improve quality of life (QOL). However, patients may also experience nausea and vomiting as a debilitating side effect of radiation (1). Incidence rate of radiotherapy-induced nausea and vomiting (RINV) is approximately 50-80% of patients receiving radiation treatment (2). Severity of RINV depends on patient and radiation related factors such as treatment volume, overall dose, current chemotherapy, and pre-existing nausea and vomiting (1). RINV may lead to delayed treatment, fear of treatment, and reduced overall QOL (2,3). RINV occurs in two phases; the acute phase immediately after radiotherapy, as well as a delayed phase (1). The Rapid Response Radiotherapy Program (RRRP) is a specialized clinic that provides immediate radiotherapy for palliative cancer patients.

There is extensive research investigating chemotherapy induced nausea and vomiting (CINV), however there is limited data on RINV (3). It is known that the mechanisms underlying CINV are very similar to RINV, as well as the treatment of these symptoms (2). Radiation treatment damages the gastrointestinal mucosa, which subsequently releases serotonin and initiates RINV through binding to 5-hydroxytryptamine-3 (5-HT3) receptors. The most commonly recommended antiemetic for the prophylaxis of RINV are 5-HT_3 receptor antagonists (RA) which prevent the binding of serotonin, and therefore RINV (2,3).

Methods

A retrospective review of the literature was obtained including all research published from the RRRP involving RINV. There were no exclusion criteria, and RINV data was collected from 2010-present including review articles. A main focus of the RRRP research is the effectiveness and optimal timing of 5-HT_3 RAs in the prophylaxis or rescue of RINV.

Results

Salvo et al. (3) conducted a systematic review of the literature in 2012 comparing the efficacy of 5-HT_3 RAs with anti-emetic medications or placebo in randomized controlled trials. Nine trials were identified and included in the review. Majority of the studies reviewed reported superiority of 5-HT_3 RAs when compared with other antiemetic medications or placebo. Two studies reported no significant difference in effectiveness; however these trials had very small sample sizes. Studies reviewed which compared 5-HT_3 RA and other antiemetic medications commonly tested tropisetron versus metroclopramide. Prevention of emesis was statistically more effective for 5-HT3 RAs, however results of prevention of nausea were not statistically significant between treatment options, suggesting nausea is a difficult symptom to control (3).

Dennis et al. (2) also conducted a review of the RINV literature in 2011. Major antiemetic guidelines were reviewed from the Multinational Association for Supportive Care in Cancer (MASCC)/European Society of Medical Oncology (ESMO), the American Society of Clinical Oncology (ASCO), and the National Comprehensive Cancer Network (NCCN). MASC/ESMO and ASCO guidelines recommend pharmaceutical treatment depending on the site of radiation, and consequently the risk of emesis. Moderate and low emetogenic risks from radiation are the most commonly seen groups in a palliative cancer setting. For low emetogenic risk patients (cranium, lower thorax), both guidelines recommend prophylaxis or rescue with a 5-HT$_3$ RA. Treatment for moderate emetic risk (upper abdomen), as recommended by MASC/ESMO is prophylaxis with a 5-HT$_3$ RA with/without concurrent dexamethasone, and ASCO recommends prophylaxis with a 5-HT$_3$ RA alone. NCCN guidelines incorporate all sites of radiation, except whole body, into the same emetic risk category, which therefore lacks validity (2). A study included in the review conducted in Italy determined only 12.4% of patients received prophylactic antiemetic therapy, though there is limited consensus on the implication of this data due to a small amount of literature available. The review by Dennis et al. (2) concluded that radiation oncologists frequently underestimate the impact and prevalence of RINV.

Dennis et al. (4) conducted a subsequent study investigating the international patterns of practice in RINV of radiation oncologists from twelve countries across the world through a web-based survey. Six clinical radiation therapy scenarios were presented in the survey; one high risk for emesis, two moderate, and two low risk cases. Respondents ranked the case for risks of nausea and vomiting, management strategies, and if applicable chose the anti-emetic medication they would prescribe. Management strategies for RINV varied across the respondents, more prominently in the moderate and low risk cases in deciding between prophylaxis or rescue therapy (4).

Another study conducted by Dennis et al. (5) investigated radiation oncology trainee's knowledge in the appropriate management and guidelines of RINV through the same survey used previously. Only 28% of the 176 trainees were aware of the current antiemetic guidelines, and treatment strategies were more variable again in the low and moderate risk cases, as expected (5). These studies show the importance of continuing research in RINV, and developing/establishing appropriate standard antiemetic guidelines.

Presutti et al. (1) conducted a prospective study involving 19 patients from the RRRP who received palliative radiation therapy to the upper abdomen and abdominal/pelvic region. The study reported the results of the preliminary analysis. Participants received radiation for painful bone metastases in single or multiple fractions. All patients were prescribed prophylactic Ondansetron (8 mg) (5-HT$_3$ RA) with varying regimens, at the discretion of the physician, and completed daily nausea and vomiting diaries for all days during and ten days post treatment. Exclusion criteria included patients receiving concomitant chemotherapy within the study period, defined as the start of radiation until 10 days post treatment, or other anti-emetic medications. Acute phase RINV was defined as from the commencement of radiation to 24 hours after completion. The delayed phase began from completion of the acute phase (24 hours post-radiation) until 10 days following. Results showed less control of nausea and vomiting in the delayed phase when compared to the acute phase, as the amount of patients with complete prophylaxis decreased (1). Dennis et al. (6) conducted the final analysis with 59 enrolled patients, and 32 with complete follow up data from 2007-2010 (6). Twenty-four patients received single fraction radiotherapy, and 8 patients received multiple fractions, of which all received 20Gy in 5 fractions except for one patient who received 30Gy in 10 fractions. Dosing schedules of Ondansetron varied, as patients receiving single fraction radiotherapy were prescribed for a duration of 1 day (n=20), 3 days (n=2), or 5 days (n=2); and multiple fraction radiotherapy prescribed for 5 days (n=6), 10 days (n=1), or 15 days (n=1). Dosing schedules were also variable, as 42% of patients in the single fraction group, and 12% of the multiple fraction group took Ondansetron once daily, as opposed to twice daily dosing. Patients were distinguished as a moderate risk for RINV if radiation included one portion of the upper abdomen (T11-L3 inclusive). Low emetogenic risk was determined to be radiation targeting or involving the pelvis (6). Similar results to Presutti et al. (1) were concluded after final analysis (1,6). Complete prophylaxis of nausea in the moderate risk emetogenic group was achieved by 56% and 31% of patients in the acute and delayed phase respectively for the single fraction group; 71% and 43% for the multiple fraction group. For the low risk emetogenic group, 50% and 43% for single fraction; 100% and 100% for multiple fractions. Complete prophylaxis of vomiting in the moderate risk emetogenic group was achieved by 69% and 44% of patients in the acute and delayed phase respectively for the single fraction group; 57% and 57% for the multiple fraction group. In the low risk emetogenic group, 100% and 57% for single fraction; 100% and 100% for multiple fractions. The authors concluded that despite prophylaxis of RINV with Ondansetron, patients still experienced nausea and vomiting, with higher rates of incidence in the delayed phase (6). Conclusions were lacking in delayed RINV in the systematic review by Salvo et al. (3). Of the studies reviewed, a significant limitation of the data collection was the absence of knowledge for the delayed phase (3). A review of the RINV literature in 2011 by Dennis et al. (2) concluded that despite 5-HT$_3$ RA being recommended for prophylaxis, optimal timing and duration are unknown. Twenty-five trials were reviewed in a subsequent study by Dennis et al. (7) to determine optimal timing and duration of 5-HT$_3$ RAs. It was determined that 5-HT$_3$ RAs were most commonly prescribed for the duration of radiotherapy, but complete control of nausea especially, was low across the majority of trials (7).

Research is lacking in a quality of life questionnaire specific to the RINV setting. One of the most commonly used tools used in the RRRP and past studies is the Functional Living Index of Emesis (FLIE). Only two of the nine trials reviewed by Salvo included some measure of QOL, and one study required patients to complete the FLIE preceding and following radiation treatment. The second study used the European Organisation of Cancer Treatment Quality of Life Questionnaire – Core 30 (EORTC QLQ-C30), a general quality of life tool for cancer patients. Results appeared to show a slight increase in QOL of patients who received treatment with 5-HT3 RAs (3). Haid et al. (8) created a self-reported daily diary to assess for nausea, vomiting, and use of rescue medications based on the MASCC Antiemesis Tool (MAT). Thirty-five patients were accrued and required to complete the daily diary for fifteen days, and the FLIE twice a week during the study period, and a debriefing questionnaire, with no telephone follow up calls. Eligible patients had irradiation to the abdomen, abdomen/pelvis, cranium, or esophagus. However, only four patients completed all follow-ups and the authors concluded this likely occurred due to a lack of follow-up calls throughout the study, and complex instructions and assessments (8).

Discussion

As determined by the literature, there are several guidelines that recommend the use of anti-emetic medications for the prophylaxis of RINV. However, as determined by Dennis et al. (4,5) in 2011 and 2012, a low percentage of physicians are aware of the current guidelines. Further education in these guidelines, especially in radiation oncology trainees, may help in reducing rates of RINV through appropriate prophylactic prescriptions and awareness (4,5). The most commonly used agent for the prophylaxis of RINV has been determined to be 5-HT$_3$ RAs, though despite the use of these medications, nausea and vomiting are still common. Future research should focus on improving the control of nausea and vomiting, particularly in the delayed phase (1,3,6). Determination of optimal timing and duration of 5-HT$_3$ RAs may assist in the control of the delayed phase, but is still unknown (7). The results of these studies show that complete control of nausea is difficult to obtain, therefore complete control of vomiting may be an important endpoint in future studies as this can be viewed as a serious side effect by patients (7). Ondansetron was the most commonly used 5-HT$_3$ RA, and upcoming alternatives may be influential on future research. Specific assessments for measuring QOL and RINV related symptoms have not been standardized. Past prospective studies in the RRRP have used assessments such as the FLIE, and designed new diaries with significant limitations. Such as the diary used by Haid et al. (8) resulted in a very low compliance rate. We have been developing a revised daily diary that is applicable for palliative cancer patients, yet optimal in collecting incidences of nausea, vomiting, and use of rescue medication. The use of follow-up calls and reminders may also elevate compliance rate in future prospective studies (8).

Conclusion

RINV still occurs in a significant proportion of palliative cancer patients receiving moderately or low emetogenic radiotherapy. Complete control of nausea has historically been lower than vomiting, suggesting it to be a more difficult symptom to prevent. Further investigation should focus on the use of other 5-HT$_3$ RAs, or use in combination with other medications. Research into the optimal timing and duration of 5-HT$_3$ RA is important to consider so the control of delayed phase RINV can be elevated. A specific QOL questionnaire and daily diary for assessing RINV is important to record symptoms, as well as decrease patient burden and optimize compliance.

Acknowledgments

We thank the generous support of Bratty Family Fund, Michael and Karyn Goldstein Cancer Research Fund, Joseph and Silvana Melara Cancer Research Fund, and Ofelia Cancer Research Fund.

References

[1]   Presutti R, Nguyen J, Holden L, DeAngelis C, Culleton S, Mitera G, et al. Radiation-induced nausea and vomiting in a palliative radiotherapy clinic: A preliminary analysis. J Pain Manag 2010;3(3):301-7.

[2]   Dennis K, Maranzano E, De Angelis C, Holden L, Wong S, Chow E. Radiotherapy-induced nausea and vomiting. Expert Rev Pharmacoecon Outcomes Res 2011;11(6):685-92.

[3]   Salvo N, Doble B, Khan L, Amirthevasar G, Dennis K, Pasetka M, et al. Prophylaxis of radiation-induced nausea and vomiting using 5-hydroxytryptamine-3 serotonin receptor antagonists: a systematic review of randomized trials. Int J Radiat Oncol Biol Phys 2012;82(1):408-17.

[4]   Dennis K, Zhang L, Lutz S, van Baardwijk A, van der Linden Y, Holt T, et al. International patterns of practice in the management of radiation therapy-induced nausea and vomiting. Int J Radiat Oncol Biol Phys 2012;84(1):e49-60.

[5]   Dennis K, Zhang L, Lutz S, van der Linden Y, van Baardwijk A, Holt T, et al. International radiation oncology trainee decision making in the management of radiotherapy-induced nausea and vomiting. Support Care Cancer 2013 Feb 26. [EPub ahead of print]

[6]   Dennis K, Nguyen J, Presutti R, DeAngelis C, Tsao M, Danjoux C, et al. Prophylaxis of radiotherapy-induced nausea and vomiting in the palliative treatment of bone metastases. Support Care Cancer 2012;20(8):1673-78.

[7]   Dennis K, Makhani L, Maranzano E, Feyer P, Zeng L, DeAngelis C, et al. Timing and duration of 5-HT3 receptor antagonist therapy for the prophylaxis of radiotherapy-induced nausea and vomiting: a systematic review of randomized and non-randomized studies. J Radiat Oncol, in press.

[8]   Haid V, Kumar K, Al Duhaiby E, Pang J, DeAngelis C, Pasetka M, et al. Evaluation of a daily diary for assessing the prevalence of radiation-induced emesis (RIE). J Pain Manag 2012;5(3):237-44.

In: Pain Management Yearbook 2013
Editor: Joav Merrick

ISBN: 978-1-63117-944-0
© 2014 Nova Science Publishers, Inc.

Chapter 25

Review of bone metastases research in the Rapid Response Radiotherapy Program (RRRP)

Breanne Lechner, BSc(C), Natalie Pulenzas, BSc(C),
Nemica Thavarajah, BSc(C) and Edward Chow, MBBS*

Rapid Response Radiotherapy Program, Department of Radiation Oncology,
Odette Cancer Centre, Sunnybrook Health Sciences Centre, University of Toronto,
Toronto, Ontario, Canada

Abstract

Bone metastases are a common occurrence in patients with advanced cancer. Complications of bone metastases can include pain, hypercalcemia, pathological fractures, spinal instability, spinal cord compression and immobility. Palliative radiotherapy (RT) is a well-established and effective treatment option for symptomatic bone metastases. The Rapid Response Radiotherapy Program (RRRP) provides timely RT for palliative cancer patients, focusing on quality of life (QOL) as an important endpoint. This paper reviewed the past research conducted in the RRRP on bone metastases. Studies in the RRRP have focused on topics including QOL in patients with bone metastases, the incidence and methods to prevent pain flare following RT, optimal treatment regimens for bone metastases and various patient population subgroups.

Keywords: Bone metastases, quality of life, pain flare, radiotherapy

* Correspondence: Professor Edward Chow MBBS, MSc, PhD, FRCPC, Department of Radiation Oncology, Odette Cancer Centre, Sunnybrook Health Sciences Centre, 2075 Bayview Avenue, Toronto, ON Canada. Email: Edward.Chow@Sunnybrook.ca.

Introduction

Bone metastases are a common occurrence in patients with advanced cancer, and are found in 70%-85% of patients at autopsy (1). Metastases to the bone are particularly common in patients with primary breast, lung and prostate carcinomas (1). The morbidity associated with metastatic bone disease includes pain, hypercalcemia, pathological fractures, spinal instability, spinal cord compression, and immobility (2). Pain is the most prevalent symptom of bone metastases and is experienced by 60-70% of patients (3). Symptoms of bone metastases can have a significant negative impact on patients' quality of life (QOL). Palliative radiotherapy (RT) is a well-established and effective treatment option for symptomatic bone metastases (3). The overall pain response rate is approximately 80% (4-7). Controversy over the optimal treatment schedules and fractionation of RT still exists, with patterns of practice in radiation oncologists consistently showing reluctance to adopt single fraction as a preferred practice despite research demonstrating the equivalence of single and multiple fractions for pain relief in uncomplicated bone metastases (7). A significant side effect associated with RT is pain flare. Pain flare is a temporary worsening of pain in the treated bony metastatic site following RT (3). Treatment for the prophylaxis of pain flare is an important topic of research in the field of radiation oncology. Promising research has been conducted on the use of the corticosteroid dexamethasone for the prophylaxis of pain flare following RT to bone metastases (8, 9).

There have been many studies that have focused on patients with bone metastases in the Rapid Response Radiotherapy Program (RRRP) at the Sunnybrook Odette Cancer Centre. The RRRP is a specialized clinic developed in 1996 to provide timely palliative RT with the purpose of improving or maintaining QOL in patients with advanced cancer (6). Extensive research regarding all aspects of palliative RT has been conducted in the RRRP since its establishment. This paper reviews the past research in the RRRP examining various aspects of bone metastases research.

Methods

A literature search was conducted to identify studies investigating bone metastases in cancer patients conducted in the RRRP from 2000 to present. All publications pertaining to patients with metastatic bone disease were included. The methods and results of the studies were summarized, and important areas of bone metastases research were discussed in detail.

Results

Studies examining the impact of bone metastases on QOL, the incidence of pain flare, the use of dexamethasone for pain flare prevention, bone metastases treatment regimens, and various patient population subgroups were examined.

Quality of life

Patients with bones metastases are often very symptomatic, and thus the improvement of QOL is a very important treatment outcome. One central area of research in the RRRP is the development of tools to assess QOL. A literature review by Tharmalingam et al. (2), published in 2008, focused specifically on QOL measurement in bone metastases patients. This review included any studies measuring QOL in patients with bone metastases from 1966 to June 2006, which resulted in 47 relevant trials identified (2). A total of 24 different instruments were used to evaluate QOL including pain assessment scales, validated QOL instruments, and study-designed questionnaires (2). Most studies employed study designed questionnaires (ten of the studies) or the European Organization for Research and Treatment of Cancer (EORTC) Core Questionnaire (EORTC-C30) (ten of the studies). The Functional Assessment of Cancer Therapy-General questionnaire (FACT-G) was used to evaluate QOL in five of the studies, the Edmonton Symptom Assessment System (ESAS) was used in four of the studies, and the Brief Pain Inventory (BPI) was used in four of the articles. The use of a variety of study-designed assessments did not allow for outcome comparison between studies. The authors of this review concluded that these results demonstrate the need for a standard instrument specific to bone metastases incorporating pain, skeletal complications, and psychosocial domains to assess QOL (2).

In 2009, a study published by Chow et al. (10) supported the development of a bone metastases module to supplement the EORTC QLQ-C30 or the EORTC Palliative Quality of Life Questionnaire (QLQ C15-PAL) for patients with bone metastases. Phases one and two of module development were conducted in Canada, Australia, and Germany in accordance with EORTC QOL group guidelines. Phase one involved identifying relevant health-related quality of life (HRQOL) issues for patients with bone metastases by reviewing the Medline and Psych info databases, existing HRQOL questionnaires for bone metastases, and interviews of patients and health care professionals. This study found 61 health-related quality of life (HRQOL) issues generated from 152 health care professionals and 413 patients. In Phase two, a list of these issues was presented to health care professionals and patients to determine which items were most relevant. This resulted in the construction of a 22 item provisional module. Phase three involved further testing in 170 patients from nine countries, which resulted in the twenty-two item bone metastases module (QLQ-BM22). This BM22 module contained symptom scales, with five painful site items and three pain characteristic items, and also functional scales, with eight functional interference items and six psychosocial aspects. The study successfully developed the EORTC QLQ-BM22 module to measure HRQOL in cancer patients with bone metastases. This single module was developed to facilitate reliable comparisons in bone metastases clinical trials.

Further research was conducted to test the reliability and validity of the EORTC QLQ-BM22 internationally by Chow et al. (11). A total of 400 patients undergoing a variety of treatments for bone metastases were accrued from March 2010 to January 2011 in seven countries including Brazil, Canada, Cyprus, Egypt, France, India, and Taiwan. The QLQ-BM22 was administered with the QLQ-C30 at baseline and at a one month follow-up. A debriefing questionnaire was administered to determine patient acceptability and understanding. Multi-trait scaling analyses confirmed 4 scales in the 22-item module. The scales were able to discriminate between clinically distinct patient groups, such as patients with varying performance status. The QLQ-BM22 was well received in all seven countries and the majority of patients did not recommend any significant changes from the module in its current form. The results of this study confirmed the validity, reliability, cross cultural applicability, and sensitivity of the EORTC QLQ-BM22 (11).

Further study by Zeng et al. (12) aimed to establish the minimal clinically important difference (MCID) for the EORTC QLQ-BM22 to aid in determining the relevance of QOL changes after treatment and in sample size determination in clinical trials. A total of 93 out of the 400 patients enrolled with bone metastases across seven countries completed the QLQ-BM22 and the QLQ-C30 at baseline and at a one month follow up and had performance status assessed at both time points. The MCID was calculated for each QOL scale for determining improvement and deterioration using both an anchor-based, which used performance status, and a distribution-based approach. Improvements of 30.5, 20.1, 30.5, and 19.6 in the pain, painful site, painful characteristic, and functional interference scales, respectively, demonstrated clinical relevance. Decreases of 12.4, 22.4, and 13.5 in emotional functioning, global health status, and financial issues, respectively, were required to represent clinically relevant deterioration. MCIDs for improvement were closest to 0.5 standard deviations, while for deterioration, closer to 0.3 standard deviations on the QLQ-BM22. These results suggest that a clinically meaningful improvement requires a greater change in QOL than a meaningful deterioration for the QLQ-BM22. For the QLQ-C30, the MCIDs were similar for improvement and deterioration. Ultimately, this study presented a set of MCIDs for the QLQ-BM22, though the study is limited by a small sample size and the use of only one anchor (12).

An additional study in the RRRP conducted by Campos et al. (13) tested the reliability of patient perceptions in important bone metastases QOL items. In 2005, 130 patients completed the EORTC QLQ-BM61, the 61 item QOL questionnaire precursor to the QLQ-BM22, and 27 of the patients were re-approached when they returned to clinic between 2007 and 2008. For each item of the QLQ-BM61, patients indicated if it was relevant to be included in the final version of the bone metastases questionnaire. Additionally, any treatment the patient received between baseline and re-approach was collected. There was no significant change in the items that patients selected for the final questionnaire between baseline and re-approach, indicating that patient perceptions of relevant QOL items did not change over time, which showed good reliability of patients' perceptions of important QOL issues. It was found that 10 of the 61 items had a significant value when assessing the relationship of the change in items patients selected and complications and treatment. This indicated that increased complications of disease and changes in treatment can affect patients' perceptions of important QOL items. This research is important to keep in mind as many QOL measurement tools are based on patient perceptions of generated QOL issues (13).

In 2009, a study by Chow et al. (14) was completed to validate what constitutes a meaningful change in pain scores following palliative RT for bone metastases. A total of 178 patients treated with external beam RT scored their worst pain on a scale of zero to ten before treatment, daily during treatment, and for ten days after RT as well as indicating if their pain was "worse", "the same", or "better" compared to pre-treatment. A total of 1431 pain scores were obtained. The results demonstrated that patients perceived an improvement in pain when their self-reported pain score decreased by at least two points. The authors concluded that this study validated the previous finding that a meaningful change in pain score is represented by a decrease in patient self-reported pain score by at least two points. This was an important confirmation for the use of pain scores in clinical trial endpoints for partial treatment responses (14).

A literature review by Presutti et al. (15) focused on examining bone metastases and QOL, addressing previous clinical trials assessing QOL in bone metastases patients receiving palliative RT. This review included aforementioned studies by the RRRP in the development of the EORTC QLQ-BM22 and further analyzed the development process. This review also examined the relevant international research on randomized trials examining single versus multiple fractions of RT for patients with bone metastases assessing QOL. Additionally, the review included external research on the development of the of the 16-item Functional Assessment of Cancer Therapy-Bone Pain (FACT-BP) scale to assess cancer related bone pain. The FACT-BP showed high internal consistency and was closely correlated with the pain intensity scales of the BPI, thus the FACT-BP was found to be a robust tool for assessing cancer related bone pain. Ultimately this review by Presutti et al. (15) concluded that QOL is a valuable endpoint in clinical trials for determining the success of an intervention for bone metastases.

An additional study in the RRRP published in 2011 examined the reported rates and predictive factors for sleep disturbance in patients with bone metastases (16). A total of 400 patients with symptomatic bone metastases treated with palliative RT were enrolled between May 2003 and June 2007, of which 235 completed all follow up points. The BPI questionnaire and analgesic consumption were recorded at baseline, and follow up BPI was completed post RT at week four, eight, and twelve. Ordinal logistic regression analysis was used to search for the relationship between sleep disturbance and other covariates. At baseline, 99 (25%) of patients had moderate sleep disturbance and 144 (36%) of patents had severe sleep disturbance. There was improvement in sleep scores for both responders and non-responders at week four and week eight, but scores worsened for non-responders at week twelve. Age, Karnofsky Performance Scale (KPS), pain score, and lung primary were the significant variables associated with sleep disturbance (16).

Research by Zeng et al. (17) assessed the levels of functional interference caused by pain after treatment with conventional RT using the BPI. After RT, a total of 159, 129, and 106 patients completed the BPI over the phone at week four, eight, and twelve respectively. To assess the validity of the BPI, Cronbach's alpha, confirmatory factor analysis, and discriminant validity tests were performed. One-way analysis of variance was used to compare BPI scores. The combination of different analyses confirmed the validity of the BPI over the telephone since reasonably high levels of internal consistency, composite reliability, and convergent validity were present at weeks four, eight, and twelve. Functional interference scores were worse in patients with lower skeletal pain, thus functional interference may be inherently higher in patients with pain in the lower body. After treatment with RT, there was no longer a statistically significant difference between patients with upper and lower body pain, thus RT reduces functional interference due to pain regardless of location on the body (17).

A study by Dennis et al. (18) aimed to determine the efficacy of RT for the palliation of pain from bone metastases among patients in their last three months of life. This study reviewed past ESAS and BPI databases compiled from patients with bone metastases receiving palliative RT, identifying patients who died within three months of receiving RT. From a total of 918 patients, 232 dying within three months of beginning treatment were identified. A pain response was evaluable for the 109 (47%) patients with available follow-up information. The overall response rates were 70% at one month and 63% at two months, which included complete and partial responses in accordance with the International Bone

Metastases Consensus definitions. Patients responding to treatment at one month reported significantly less interference due to pain in their general activity, walking ability, normal work, and enjoyment of life than patients not responding to treatment. Thus, it was concluded that despite being near the end of life, patients responding to palliative RT for painful bone metastases may benefit from improvement of functional abilities prior to passing away in addition to pain relief alone.

Pain flare

Pain flare is defined as a temporary worsening of pain in radiated bony metastatic sites immediately after RT (19). The incidence of pain flare following palliative RT for bone metastases is an area of interest for research in the RRRP.

An initial study conducted by Chow et al. (20) in 2005 examined the incidence of pain flare following RT by recording patients' daily pain scores and oral morphine equivalent dose. Pain flare was defined as a two point increase in pain score compared to baseline with no decrease in analgesic intake, or a 25 % increase in analgesic intake with no decrease in pain score. This study resulted in an overall incidence of pain flare ranging from 2% to 16%. This finding added to the results of previous studies, with a wide range of reported incidence of pain flare in the literature spanning from 2% to 44%. A joint study was thus initiated to further investigate the incidence of pain flare.

Hird et al. (1) conducted a multicenter study to more definitively determine the incidence of pain flare in patients with bone metastases being treated with RT. A total of 111 patients with painful bone metastases, the majority of which received either 8Gy in one fraction (64%) or 20Gy in five fractions (25%), were enrolled. Overall, pain flare occurred in 44 of the 111 patients (40%) during RT and within ten days following RT. Patients treated with a single 8Gy fraction reported pain flare incidence of 39% (27/70) and for those treated with multiple fractions the incidence was 41% (17/21). Pain flare occurred within the first five days following RT in 80% of all evaluable patients. Thus, this study was able to document the incidence of pain flare in patients with bone metastases receiving RT.

Additional investigations regarding pain flare in the RRRP examined the incidence of pain flare, its impact on patients, and prophylaxis of pain flare. Results of previous investigations, including those previously mentioned, were reviewed by Presutti et al. (19). The review also included a study by Hird et al. (3) published in 2009 that involved administering a five item Pain Flare Qualitative Questionnaire to 35 patients, 13 of which completed the questionnaire. Overall, 10/13 (77%) of patients indicated some level of functional interference due to the pain flare experienced. More than three quarters of the patients had to increase their pain medications in order to cope with pain flare. Despite this, still 9/13 (69%) of the patients failed to achieve adequate pain control. It was stated by 11/13 (85%) of patients that they would prefer the prevention of the pain flare as opposed to management with pain medication. One significant limitation of this study was the small sample size.

Dexamethasone

One treatment option for the prophylaxis of pain flare is the prescription of dexamethasone, a corticosteroid, prior to treatment. Essential research has been done in the RRRP regarding dexamethasone and its ability to reduce the instance of pain flare in patients receiving RT for bone metastases. Initially, a pilot study was published in 2007 examining dexamethasone for the prophylaxis of radiation-induced pain flare, which included 33 patients. Dexamethasone was found to be well tolerated, though further investigation was indicated to confirm the efficacy of dexamethasone in preventing pain flare (8). Subsequently, a phase two study was completed in the RRRP and published in 2009 by Hird et al. (21). Patients with bone metastases treated with a single 8Gy were prescribed 8mg of dexamethasone just before palliative RT and for three consecutive days after treatment. Worst pain score and analgesic consumption converted into total daily oral morphine equivalents were collected at baseline and daily for ten days after treatment. A total of 41 patients were evaluable. The overall incidence of pain flare was 9/41 (22%) within ten days of completing RT. Most (55%) of these pain flares occurred on day five. It was concluded that dexamethasone is effective in the prophylaxis of RT-induced pain flare after palliative RT for bone metastases, though further randomized studies are necessary to confirm this finding.

Treatment Regimens

The optimal regimen for palliative RT of bone metastases has been the subject of much debate throughout the literature. A significant amount of research has been conducted in the RRRP regarding single versus multiple fractionation schedules for RT. A review by Culleton et al. (22) examined conventional RT to bone metastases in the literature, specifically focusing on studies comparing a single fraction (SF) versus multiple fractions (MF). The most common treatment schedules delivered for palliation of bone metastases include single 8Gy treatment and multi-fractioned low dose regimes consisting most commonly of 20Gy in five fractions and 30Gy in ten fractions. Upon review of past meta-analyses and studies with a variety of endpoint definitions used, it was evident that an international consensus on endpoint definitions was needed. In response to the need for endpoint definition for future trials, the International Bone Metastases Consensus working party was established in 2000 to reach a consensus. Conclusions that the party agreed upon were published in 2002 by Chow et al. (23). One of the most important findings was the definition of complete response as a pain score of zero at the treated site with no concomitant increase in analgesic intake, and partial response as pain reduction of two or more points on a scale of ten without increase in analgesic intake or analgesic reduction of 25% or more without an increase in pain score (23). This international consensus was updated again in research published by Chow et al. in 2011 (24). Changes from the original consensus included the suggestion that only worst pain at the index site should be measured, not average pain in addition to worst pain. Also, the more recent consensus suggested the use of an additional response category, indeterminate response, to represent cases that could not be classified as complete response, partial response, or pain progression. In 2004, a study in the RRRP was conducted comparing response rates from palliative RT of bone metastases employing the international consensus endpoints and traditional endpoints for 518 patients. It was found that the international consensus endpoints lowered the complete and partial response rates compared to the traditional endpoints and more accurately reflected the true efficacy of radiation (25). In 2007, a systematic review was conducted of randomized palliative RT trials updating previous meta-analyses (7). The purpose of this study was to compare response rates for trials evaluating SF versus MF regimens. A total of 16 randomized trials were identified, and the overall SF response rate was 58% which was similar to the MF response rate, at 59 %. The complete response rates were found to be 23% for a SF and 24% for MF with no significant differences between the two groups. This review was updated in 2011 by Chow et al. (26). In total, 25 randomized controlled trials were identified. The overall response rate was similar in patients receiving SF (1696 of 2818; 60%) and MF (1711 of 2799; 61%). Complete response rates were 620 of 2641 (23%) in the SF arm and 634 of 2622 (24%) in the MF arm. No significant difference was seen in overall or complete response rates. Retreatment rates favored patients in the MF arm, where the likelihood of requiring re-irradiation was 2.6-fold greater in the SF arm. Thus, it was concluded that SF and MF regimens provided equal pain relief; however, significantly higher retreatment rates occurred in those that received a SF.

In 2006, our group conducted a study to examine how patients categorize their pain with both the verbal descriptor scale and eleven-point visual analogue scale (27). It was found that patients scored pain as 'mild' if pain was equal to four or less, 'moderate' if pain was between five and seven, and 'severe' if pain was equal to eight or more (27). Similarly in 2007, Li et al. (28) also conducted a study to establish cut off points for 'mild', 'moderate', and 'severe' pain by grading pain intensity with functional interference using the BPI. The optimal cut points were 1-4 for mild pain, 5-6 for moderate and 7-10 for severe pain. Li et al. (29) also conducted a study, published in 2008, to determine the most appropriate time to evaluate the response to palliative RT for bone metastases. It was concluded that two months was the most appropriate time to measure response rates because maximum pain relief may take more than one month for some patients to achieve, and attrition is a major problem after two months.

Another important topic addressed in the review by Culleton et al. (22) was the examination of patterns of practice. In 2000, the results of a survey of 172 Canadian radiation oncologists made up of case scenarios were published by Chow et al. (30). The most common dose prescribed was 20Gy in five fractions (72%) followed by 8Gy in one fraction (16%). It was found that 70% of practitioners used standard dose fractions to palliate painful bone metastases irrespective of site and tumor type. When evaluating the pattern of practice in the RRRP from 1999 to 2005, there was a significant increase in the prescription of SF for bone metastases. The noted increase in SF went from 51% in 1999 to 66% in 2005 (31). In 2008, a survey was distributed internationally to 962 practicing radiation oncologists (32). It was found that a SF was used most often by the Canadian Association of Radiation Oncology (CARO) members but overall, the most common palliative dose prescribed in all cases was 30Gy in ten fractions. SF regimens were prescribed most often frequently by Canadian Association of Radiation Oncology (CARO) members and they were two to three times more likely to recommended it when compared with American Society for Radiation Oncology (ASTRO) members who overall, were the least likely to use a SF. This international survey concluded that despite evidentiary support, SF has not been widely accepted as a treatment for uncomplicated painful bone metastases (32).

Recently, a review by Dennis et al. (33) was conducted to determine the optimal dose of SF conventional palliative RT for the relief of pain caused by bone metastases. Relevant randomized controlled trials were included. A total of 26 articles were found for review, and

24 trials cumulatively randomized 3233 patients to 28 SF arms: two arms received 4Gy, one 5Gy, one 6Gy, twenty-two 8Gy, one 10Gy and one 8–15Gy. Efficacy endpoints and pain assessment times varied. In general, higher doses produced better pain response rates. In trials that directly compared different SF doses, 8Gy was statistically superior to 4Gy. Also, 8Gy was by far the most commonly administered SF dose within 24 randomized trials of conventional RT for the palliation of bone metastases. Thus, the authors concluded that 8Gy should be the standard dose against which future treatments are compared due to its reproducible pain response rate and its established safety profile (33).

In addition to studies regarding palliative RT for bone metastases, research completed in the RRRP has analyzed various methods for the detection and treatment of bone metastases. A review by Bedard et al. (34) examined the literature to evaluate the accuracy, specificity, and sensitivity of Positron Emission Tomography (PET) used in the diagnosis of bone metastases. Out of the 44 publications identified, all studies except for one demonstrated that PET scan with the use of fluorodexyglucose (FDG) is superior to a bone scan. While FDG detects osteolytic lesions with great accuracy, it is unsuccessful in detecting osteoblastic lesions suggesting use for other modalities.

A review by Culleton et al. (35) examined the clinical benefits of combining bisphosphonates with RT for the treatment of bone metastases. A search of publications from 1950 to 2008 identified thirteen relevant studies. Three studies were in-vitro cell studies, which found a significant synergistic effect when the treatments were combined, by means of a reduction in cell viability via induced apoptosis. Two of the studies involved animal tumor models which found that combined treatment may lead to improved mineralization compared to RT alone. The remaining eight were human studies. Two of the human studies were randomized trials comparing combination therapy versus a placebo and RT, which both showed greater long term benefits in the arm that received both RT and bisphosphonates in terms of recalcification and the development of new bony lesions. Thus, the authors concluded that this preliminary evidence demonstrates that patients with bone metastases may significantly benefit from treatment with bisphosphonates and RT concurrently.

Patient populations

Research in the RRRP has also focused on various patient populations affected by bone metastases and RT for these patient populations. A study by Hird et al. (36) was completed to examine if bone metastases from gastrointestinal (GI) cancers show response rates similar to those of bone metastases from other primary cancers after RT in the RRRP. A total of 69 patients with bone metastases from GI primaries who received palliative RT in the RRRP clinic during 1999 to 2006 were identified, patients between 1999-2003 were assessed with the ESAS and patients from 2003-2006 were assessed with the BPI. Response rates for this cohort of metastatic GI cancer patients were then compared to rates for 479 patients receiving palliative RT for bone metastases from other primary cancer sites. No statistically significant differences were observed in RT response rates for bone metastases from GI cancers than from other primary cancer sites.

A study by Campos et al. (37) was published in 2010 that examined the efficacy of palliative RT in relieving metastatic bone pain in elderly patients. The response to RT for palliation of metastatic bone pain was evaluated in 558 patients between 1999 and 2008. No significant difference was found in the response rate in patients aged ≥ 65, ≥ 70, and ≥ 75 years compared with younger patients at one, two, and three months after RT. The response was found to be significantly related to the performance status of the patient. Elderly patients should be referred for palliative RT for their painful bone metastases, regardless of age, because they receive equal benefit from treatment.

A study conducted by Culleton et al. (38) evaluated the effect of gender on symptoms among patients with bone metastases controlling for gender-specific malignancies. This retrospective review included 900 patients who received palliative RT and completed the ESAS (n=508) or the BPI (n=392) from 1999 to 2004 at baseline and follow up. In all patients who completed the ESAS, females had significantly greater severity of tiredness, nausea, depression, anxiety, and breathlessness. In sub-analysis when gender-specific primary cancers were removed, no significant differences in ESAS symptoms were found between genders. The BPI walking ability item was significantly worse for females in both the overall and sub-analysis. Females had worse symptoms at follow up prior to the removal of gender specific primaries in both the ESAS and BPI. Conclusions of this study resolved that gender-specific cancers may significantly bias gender studies of cancer-related symptoms when primary tumor type is not taken into account.

Zeng et al. (39) published a study to compare functional interference and pain response outcomes using the BPI for patients treated with palliative RT to spine versus non-spine bones. A total of 386 patients were analyzed, 62% were treated with a SF, 38% with MF. Pain and functional interference scores significantly improved over time in both spine and non-spine sites. At three months, 42% of all patients had a partial response, and 25% had a complete response. Location of bone metastases and RT dose were not predictive factors for pain response or functional interference following radiation treatment.

Discussion

An extensive amount of research has been conducted in the RRRP regarding all aspects of treatment for bone metastases. Studies in the RRRP have focused on QOL in bone metastases patients, optimal treatment regimens, pain flare and its prophylaxis with dexamethasone, and the comparison of different patient populations. Many significant findings have been established based on research in the RRRP.

In terms of QOL research in patients with bone metastases, studies in the RRRP have been successful in defining standards for future clinical trials. In coordination with the EORTC, a bone metastases specific module, the QLQ-BM22, was developed and validated to assess QOL in patients with bone metastases using questions specifically relevant for patients with bone metastases (10). Additionally, research in the RRRP has helped to establish standardized methods of assessing partial and complete response to RT, definitions of meaningful changes in pain scores, and associating verbal descriptors with analogue scales (12, 14, 23). These findings have great significance for future research by allowing large scale reviews and analyses to yield comparable studies and significant results.

Research in the RRRP has also analyzed patterns of practice for RT by radiation oncologists and has compared different fractionation schedules for RT. Research in the RRRP has demonstrated that despite evidence demonstrating SF as equivalent to MF in pain response rate, many practicing radiation oncologists still prescribe MF (7, 26, 32). Research in this area is of great clinical importance, as it would be ideal to balance fewer appointments for patients with efficacy of treatment. Current research in the RRRP is examining the results of patients randomized to either a SF or MF to determine equivalence between the two fractionation schedules on pain relief in re-irradiation.

Another important area of research in the RRRP has investigated pain flare following RT and the prevention of pain flare with the use of steroids. Previous pilot and phase two studies in the RRRP have demonstrated promising results for the use of dexamethasone in pain flare prevention (8, 21). Currently, a randomized trial in the RRRP is underway to assess the efficacy of dexamethasone in the prophylaxis of radiation-induced pain flare when compared with a placebo.

Conclusion

There has been an ample amount of research on bone metastases conducted in the RRRP. Substantial work has been accomplished over the years in the RRRP to aid in the development of a bone metastases specific QOL module, establish standard definitions for RT response and pain assessment, determine ideal RT treatment schedules, and prevent or treat pain flare in patients with bone metastases receiving RT. Further research concerning bone metastases is underway in the RRRP, and should continue to investigate optimal treatment regimens and methods to diminish pain flare in patients with bone metastases treated with RT.

Acknowledgments

We thank the generous support of Bratty Family Fund, Michael and Karyn Goldstein Cancer Research Fund, Joseph and Silvana Melara Cancer Research Fund, and Ofelia Cancer Research Fund.

References

[1] Hird A, Chow E, Zhang L, Wong R, Wu J, Sinclair E, et al. Determining the incidence of pain flare following palliative radiotherapy for symptomatic bone metastases: Results from three canadian cancer centers. Int J Radiat Onc Biol Phys 2009;75(1):193-7.

[2] Tharmalingam S, Chow E, Harris K, Hird A, Sinclair E. Quality of life measurement in bone metastases: A literature review. J Pain Res 2008;1:49-58.

[3] Hird A, Wong R, Flynn C, Hadi S, De Sa E, Zhang L, et al. Impact of pain flare on patients treated with palliative radiotherapy for symptomatic bone metastases. J Pain Manage 2009;2(4):401-6.

[4] Chow E, Wong R, Hruby G, Connolly R, Franssen E, Fung KW, et al. Prospective patient-based assessment of effectiveness of palliative radiotherapy for bone metastases. Radiother Oncol 2001;61(1):77-82.

[5] Berk L. Prospective trials for the radiotherapeutic treatment of bone metastases. Am J Hospice Palliat Med 1995;12(4):24-8.

[6]   Arcangeli G, Giovinazzo G, Saracino B, D'Angelo L, Giannarelli D, Arcangeli G, et al. Radiation therapy in the management of symptomatic bone metastases: The effect of total dose and histology on pain relief and response duration. Int J Radiat Oncol Biol Phys 1998;42(5):1119-26.

[7]   Chow E, Harris K, Fan G, Tsao M, Sze WM. Palliative radiotherapy trials for bone metastases: A systematic review. J Clin Oncol 2007;25(11):1423-36.

[8]   Chow E, Loblaw A, Harris K, Doyle M, Goh P, Chiu H, et al. Dexamethasone for the prophylaxis of radiation-induced pain flare after palliative radiotherapy for bone metastases: A pilot study. Support Care Cancer 2007;15(6):643-7.

[9]   Hird A, Zhang L, Holt T, Fairchild A, DeAngelis C, Loblaw A, et al. Dexamethasone for the prophylaxis of radiation-induced pain flare after palliative radiotherapy for symptomatic bone metastases: A phase II study. Clin Oncol (R Coll Radiol) 2009;21(4):329-35.

[10]   Chow E, Hird A, Velikova G, Johnson C, Dewolf L, Bezjak A, et al. The European Organisation for Research and Treatment of Cancer quality of life questionnaire for patients with bone metastases: The EORTC QLQ-BM22. Eur J Cancer 2009;45(7):1146-52.

[11]   Chow E, Nguyen J, Zhang L, Tseng LM, Hou MF, Fairchild A, et al. International field testing of the reliability and validity of the EORTC QLQ-BM22 module to assess health-related quality of life in patients with bone metastases. Cancer 2012;118(5):1457-65.

[12]   Zeng L, Chow E, Zhang L, Tseng LM, Hou MF, Fairchild A, et al. An international prospective study establishing minimal clinically important differences in the EORTC QLQ-BM22 and QLQ-C30 in cancer patients with bone metastases. Support Care Cancer 2012;20(12):3307-13.

[13]   Campos S, Zhang L, Chow E. Determining reliability of patient perceptions of important bone metastases quality of life issues. J Pain Manage 2009;2(4):453-64.

[14]   Chow E, Hird A, Wong R, Zhang L, Wu J, Barbera L, et al. Validation of meaningful change in pain scores in the treatment of bone metastases. J Pain Manage 2009;2(4):407-11.

[15]   Presutti R, Nguyen J, Hird A, Fairchild A, Clemons M, Kerba M, et al. Bone metastases and quality of life. J Pain Manage 2011;4(1):117-31.

[16]   Khan L, Uy C, Nguyen J, Chow E, Zhang L, Zeng L, et al. Self-reported rates of sleep disturbance in patients with symptomatic bone metastases attending an outpatient radiotherapy clinic. J Palliat Med 2011;14(6):708-14.

[17]   Zeng L, Sahgal A, Zhang L, Koo K, Holden L, Jon F, et al. Patterns of pain and functional improvement in patients with bone metastases after conventional external beam radiotherapy and a telephone validation study. Pain Res Treat 2011; 601720.

[18]   Dennis K, Wong K, Zhang L, Culleton S, Nguyen J, Holden L, et al. Palliative radiotherapy for bone metastases in the last 3 months of life: Worthwhile or futile? Clin Oncol (R Coll Radiol) 2011;23(10):709-15.

[19]   Presutti R, Hird A, DeAngelis C, Fairchild A, Holt T, Loblaw A, et al. Palliative radiotherapy of bone metastases and pain flare. J Pain Manage 2011;4(1):105-1.

[20]   Chow E, Ling A, Davis L, Panzarella T, Danjoux C. Pain flare following external beam radiotherapy and meaningful change in pain scores in the treatment of bone metastases. Radiother Oncol 2005;75(1):64-9.

[21]   Hird A, Zhang L, Holt T, Fairchild A, DeAngelis C, Loblaw A, et al. Dexamethasone for the prophylaxis of radiation-induced pain flare after palliative radiotherapy for symptomatic bone metastases: A phase II study. Clin Oncol (R Coll Radiol) 2009;21(4):329-35.

[22]   Chow E, Culleton S, Kwok S. Conventional radiation treatment and bone metastases. J Pain Manage 2010;4(1):23-32.

[23]   Chow E, Wu JS, Hoskin P, Coia LR, Bentzen SM, Blitzer PH. International consensus on palliative radiotherapy endpoints for future clinical trials in bone metastases. Radiother Oncol. 2002 Sep;64(3):275-80.

[24]   Chow E, Hoskin P, Mitera G, Zeng L, Lutz S, Roos D, et al. Update of the international consensus on palliative radiotherapy endpoints for future clinical trials in bone metastases. Int J Radiat Oncol Biol Phys 2012 ;82(5):1730-7.

[25] Chow E, Davis L, Holden L, Schueller T, Wong R, Hayter C, et al. A comparison of radiation therapy outcomes of bone metastases employing international consensus endpoints and traditional endpoints. Support Cancer Ther 2004;1(3):173-8.

[26] Chow E, Zeng L, Salvo N, Dennis K, Tsao M, Lutz S. Update on the systematic review of palliative radiotherapy trials for bone metastases. Clin Oncol (R Coll Radiol) 2012;24(2):112-24.

[27] Chow E, Doyle M, Li K, Bradley N, Harris K, Hruby G, et al. Mild, moderate, or severe pain categorized by patients with cancer with bone metastases. J Palliat Med 2006;9(4):850-4.

[28] Li KK. Harris K. Hadi S. Chow,E. What should be the optimal cut points for mild, moderate, and severe pain? J Palliat Med 2007;10(6):1338-46.

[29] Li KK, Hadi S, Kirou-Mauro A, Chow E. When should we define the response rates in the treatment of bone metastases by palliative radiotherapy? Clin Oncol (R Coll Radiol) 2008;20(1):83-9.

[30] Chow E, Danjoux C, Wong R, Szumacher E, Franssen E, Fung K, et al. Palliation of bone metastases: A survey of patterns of practice among Canadian radiation oncologists. Radiother Oncol 2000;56(3):305-14.

[31] Bradley NM, Husted J, Sey MS, Sinclair E, Li KK, Husain AF, et al. Did the pattern of practice in the prescription of palliative radiotherapy for the treatment of uncomplicated bone metastases change between 1999 and 2005 at the rapid response radiotherapy program?. Clin Oncol (R Coll Radiol) 2008;20(5):327-36.

[32] Fairchild A, Barnes E, Ghosh S, Ben-Josef E, Roos D, Hartsell W, et al. International patterns of practice in palliative radiotherapy for painful bone metastases: Evidence-based practice?. Int J Radiat Oncol Biol Phys 2009;75(5):1501-10.

[33] Dennis K, Makhani L, Zeng L, Lam H, Chow E. Single fraction conventional external beam radiation therapy for bone metastases: A systematic review of randomised controlled trials. Radiother Oncol 2013;106(1):5-14.

[34] Bedard G, Zeng L, Lam H, Lauzon N, Hicks K, Chow E. Positron emission tomography and bone metastases – A review of the literature. J Pain Manage 2012;5(4):331-345.

[35] Culleton S, Hird A, Nguyen J, Emmenegger U, Verma S, Simmons C, et al. Bisphosphonates in combination with radiotherapy for the treatment of bone metastases: A literature review. J Pain Manage 2009;2(4):375-8.

[36] Hird A, Chow E, Yip D, Ross M, Hadi S, Flynn C, et al. After radiotherapy, do bone metastases from gastrointestinal cancers show response rates similar to those of bone metastases from other primary cancers? Curr Oncol 2008;15(5):219-25.

[37] Campos S, Presutti R, Zhang L, Salvo N, Hird A, Tsao M, et al. Elderly patients with painful bone metastases should be offered palliative radiotherapy. Int J Radiat Oncol Biol Phys 2010;76(5):1500-6.

[38] Culleton S, Dennis K, Koo K, Zhang L, Zeng L, Nguyen J, et al. Gender difference in symptom presentations among patients with bone metastases in gender-specific and gender-neutral primary cancers. World J Oncol 2011;2(3):102-112.

[39] Zeng L, Chow E, Zhang L, Culleton S, Holden L, Jon F, et al. Comparison of pain response and functional interference outcomes between spinal and non-spinal bone metastases treated with palliative radiotherapy. Support Care Cancer 2012;20(3):633-9.

In: Pain Management Yearbook 2013
Editor: Joav Merrick

ISBN: 978-1-63117-944-0
© 2014 Nova Science Publishers, Inc.

Chapter 26

Surgery for pelvic pain in endometriosis

Paul J Yong*, MD, PhD, FRCSC, Innie Chen, MD, FRCSC,
Catherine Allaire, MDCM, FRCSC,
and Christina Williams, MD, FRCSC

Department of Obstetrics and Gynaecology, University of British Columbia and
the BC Women's Centre for Pelvic Pain and Endometriosis, Vancouver,
British Columbia, Canada

Abstract

Endometriosis is a common cause of pelvic pain including dysmenorrhea, chronic pelvic pain, dyspareunia, and dyschezia. Placebo-controlled, blinded, randomized controlled trials have shown that surgery for endometriosis can improve pelvic pain. However, successful surgical management of endometriosis for pelvic pain requires careful selection of the right procedures in appropriately selected patients. In order to make this selection, we first review pre-operative management. We then discuss issues for the different types of surgery: conservative surgery (ablation or excision), adjunct procedures (such as insertion of levonorgestrel-releasing IUD, presacral neurectomy, and ovarian or uterine suspension), and definitive surgery (hysterectomy +/- bilateral salpingo-oophorectomy). Also considered are patients with previous surgery, age and fertility considerations, and sensitization with hyperalgesia and chronic pain syndrome. This information synthesized to help decide whether a patient is a surgical candidate, and if so, which surgery should be offered.

Keywords: Laparoscopy, pelvic pain, endometriosis

* Correspondence: Paul Yong, MD, PhD, FRCSC, Assistant Professor, Department of Obstetrics and Gynaecology, University of British Columbia, Vancouver, Canada. E-mail: pyong@cw.bc.ca.

Introduction

Endometriosis affects approximately 10% of reproductive aged women and can cause pelvic pain including dysmenorrhea, chronic pelvic pain, dyspareunia, and dyschezia (1, 2). It is defined as the endometrial tissue from the inside of the uterus, being found outside of the uterus as superficial implants or deep implants (invasive > 5mm) on the peritoneum, ovaries, bowel, bladder or other organs (1, 2). The successful surgical management of endometriosis for pelvic pain depends on a number of patient-specific factors such as previous surgery, age and desire for fertility. Another patient-specific factor is the presence of neural sensitization. It is thought that endometriosis leads to pain by activating peripheral sensors (nerves), which signal through the spinal cord to the brain, where the signals can be perceived as pain (3-7). In some cases, endometriosis can lead to sensitization: consisting of peripheral sensitization (of the peripheral nerve sensors), central sensitization (of the pathways in the spinal cord and brain), and cross-sensitization (of other structures in the pelvis, such as the bladder, bowel, and musculoskeletal system) (3-7). Sensitization results in a chronic pain syndrome, symptoms in multiple body systems (e.g., bowel, bladder, and musculoskeletal), and hyperalgesia and allodynia on examination (3-7). Thus, a patient can have a myriad of symptoms and findings due to sensitization, but with endometriosis as the underlying cause.

Depending on these patient-specific factors, surgery for endometriosis can be conservative or definitive, with or without adjunct procedures. We define conservative surgical treatment as either excision of endometriosis or ablation of endometriosis. Placebo-controlled, blinded, randomized controlled trials (RCTs) have demonstrated that conservative laparoscopic treatment of endometriosis results in significantly greater pain relief compared to diagnostic laparoscopy only (8). Adjunct surgical treatments include insertion of the levonorgestrel-releasing IUD, presacral neurectomy, ovarian suspension, and uterine suspension. Definitive surgical management is hysterectomy with or without unilateral salpingo-oophorectomy or bilateral salpingo-oophorectomy (BSO).

In this paper, we review the above considerations in the surgical management of endometriosis, with the goal of choosing the right surgery in the patient with endometriosis and pelvic pain.

Pre-operative assessment and management

For women with symptoms of endometriosis, empiric medical management is first-line (1). Medical management with hormonal suppression can provide significant symptom relief for an extended period of time and allow the patient to avoid an invasive procedure. Moreover, up to 50% of patients undergoing conservative surgical treatment of endometriosis will have a re-operation by 5 years (9). Thus, conservative surgical treatment alone cannot be considered a long-term solution in many cases. Furthermore, the fertility benefits of conservative surgical treatment have only been studied up to 9-12 months in RCTs (10), and therefore patients may want to postpone laparoscopic surgery to a time they desire pregnancy. There are also unintended consequences of surgery, such as post-operative adhesions or development of chronic pain from surgical incisions.

However, patients who fail medical management or who are having problems with side-effects may be candidates for conservative surgery. To decide whether a patient should be offered laparoscopy, we perform detailed history taking (with the aid of standardized and validated questionnaires) and physical examination. Physical assessment includes screening musculoskeletal exam (e.g., for pelvic girdle pain) (4,11), abdominal exam (including Carnett's test for abdominal wall pain) (12), digital pelvic exam for nodularity (thickening due to deep endometriosis), and endovaginal ultrasound (EVUS)-assisted pain mapping (13). EVUS-assisted pain mapping begins with single-digit pelvic exam to look for tenderness: we palpate the levator ani, bladder base, cervix and uterus, and then the para-cervical (adnexal) regions, both uterosacrals and cul-de-sac. This is then repeated with an EVUS probe to palpate the same areas, using the ultrasound to visualize the pelvic organs and confirm the areas being palpated and found to be tender. EVUS is also used to look for nodules of deep endometriosis and for ovarian endometriosis cysts (endometriomas). Putting together information from the history and physical, we estimate the probability the patient has endometriosis (14), allowing the clinician and patient to decide whether laparoscopy is a reasonable option.

On history, moderate-to-severe dysmenorrhea alone is a significant risk factor for endometriosis (14), and in itself, could be considered an indication for laparoscopy in patients who have failed medical management. The presence of chronic pelvic pain, deep dyspareunia, dyschezia, and/or infertility, also provides indications for offering laparoscopy (14). Some of these women will have been referred with marked symptoms from other visceral organs (e.g., diarrhea and/or constipation, and urinary frequency and urgency) and have been told that endometriosis is unlikely. However, even if patients have concurrent symptoms in other body systems, we do not consider this to be contraindication to offering laparoscopy as long as dysmenorrhea or other gynaecologic symptoms are present.

It is recognized that symptoms in other body systems can be the result of cross-sensitization in the sensitized patient (7). In particular, studies have found that conditions such as irritable bowel syndrome (IBS) or painful bladder syndrome (PBS) can co-exist with endometriosis (15,16). On examination, most patients with dysmenorrhea and/or other gynaecologic symptoms will have findings on pelvic exam (nodularity and/or tenderness). Patients who have a combination of moderate-to-severe dysmenorrhea and tenderness or nodularity on exam are very likely to have endometriosis and are good candidates for laparoscopy (14).

Conservative surgery and adjunct procedures

In women who choose surgery, laparoscopy is preferred to laparotomy because greater magnification allows recognition of subtle lesions and more precise treatment, and there is reduced trauma to tissues and adhesion formation. However, there is controversy about the type of conservative laparoscopic treatment: that is, whether excision of endometriosis and ablation of endometriosis differ in outcomes. Two RCTs showed no significant differences between excision and ablation although they were limited by sample size (17, 18). It is likely that both modalities are equivalent for most superficial endometriosis, as ablation should be able to completely destroy such superficial lesions. However, there may be a difference for deep endometriosis, which may not be completely destroyed by ablation. For ovarian endometriosis cysts, excision results in lower recurrence rates than ablation (1).

In our experience, three to four laparoscopic ports are necessary for safe and complete treatment of endometriosis. The extra instruments allow retraction of bowel away from the operative site and placement of tissues on stretch which aides with excisional procedures. We prefer excision over ablation for several reasons. First, it allows for histological confirmation in all suspected sites of endometriosis. Second, excision allows treatment of endometriosis near or on visceral structures (e.g., ureter, bladder, bowel), by incising the peritoneum and mobilizing the structure away from the lesion. We use monopolar electrosurgery and a micro-needle tip instrument. Brief pulses of energy are used to ensure safety. All suspected lesions are excised, including very subtle or atypical areas, with particular focus on those structures that were tender on EVUS-assisted pain mapping. Using these procedures, we found a re-operation rate of 10% in a cross-sectional study of our patients (19). Other energy modalities (e.g., laser) are expected to be equivalent. Cold excision of endometriosis (with scissors in the absence of energy) can be considered when very near the ureter or bowel, or for excision of ovarian endometriosis cysts where electrosurgery can damage adjacent ovarian tissue. However, cold excision will result in more bleeding which may negatively impact visualization and may be more adhesiogenic.

For endometriosis on the pelvic sidewall, the ovaries can often hinder visualization. An instrument can be used to retract ovary, or an ovarian suspension suture placed (20). We use a suture on a straight needle, which is put directly through the abdominal wall into the peritoneal cavity. The needle is then put through the ovarian cortex, and back out through the abdomen wall about 2 cm from the entry point. The suture is pulled up to put the ovary on tension, lifting it towards the abdominal wall and off the pelvic sidewall, and then clamped externally at the abdomen. This saves one instrument from being used only for retraction. We will often tie the suture at the end of the case, suspending the ovaries off the sidewall, and cut the sutures at 1 week post-op. We believe this prevents the ovaries from attaching to an inflamed peritoneal resection site, and allows the peritoneum to heal over before the suspension suture is cut. Patients will feel a pulling sensation with the suspension suture, but this disappears once the suture is cut. There is a RCT in-progress evaluating ovarian suspension (21).

Uterine suspension has been studied in the context of symptomatic uterine suspension retroversion, showing good symptom relief in observational studies, particularly for dyspareunia (22-24). If patients are found to have a tender retroverted fundus in the cul-de-sac on pre-operative exam, then we offer uterine suspension at the time of surgery. Uterine suspension can also be considered intra-operatively to aid in retraction, by placing a suture through the fundus and then to abdominal wall, similar to the ovarian suspension suture. However, we find that this is rarely necessary, as modern uterine manipulators offer excellent retraction.

For patients who have a radiologic evidence of adenomyosis, significant dysmenorrhea, central chronic pelvic pain, and/or significant cervical or uterine tenderness, we offer insertion of the levonorgestrel-releasing IUD at the time of surgery because these findings suggest an uterine origin of the pain. The endometriumal inside the uterus is known to be abnormal in endometriosis (25), and is not accessible by laparoscopy; thus, the levonorgestrel-releasing IUD is an attempt to treat the uterine endometrium. RCTs support the use of the levonorgestrel-releasing IUD in combination with surgery (26). If endometriosis lesions are present centrally (e.g., above or below the uterus), they may also contribute to dysmenorrhea-type pain (27-28) and thus conservative surgery alone may also improve dysmenorrhea symptoms to some degree (29).

Procedures in patients with prior conservative surgery

In the patient who had a previous laparoscopy with conservative treatment of endometriosis, and who presents with recurrence of symptoms, we perform detailed pre-operative assessment as above. It is important to rule out other conditions that may be causing symptoms mimicking endometriosis, including IBS, PBS, abdominal wall pain, and pelvic girdle pain. However, even if tenderness is found on pain mapping, it may not be 100% predictive of a recurrence of endometriosis. In these circumstances, a repeat exam on another day to ensure the findings are reproducible can be very helpful. Even if reproducible, tenderness in these regions can indicate recurrent endometriosis, but can also be due to referred pain from other structures (e.g., referred from the musculoskeletal system). In these circumstances, it is prudent to offer medical management first, and laparoscopy only if pain persists. Exceptions to this rule would include patients whose previous laparoscopic treatment of endometriosis was clearly incomplete (as noted on the operative note, e.g., lesions near the ureter left untreated) or who have palpable nodularity (deep endometriosis) or an ovarian endometriosis cyst on ultrasound.

For patients with a previous conservative laparoscopic treatment of endometriosis, and who have a recurrence of symptoms, fail medical management and opt for repeat conservative laparoscopy, the use of adjunct surgical procedures should be considered. In patients with adenomyosis, significant dysmenorrhea, central chronic pelvic pain, and/or cervical and uterine tenderness on exam, the levonorgestrel-releasing IUD can be offered. If the patient has previously tried the levonorgestrel-releasing IUD but did not improve, then presacral neurectomy (30-31) can be offered for those who desire uterine conservation and future fertility. Patients should be counseled about the risk of bowel and bladder dysfunction (e.g., constipation and urinary urgency) with presacral neurectomy (31).

Definitive surgery and its impacts

Some younger women with previous conservative laparoscopy for endometriosis, and who have a recurrence of symptoms and fail medical management, may desire more definitive management (hysterectomy +/- BSO). In these circumstances, it is important to again rule out other conditions that may be causing their symptoms. GnRH agonists can be offered for both diagnostic and therapeutic purposes: if symptoms are markedly better with amenorrhea achieved with GnRH agonist, then definitive surgery is expected to be more beneficial. We ask young patients to meet with our reproductive counselor and to write a letter clearly explaining their understanding of the procedure and its implications. For hysterectomy, there is the loss of fertility, including assisted fertility (except with IVF and a surrogate).

If the patient is parous, then hysterectomy is more reasonable, but there will be a few nulliparous patients who will request hysterectomy at a young age. If hysterectomy is likely to be helpful and other conditions have been ruled-out (or treated), and if they understand the implications and that it cannot be 100% guaranteed that their pain will be completely cured, then hysterectomy can be offered. Hysterectomy is effective for endometriosis, with one study found a re-operation rate of 13.4% at 5 years after hysterectomy for endometriosis (9). In almost all cases, hysterectomy can be done laparoscopically. Even if the hysterectomy could be done completely vaginally, it is important that the procedure be laparoscopic-assisted in order to treat any concurrent endometriosis.

Performing a hysterectomy and leaving behind residual endometriosis (especially with ovarian conservation) is less likely to be effective (32). We also prefer to remove the cervix, as we have anecdotally seen the cervix become a source of pelvic pain in some patients after supracervical/subtotal hysterectomy.

A small proportion of younger women will ask for salpingo-oophorectomy in addition to hysterectomy. If much of the pain is lateralizing (i.e., right- or left-sided), then unilateral salpingo-oophorectomy can be offered, especially if the adnexa is tender on EVUS-assisted pain mapping. A few younger patients will desire "pelvic silence" with hysterectomy BSO. We discourage this for a number of reasons. First, one study found that although adding BSO to hysterectomy somewhat reduced the risk of reoperation at 5 years (to ~10%), this benefit was not observed for ages 30-39 years (9). The second consideration is the importance of ovarian function for cardiovascular, bone, and mental health, as well as for survival (33). However, there will the occasional younger patient with known endometriosis who has failed all other treatments who will still want hysterectomy BSO. If the patient is parous, then the decision is a little easier, but some patients will be nulliparous.

We again ask the patient to meet with our reproductive counselor and to write a clear letter describing understanding of all the implications, specifically the consequences of surgical menopause, the need for HRT until approximately age 50 years, and the total loss of fertility (including IVF and surrogacy being no longer an option). Sometimes a phone appointment with the patient's family physician can provide additional insight. Ultimately, if the patient has endometriosis and desires hysterectomy BSO, and the procedure likely to be helpful, we will allow the patient to make the choice although BSO will be discouraged.

For older women, conservative laparoscopy can be offered, whether or not they have had a previous conservative laparoscopy of endometriosis, with similar considerations as for younger patients. However, hysterectomy is more readily offered in the older population, especially for those experiencing dysfunctional bleeding.

Unilateral oophorectomy can also be more liberally considered in this population, particularly if the pain is lateralizing and the adnexa is tender on pain mapping. If the patient is in their mid- to-late 40's (and certainly, if in their 50's), then BSO can be offered at the same time. We learn towards ovarian conservation in the early 40's, as there may be a health and survival benefit (33), although BSO can be done in this age group if the endometriosis and symptoms are significant and the patient desires definitive surgery.

Procedures in patients with previous hysterectomy

For patients who had a previous hysterectomy with or without unilateral salpingo-oophorectomy or BSO, and who have recurrence of symptoms, detailed assessment is required to rule-out or treat other causes such as IBS, PBS, or musculoskeletal dysfunction. If endometriosis is suspected – such as patients in whom endometriosis was not completely treated at the time of hysterectomy, who have focal tenderness or palpable nodularity at the vault, or who have an endometrioma in a conserved ovary – these patients can be offered laparoscopy. Excision is recommended, as anatomy can be distorted, often requiring careful dissection and mobilization of the ureter and other structures in order to safely treat the recurrent endometriosis. In addition to recurrence of endometriosis, post-operative adhesions can also cause of pain (especially if the hysterectomy was done by laparotomy), residual ovaries can be entrapped (or retroperitoneal), or an ovarian remnant can be left behind after a previous attempted BSO (diagnosed by pre-menopausal FSH/estradiol and/or ultrasound). These causes can also be treated at the time of laparoscopy.

Sensitized patient

The sensitized patient, regardless of age, presents a clinically challenging scenario. In most circumstances, we recommend multidisciplinary care before considering surgery. Such patients usually have global hyperalgesia on pain mapping, and it must be explained to the patient that surgery is not optimal when much of the tenderness on exam is due to neural sensitization. The only exception may be the patient who has never had a laparoscopy and in whom endometriosis is suspected. Such patients can be offered laparoscopy to make the diagnosis and to treat it, in combination with multidisciplinary care. However, it should be explained that surgery in the sensitized state may mean a more difficult recovery and perhaps even a poorer clinical response.

We utilize the following multidisciplinary care for sensitized patients. For those with IBS, recommendations include dietary changes (with the help of a dietician), tricyclics (first-line nortriptyline), pinaverium bromide (Dicetel, a gastrointestinal calcium channel blocker), and referral for colonoscopy if there are risk factors for other bowel conditions (e.g., family history of colon cancer and hematochezia). For those with PBS, recommendations include dietary changes ("interstitial cystitis diet"), tricyclics, Elmiron, anti-histamines, and referral for cystoscopy if there are risk factors for bladder pathology (e.g., history of smoking and hematuria). Referral to an urologist with expertise in PBS can also provide bladder instillation therapies.

Even for patients without IBS or PBS, tricyclics can be helpful to reduce nerve sensitization. Other neuromodulatory medications that we use include gabapentin, pregabalin, and duloxetine. These neuromodulators may not only be helpful for reducing sensitization and ameliorating symptoms, but if continued in the peri-operative period, may assist with reducing post-operative pain and surgical recovery. Muscle relaxants can also be helpful. For example, vaginal diazepam (compounded) 2.5-10mg every 8 hours as needed can be well tolerated and effective for sensitized patients who have myofascial pelvic pain, pelvic floor tenderness, and/or vaginismus on examination.

Physiotherapy is critical for sensitized patients (11, 34-35). This includes specific recommendations for pelvic girdle pain [11]. Abdominal wall myofascial trigger points can be treated with manual therapy. Treatment of vaginismus and a tender pelvic floor can also be very helpful. Physiotherapy also helps patient to reduce kinesiophobia and appropriately increase activity. It is unclear if physiotherapy is best employed before and/or after surgery in sensitized patients. Pre-operative physiotherapy should help to decrease sensitization, and therefore may improve post-op pain with quicker recovery. Alternatively, physiotherapy post-operatively may help with reducing any residual sensitization after removal of the underlying cause of the sensitization (i.e., endometriosis).

We also employ small group workshops for cognitive behavioural therapy (CBT) and mindfulness meditation, in order to reduce sensitization (36, 37). Pre-operative CBT and mindfulness can be useful in patients with acute anxiety, depression, and/or catastrophizing. If these factors can be reduced before surgery, in particular catastrophizing and pre-operative pain due to sensitization, the success of surgery is likely to be increased specifically a reduction in post-surgical pain (38). CBT and mindfulness post-operatively can help patients prevent recurrence of sensitization in the future. There is also a social work element to surgery for endometriosis and pelvic pain. Part of patient optimization is to try to connect patients to community resources, especially for patients that are isolated and unable to work. If a patient's social situation has been stabilized, surgery is more likely to be successful and the post-operative recovery to be easier.

We also employ various needling procedures, such as trigger point infiltration with local anesthetic (4), dry needling and intra-muscular stimulation (IMS) (4), and prolotherapy (39), although these procedures require more study. Specifically, it is unclear whether these therapies are effective in endometriosis and pelvic pain, and whether they should be pursued pre- and/or post-operatively.

Conclusion

In conclusion, choosing the right surgery in the appropriate patient is critical in endometriosis and pelvic pain. Factors important in this decision making include conservative or definitive surgery, age, desire for fertility, previous surgery, and sensitization. More research is needed to guide peri-operative decision making in endometriosis surgery.

References

[1]   Leyland N, Casper R, Laberge P, Singh SS; SOGC. Endometriosis: diagnosis and management. J Obstet Gynaecol Can 2010;32(7Suppl2):S1-S32.
[2]   Koninckx PR, Ussia A, Adamyan L, Wattiez A, Donnez J. Deep endometriosis: definition, diagnosis, and treatment. Fertil Steril 2012;98(3):564-71.
[3]   Jarrell JF, Vilos GA, SOGC. Consensus guidelines for the management of chronic pelvic pain. J Obstet Gynaecol Can 2005;27(8):781–801.

[4]   Jarrell JF, Vilos GA, SOGC. Consensus guidelines for the management of chronic pelvic pain. J Obstet Gynaecol Can 2005;27(9):869–87.

[5]   Fraser IS. Mysteries of endometriosis pain: Chien-Tien Hsu Memorial Lecture 2009. J Obstet Gynaecol Res 2010;36(1):1-10.

[6]   Stratton P, Berkley KJ. Chronic pelvic pain and endometriosis: translational evidence of the relationship and implications. Hum Reprod Update 2011;17(3):327-46.

[7]   Malykhina AP. Neural mechanisms of pelvic organ cross-sensitization. Neuroscience 2007;149:660-72.

[8]   Jacobson TZ, Duffy JMN, Barlow D, Koninckx PR, Garry R. Laparoscopic surgery for pelvic pain associated with endometriosis. Cochrane Database Syst Rev 2009;4:CD001300.

[9]   Shakiba K, Bena JF, McGill KM, Minger J, Falcone T. Surgical treatment of endometriosis: A 7-year follow-up on the requirement for further surgery. Obstet Gynecol 2008;111(6):1285-92.

[10]   Jacobson TZ, Duffy JMN, Barlow D, Farquhar C, Koninckx PR, Olive D. Laparoscopic surgery for subfertility associated with endometriosis. Cochrane Database Syst Rev 2010;1:CD001398.

[11]   Vleeming A, Albert AB, Ostgaard CH, Sturesson B, Stuge B. European guidelines for the diagnosis and treatment of pelvic girdle pain. Eur Spine J 2008;17:794–819.

[12]   Suleiman S, Johnston DE. The abdominal wall: an overlooked source of pain. Am Fam Physician 2001;64:431-8.

[13]   Yong PJ, Sutton C, Suen M, Williams C. Endovaginal ultrasound-assisted pain mapping in endometriosis and chronic pelvic pain. J Obstet Gynaecol, in press.

[14]   Whitehill K, Yong PJ, Williams C. Clinical predictors of endometriosis in the infertility population: is there a better way to determine who needs a laparoscopy? J Obstet Gynaecol Can 2012;34(6):552-7.

[15]   Seaman HE, Ballard KD, Wright JT, de Vries CS. Endometriosis and its coexistence with irritable bowel syndrome and pelvic inflammatory disease: findings from a national case-control study—Part 2. BJOG 2008;115(11):1392-6.

[16]   Paulson JD, Delgado M. The relationship between interstitial cystitis and endometriosis in patients with chronic pelvic pain. JSLS 2007;11(2):175-81.

[17]   Wright J, Lotfallah H, Jones K, Lovell D. A randomized trial of excision versus ablation for mild endometriosis. Fertil Steril 2005;83(6):1830-6.

[18]   Healey M, Ang WC, Cheng C. Surgical treatment of endometriosis: a prospective randomized double-blinded trial comparing excision and ablation. Fertil Steril 2010; 94(7):2536-40.

[19]   Taylor E, Williams C. Surgical treatment of endometriosis: location and patterns of disease at reoperation. Fertil Steril 2010;93(1):57-61.

[20]   Abuzeid MI, Ashraf M, Shamma FN. Temporary ovarian suspension at laparoscopy for prevention of adhesions. J Am Assoc Gynecol Laparosc 2002; 9(1):98-102.

[21]   Hoo WL, Saridogan E, Cutner A, Pandis G, Jurkovic D. Effectiveness of ovarian suspension in preventing post-operative ovarian adhesions in women with pelvic endometriosis: a randomised controlled trial. BMC Women's Health 20011;11:14.

[22]   Batioglu S, Zeyneloglu HB. Laparoscopic placation and suspension of the round ligament for chronic pelvic pain and dyspareunia. J Am Assoc Gynecol Laparosc 2000;7(4):547-51.

[23]   Ou CS, Liu YH, Joki JA, Rowbotham R. Laparoscopic uterine suspension by round ligament placation. J Reprod Med 2003;47(3):211-6.

[24]   Perry CP, Presthus J, Nieves A. Laparoscopic uterine suspension for pain relief: A multicenter study. J Reprod Med 2005;50(8):567-70.

[25]   Carvalho L, Podgaec S, Bellodi-Privato M, Falcone T, Abrão MS. Role of eutopic endometrium in pelvic endometriosis. J Minim Invasive Gynecol 2011;18(4):419-27.

[26]   Abou-Setta AM, Al-Inany HG, Farquhar C. Levonorgestrel-releasing intrauterine device (LNG-IUD) for symptomatic endometriosis following surgery. Cochrane Database Syst Rev 2006;4:CD005072.

[27]   Burney RO, Giudice LC. Pathogenesis and pathophysiology of endometriosis. Fertil Steril 2012;98(3):511-9.

[28]   Brosens IA. Endometriosis – a disease because it is characterized by bleeding. Am J Obstet Gynecol 1997;176(2):263-7.

[29]   Roman JD. Surgical treatment of endometriosis in private practice: cohort study with mean follow-up of 3 years. J Minim Invasive Gynecol 2010;17(1):42-6.

[30]   Yeung PP Jr, Shwayder J, Pasic RP. Laparoscopic management of endometriosis: comprehensive review of best evidence. J Minim Invasive Gynecol 2009;16(3):269-81.

[31]   Proctor M, Latthe P, Farquhar C, Khan K, Johnson N. Surgical interruption of pelvic nerve pathways for primary and secondary dysmenorrhoea. Cochrane Database Syst Rev 2005;4:CD001896.

[32]   Clayton RD, Hawe JA, Love JC, Wilkinson N, Garry R. Recurrent pain after hysterectomy and bilateral salpingo-oophorectomy for endometriosis: evaluation of laparoscopic excision of endometriosis. Br J Obstet Gynaecol 1999;106(7):740-4.

[33]   Erekson EA, Martin DK, Ratner ES. Oophorectomy: the debate between ovarian conservation and elective oophorectomy. Menopause 2013;20(1):110-4.

[34]   Apte G, Nelson P, Brismee JM, Dedrick G, Justiz R 3rd, Sizer PS Jr. Chronic female pelvic pain – part 1: clinical pathoanatomy and examination of the pelvic region. Pain Pract 2012;12(2):88-110.

[35]   Apte G, Nelson P, Brismee JM, Dedrick G, Justiz R 3rd, Sizer PS Jr. Chronic female pelvic pain – part 2: differential diagnosis and management. Pain Pract 2012;12(2):111-41.

[36]   Nash VR, Ponto J, Townsend C, Nelson P, Bretz MN. Cognitive behavioral therapy, self-efficacy, and depression in persons with chronic pain. Pain Manag Nurs 2012 Dec 27. [Epub ahead of print].

[37]   Wong SY, Chan FW, Wong RL, Chu MC, Kitty Lam YY, Mercer SW, Ma SH. Comparing the effectiveness of mindfulness-based stress reduction and multidisciplinary intervention programs for chronic pain: a randomized comparative trial. Clin J Pain 2011;27(8):724-34.

[38]   Pinto PR, McIntyre T, Almeida A, Arauljo-Soares V. The mediating role of pain catastrophizing in the relationship between presurgical anxiety and acute postsurgical pain after hysterectomy. Pain 2012;153(1):218-26.

[39]   Goswami A. Prolotherapy. J Pain Palliat Care Pharmacother 2012;26(4):376-8.

In: Pain Management Yearbook 2013
Editor: Joav Merrick

ISBN: 978-1-63117-944-0
© 2014 Nova Science Publishers, Inc.

Chapter 27

Mindfulness training does not reduce inflammatory cytokine levels in chronic tension-type headache

Stuart Cathcart, PhD[*1]*, Chris Della Vedova, PhD*[2],
Maarten Immink, PhD[3]*, Michael Proeve, PhD*[4]
and John Hayball, PhD[2]

[1]Centre for Applied Psychology, Faculty of Health, University of Canberra
[2]School of Pharmacy and Medical Sciences, University of South Australia
[3]School of Health Sciences, University of South Australia
[4]School of Psychology, University of Adelaide, Australia

Abstract

To examine effects of mindfulness training on serum pro-inflammatory cytokine levels in chronic tension-type headache (CTH) sufferers. Method: Forty-three CTH sufferers participated in a randomized wait-list controlled trial of a mindfulness intervention for headache. Serum concentrations of cytokines IL1-β, IL-2, IL-6, IL-8, IL-12, IL-18, IFN-γ, MCP-1 and TNF-α were measured before and after treatment/wait-list control conditions. Results: Repeated Measures Analysis of Variance revealed that IL1-β, IL-6, IL-8, MCP-1 and TNF-α decreased from pre to post assessments in the treatment and wait-list groups, with no group or group x time effects. Conclusions: Mindfulness training compared to a wait-list control condition does not reduce serum cytokine levels in CTH sufferers.

Keywords: Mindfulness, headache, cytokines, randomized controlled trial

---

* Correspondence: Stuart Cathcart, PhD, Centre for Applied Psychology, University of Canberra, Bruce 2601, Australia. E-mail: stuart.cathcart@canberra.edu.au.

Introduction

Mindfulness training has been reported as beneficial for reducing symptoms in several chronic pain conditions, including headache (1,2). One potential mechanism for the therapeutic effects of mindfulness may be a reduction in pro-inflammatory cytokine (PIC) levels. Cytokines are regulatory proteins secreted by numerous cells including immune cells in the periphery and microglia in the Central Nervous System (CNS). Pro-inflammatory cytokines are involved in both stress and pain processing (3,4), and are increased in several chronic pain conditions, including headache (5,6). Mindfulness-based interventions have been shown to reduce PIC levels in healthy and clinical samples (7,8), however this has not been examined in CTH sufferers to date.

Elsewhere we reported elevated PIC levels in the present sample of CTH sufferers (9), and a reduction in headache activity following mindfulness intervention (10). The present study examines if the mindfulness intervention reduced PIC levels in that sample of CTH sufferers.

Methods

Participant information has been reported in detail elsewhere (9,10). Briefly, Fifty-eight volunteers satisfying diagnosis of CTH were recruited from the general population and completed pre-treatment measures. Forty-three participants completed post-treatment measures (N=24 treatment, N=19 wait-list). Volunteers were excluded if they reported any chronic pain other than CTH, satisfied other headache diagnoses including migraine or suspected Medication Overuse Headache, or had major medical or psychiatric diagnoses concurrent or in the past 12 months. The mean age of the total sample was 45.5 years (SD=13.8), 37% were male.

Measures

Blood samples (9mL) were collected via venepuncture by a phlebotomist nurse at the School of Psychology, University of South Australia. All participants had their blood taken between 9am and 11am, to control for circadian variation in cytokine levels. Samples were collected in ethylenediaminetetracetic acid (EDTA) and serum clotting tubes, and transported in biohazard containers to the Experimental Therapeutics Laboratory, Hanson Institute. The tubes were centrifuged at 2,500 x g for 10 minutes at room temperature, and the blood components (serum, plasma, buffy coat cells) were aliquoted separately (500µL) into labelled 1.8mL cryovials (Nunc, Roskilde, Denmark). The cryovials were placed into liquid nitrogen to snap freeze, and stored at -70oC before analysis.

Determination of cytokine levels

Cytokine levels in serum samples were analyzed using an established cytometric bead array kit (FlowCytomix; Bender MedSystems, Vienna, Austria) according to the manufacturers' instructions. The kit reagents were diluted 1:2 for each run, and all samples were run in duplicate. Standard curves for each cytokine were included in each run, and sample concentrations were calculated using FlowCytomix Pro software.

Intervention

The intervention was based on Mindfulness-Based Stress Reduction (MBSR) and Mindfulness Based Cognitive Therapy (MBCT), and is detailed elsewhere (10). Delivered by one of the authors (MI), the intervention involved six 1-hour group classes held twice per week for three weeks, and 30mins daily home practice. The program was developed by some of the authors (SC, MP, MI) who are psychologists (SC, MP) with formal training and teaching, practice, and research experience in mindfulness and/or meditation.

Three formal mindfulness meditation practices were taught: 1) body scan meditation, which involves focusing on each region of the body systemically from the foot to the head, and noticing the sensations that are present with openness and curiosity; 2) formal sitting meditation, focusing on mindfulness of breath and other experiences such as sounds and thoughts; 3) three-minute breathing space, which involves three sequential steps of a) focusing awareness of present internal experiences, b) focusing awareness on the breath, and c) expanding awareness to the body as a whole.

Home practice was supported by a written instruction manual and a compact disc containing audio-recorded instructions. The program also included other activities so that participants could practice applying concepts of mindfulness to activities of daily living, recognizing nourishing and draining activities, and documenting observations and reactions to pleasant and unpleasant events.

Procedures

The study was approved by the University of South Australia Human Research Ethics Committee. Following a screening interview and provision of written consent to participate, volunteers completed questionnaires and had blood drawn for cytokine analysis. Headache sufferers were then randomly assigned to either treatment or wait-list conditions. Post-treatment measures were recorded in all CTH participants in the week following completion of the intervention by the treatment group. The wait-list control group commenced mindfulness training the following week.

Results

Repeated Measures Analysis of Variance results (table 1) yielded significant Time effects indicating a decrease from pre to post assessments for IL1-β (F (1,41) = 9.65, p < .01, η=.15), IL-6 (F (1,41) = 15.56, p < .01, η=.22), IL-8 (F (1,41) = 5.13, p < .04, η=.10), MCP-1 (F (1,41) = 10.66, p < .01, η=.17) and TNF-α (F (1,41) = 11.54, p < .01, η=.18). Group and Group x Time effects were not significant for any measure (all p>.05).

Table 1. Cytokine levels before and after mindfulness intervention and wait-list control conditions in chronic tension-type headache sufferers

Measure[1]	Mindfulness group N=24				Wait-list group N=19				Test value[2]		
	Pre		Post		Pre		Post				
	Mean	SD	Mean	SD	Mean	SD	Mean	SD	Group effect	Time effect	G x T effect
IL-1β	3.59	.53	2.57	1.95	3.56	.62	3.03	1.48	.42	9.65**	.98
IL-2	2.53	1.19	1.81	1.89	2.26	.50	2.17	1.10	.05	3.11	1.93
IL-6	15.22	1.95	10.09	7.59	14.77	1.97	12.12	5.66	.65	15.56**	1.57
IL-8	35.08	110.9	24.32	85.17	14.46	9.59	11.85	9.11	.62	5.13*	1.91
IL-12	1.74	.46	1.27	.98	1.70	.46	1.65	.88	1.27	3.63	2.28
IL-18	1.05	.93	.85	.95	.92	1.01	.70	.92	.48	1.43	.01
IFN-γ	1.66	.38	1.31	1.03	1.62	.48	1.63	.88	.91	1.44	1.57
MCP-1	223.76	99.68	159.38	151.11	278.10	153.70	230.79	203.74	2.81	10.66**	.25
TNF-α	6.40	.81	4.41	3.30	6.21	.83	5.31	2.56	.66	11.54**	1.67

[1.] Serum cytokine levels (mean fluorescent intensity) IL-1β; Interleukin 1-beta, IL-2; interleukin-2, IL-6; interleukin-6, IL-8; interleukin-8, IL-12; interleukin-12p70, IL-18; interleukin-18, IFN-γ; interferon-γ, MCP-1; Monocyte Chemoattractant Protein-1, TNF-α; Tumour Necrosis Factor-alpha.

[2.] Repeated measures analysis of variance F value, all df=1,41.

* p<.05, **p<.01.

Discussion

To our knowledge, this is the first study to examine effects of mindfulness training on pro-inflammatory cytokines in CTH sufferers. The results indicate a pre to post treatment reduction in several of the PIC's examined, in both the treatment and wait-list groups, with no difference between groups. This indicates that mindfulness training compared to a wait-list control group does not reduce PIC levels in CTH sufferers. Elsewhere we have reported that the mindfulness training reduced headache activity in this sample of CTH sufferers (10). Although we did not presently examine relationships between headache activity and PIC's, the findings suggest the therapeutic effect of the intervention previously observed was not due to a reduction in PIC levels. The results also call in to question previous uncontrolled findings of effects of mindfulness training on cytokines (e.g., 8). The cause of the decrease in PICs in the treatment and wait-list groups is unclear. One possibility is non-specific effects common to both treatment and wait-list conditions (e.g., expectancy). Alternatively, the reduction in PIC levels may be coincidental.

Limitations to the present study include the brief nature of our intervention, the lack of an active control group, and the lack of longer-term follow-up. The lack of significant findings is unlikely due to low power associated with the small sample size, since time effects were observed and there were no trends indicating a group x time effect. The above limitations withstanding, the present results indicate that mindfulness training, elsewhere shown to reduce headache activity in this sample of CTH sufferers, does not reduce PIC levels in the same sample. Replication and extension of the present results would further understanding of the importance of PICs in, and the mechanisms of mindfulness intervention for, CTH.

Acknowledgments

The authors are grateful to Nicola Galatis and Margaret Mitchell for assistance in data collection. This research was funded in part by a Medical Advances without Animals Trust grant.

This study is registered with the Australian and New Zealand Clinical Trials Registry, number ACTRN12610001039077

References

[1]   Morone NE, Greco CM, Weiner DK. Mindfulness meditation for the treatment of chronic low back pain in older adults: a randomized controlled pilot study. Pain 2008;134:310-9.

[2]   Kabat-Zinn J, Lipworth L, Burney R. The clinical use of mindfulness meditation for the self-regulation of chronic pain. J Behav Med 1985;8:163-90.

[3]   Chapman C, Tuckett R, Song C. Pain and stress in a systems perspective: Reciprocal neural, endocrine, and immune interactions. J Pain 2008;9(2):122-45.

[4]   Marchand F, Perretti M and McMahon SB. Role of the immune system in chronic pain. Nat Rev Neurosci 2005;6:521-32.

[5]   Bazzichi L, Rossi A, Massimetti G, Giannaccini G, Giuliano T, De Feo F, Ciapparelli A, Dell'Osso L, Bombardieri S. Cytokine patterns in fibromyalgia and their correlation with clinical manifestations. Clin Exp Rheumatol 2007;25:225–30.

[6]   Koçer A, Koçer E, Memişoğullari R, Domaç FM, Yüksel H. Interleukin-6 levels in tension headache patients. Clin J Pain 2010;26(8):690-3.

[7]   Koh KB, Lee Y, Beyn KM, Chu SH, Kim DM. Counter-stress effects of relaxation on proinflammatory and anti-inflammatory cytokines. Brain Behav Immun 2008;22(8):1130-7.

[8]   Carlson LE, Speca M, Faris P et al. One year pre-post intervention follow-up of psychological, immune, endocrine and blood pressure outcomes of mindfulness-based stress reduction (MBSR) in breast and prostate cancer outpatients. Brain Behav Immun 2007 21(8):1038-49.

[9]   Della-Vedova, C. Cathcart, S. Dohnalek, A., Immink, M. & Hayball, J. Peripheral interleukin-1 Beta and Interleukin-18 levels are elevated in Chronic Tension-Type Headache. Pain Res Manage, in press.

[10]   Cathcart S, Galatis N, Immink M, Proeve M, Petkov J. Brief mindfulness-based meditation for chronic tension-type headache: A randomized controlled trial. Behav Cog Psychother, in press.

In: Pain Management Yearbook 2013
Editor: Joav Merrick

ISBN: 978-1-63117-944-0
© 2014 Nova Science Publishers, Inc.

Chapter 28

The Functional Assessment of Cancer Therapy – Brain (FACT-Br) for assessing quality of life in patients with brain metastases: A comparison of recall periods

Nemica Thavarajah, BSc(C)[1], Gillian Bedard, BSc(C)[1],
Liying Zhang, PhD[1], David Cella, PhD[2],
Jennifer L Beaumont, MSc[2], May Tsao, MD[1],
Elizabeth Barnes, MD[1], Cyril Danjoux, MD[1], Arjun Sahgal, MD[1],
Hany Soliman, MD[1] and Edward Chow, MBBS[1]*

[1]Sunnybrook Health Sciences Centre, University of Toronto, Toronto, Ontario, Canada
[2]Northwestern University, Chicago, Illinois, US

Abstract

To assess the use of the Functional Assessment of Cancer Therapy - Brain (FACT-Br) to assess quality of life (QOL) in patients with brain metastases based on a recall period of 24 hours by assessing its predictive value of the past seven days. Brain metastases patients were interviewed using the FACT-General (FACT-G) and FACT-Br one week prior to treatment, and completed a follow-up assessment one month post treatment. Patients completed the questionnaires by rating items simultaneously based on the past seven days, as well as the past 24 hours. Forty patients had complete one month follow-

---

* Correspondence: Edward Chow, MBBS, MSc, PhD, FRCPC, Department of Radiation Oncology, Odette Cancer Centre, Sunnybrook Health Sciences Centre, 2075 Bayview Avenue, Toronto, Ontario, M4N 3M5 Canada. E-mail: edward.chow@sunnybrook.ca.

up data and were included in the analyses. The median age of patients was 64 years, median Eastern Cooperative Oncology Group performance status (ECOG) was 1, and the median Karnofsky Performance Status (KPS) was 80. Pearson correlations between the FACT-Br subscale scores for the past seven days and past 24 hours were all highly correlated (0.95 or greater). There was no statistically significant difference between the past seven day and past 24 hour subscale scores at both baseline and one month follow-up ($p > 0.05$). The past 24 hour subscale scores were significantly predictive of the past seven days for all FACT-G and FACT-Br subscales at baseline and one month follow-up. Thus, the FACT-G and FACT-Br can successfully be used to assess QOL based on the past 24 hours in brain metastases patients. Future clinical trials should use a 24 hour recall period for the FACT-G and FACT-Br for patients with poor neurocognitive and/or performance status, or for daily assessments based on the needs of the study.

Keywords: Quality of life, brain metastases, questionnaire, predictive value, FACT-Br, recall period

Introduction

A significant cause of morbidity and mortality in advanced cancer patients is the development of brain metastases (1). The incidence and detection of brain metastases have been on the rise as current screening techniques and imaging modalities continue to evolve (2). The development of brain metastases most commonly occurs in patients with primary cancers of the breast, lung, skin, colon, or kidneys, developing in approximately 20-40% of patients during the course of their illness (3). These patients often present with some level of neurocognitive dysfunction, including symptoms such as headaches, lack of muscle coordination, behavioural changes, speech impediments, and seizures (3-5).

Brain metastases can be managed in patients using different methods which can be categorized into symptomatic and therapeutic strategies. For instance, symptomatic strategies include the use of corticosteroids to reduce edema, and anticonvulsants to prevent seizures (2). Therapeutic strategies include whole brain radiation therapy (WBRT), stereotactic radiosurgery (SRS), neurosurgery, and chemotherapy (2). However, the treatment method selected is often dependent on patient factors including extent of extracranial disease, age, and functional status (2).

With various complications arising from brain metastases, employing therapeutic and/or symptomatic strategies can help improve overall survival and maintain quality of life (QOL) in patients. QOL is often defined as a multidimensional and subjective construct which incorporates both physical and psychosocial factors (6). QOL is commonly assessed in brain metastases patients using instruments such as the European Organisation for Research and Treatment of Cancer Quality of Life Questionnaire - Brain Neoplasm (EORTC QLQ-BN20) (used in conjunction with the QLQ-C30) and the Functional Assessment of Cancer Therapy - Brain (FACT-Br) (used in conjunction with the FACT- General (FACT-G)) (7,8). The FACT-G and FACT-Br in particular make a combined total of 50 items with subscales focusing on physical well-being (PWB), social/family well-being (SWB), emotional well-being (EWB), functional well-being (FWB), and brain metastases specific aspects of well-being (included on the FACT-Br subscale) (Appendix I) (7).

Both the FACT-Br and EORTC QLQ-BN20 involve assessing patients on various aspects of QOL based on the past seven days (7,8). However, many patients experience a decline in neurocognitive function (i.e., memory) as their disease progresses, or even in response to specific treatment regimens (i.e., WBRT) (9,10). Consequently, these patients may have difficulty recalling the past seven days when using questionnaires like the FACT-Br, and may benefit more from rating the items based on a shorter timeframe (i.e., the past 24 hours).

The purpose of this study was to assess whether the FACT-Br can be used to assess QOL in patients with brain metastases based on the past 24 hours rather than the past seven days. This will be determined by assessing the association between FACT-Br 24 hour subscale scores and the past seven days subscale scores.

Methods

Eligible patients for the study were over the age of 18 with a histologically proven cancer, able to provide written informed consent, and had documented single or multiple brain metastases. Furthermore, eligible patients were undergoing treatment regimens including neurological resection (Group A), SRS with or without WBRT (Group B), or WBRT alone (Group C). Patient demographic information was collected at baseline including primary cancer site, age, gender, number of brain metastases, Karnofsky Performance Status (KPS), Eastern Cooperative Oncology Group performance status (ECOG), and other variables as shown in Table 1.

Data collection procedure

All patient interviews were conducted in person by a trained research assistant using the FACT-Br approximately one week prior to their given treatment. All 50 items were rated by patients on a scale of 0 ('not at all') to 4 ('very much'). Each item was simultaneously rated based on both the past seven days and the past 24 hours. A follow-up assessment approximately one month (four to six weeks) following the initiation of the brain metastases specific treatment was completed with all patients. The follow-up assessment was completed over the phone or with the patient in person (if the patient was scheduled for a return visit to the clinic) using the FACT-Br.

Statistical methods

All data was analyzed using Statistical Analysis Software (SAS version 9.3 for Windows). Descriptive statistics were used to express demographic data; the mean, median, standard deviation (SD), and range for continuous variables; and proportions for categorical variables. The FACT-Br scores were analyzed using the following subscales: PWB, SWB, EWB, FWB, FACT-G total score, brain cancer subscale (BrC), and the FACT-Br total score. A higher subscale score indicated a higher extent of relevance to brain metastases patients.

Pearson correlation coefficient (r) was calculated to determine the correlation between the past 24 hour and past seven day FACT-Br subscale scores at baseline and one month follow-up. Subscale scores were considered correlated when $r \geq 0.40$. Paired t-test was conducted at baseline and one month follow-up to investigate the degree of systematic difference between the past 24 hours and the past 7 days on each FACT-G and FACT-Br subscale score. Mean difference and 95% confidence intervals (CI) were also estimated for each subscale score. $P < 0.05$ was considered statistically significant.

Results

Sixty-two patients were initially enrolled in the study and completed baseline assessment. Of these 62 patients, 40 patients completed the one month follow-up assessment and were included in the final analyses. Of the 22 patients who did not complete the one month follow-up assessment, six patients withdrew from the study, six patients deceased within the study period, and 10 patients were unable to be reached for follow-up.

Patient demographics

Patient demographics are displayed in table 1. The median age of patients was 64 years old (range: 33 to 86 years old), the median ECOG was 1 (range: 0 to 3), and the median KPS was 80 (range 40 to 90). Seventy-eight percent of patients were female, and all patients were outpatients accrued in a radiotherapy clinic. The most common primary cancer sites were the lung (58%), breast (23%), and kidney (5%). Almost half of all patients had only one brain metastasis (51%), and the majority of patients had no other sites of metastasis (60%). However, patients with sites of metastasis included the bone (16%), lymph nodes (14%), lung (11%), liver (11%), and/or adrenal gland (3%). With respect to treatment groups, 5% of patients underwent neurological resection (Group A), 60% of patients received SRS with or without WBRT (Group B), and 35% of patients received WBRT alone (Group C). Seventy-one percent of patients had prior chemotherapy, 13% had prior hormone therapy, and 40% had other prior therapies such as prior radiation therapy. Most patients were not receiving dexamethasone 24 hours prior to the baseline assessment (67%) and 47% of patients had a level of education higher than high school.

FACT-G and FACT-Br mean subscale scores

Figures 1 and 2 show the FACT-G and FACT-Br mean subscale scores for the past 24 hours and past 7 days in patients at baseline and one month follow-up.

Correlation between subscale scores for the past seven days and past 24 hours

Pearson correlations between the FACT-Br subscale scores for the past seven days and past 24 hours were all highly correlated (0.95 or greater) (see table 2).

Table 1. Patient characteristics (n=40 patients)

Age (years)		
n	40	
Mean ± SD	61.8 ± 10.5	
Median (range)	64 (33 – 86)	
KPS		
n	36	
Mean ± SD	75.8 ± 13.4	
Median (range)	80 (40 – 90)	
KPS Distribution		
40	1	(2.78%)
50	3	(8.33%)
60	2	(5.56%)
70	8	(22.22%)
80	12	(33.33%)
90	10	(27.78%)
Years from primary cancer to brain metastases		
n	37	
Mean ± SD	3.7 ± 5.8	
Median (range)	2 (0 – 28)	
Patients Group		
A - Neurosurgery	2	(5 %)
B - Radiosurgery w/wo WBRT	24	(60 %)
C - WBRT Alone	14	(35 %)
ECOG		
n	36	
Mean	1	
Median (range)	1 (0 – 3)	
0	10	(27.78%)
1	20	(55.56%)
2	5	(13.89%)
3	1	(2.78%)
4	0	(0%)
Gender		
Female	31	(77.50%)
Male	9	(22.50%)
Primary cancer site		
Lung	23	(57.50%)
Breast	9	(22.50%)
Kidney	2	(5.00%)
Colon	1	(2.50%)
Melanoma	1	(2.50%)
Others	3	(7.50%)
Age (years)		
n	40	
Unknown	1	(2.50%)
Accrual		
Radiotherapy clinic	40	(100 %)

Table 1. (Continued)

Out/In-patients		
Outpatient	40	(100 %)
Inpatient	0	(0%)
Education Level		
Elementary School	1	(2.63%)
High School	19	(50.00%)
College	3	(7.89%)
University	12	(31.58%)
Masters	2	(5.26%)
PhD	1	(2.63%)
Employment Status		
Retired	20	(50.00%)
Employed	13	(32.50%)
Unemployed	7	(17.50%)
Number of Brain Metastases		
1	20	(51.28%)
2-3	7	(17.94%)
>3	12	(30.77%)
Other Site of Metastases		
Bone	6	(16.22%)
Lung	4	(10.81%)
Liver	4	(10.81%)
Lymph node	5	(13.51%)
Adrenal	1	(2.70%)
None	24	(60.00%)
Previous Chemotherapy		
No	11	(28.95%)
Yes	27	(71.05%)
Previous Hormone Therapy		
No	33	(86.84%)
Yes	5	(13.16%)
Previous Other therapies		
No	24	(60 %)
Yes	16	(40 %)
Baseline Dexamethasone Dose		
16 mg	1	(3 %)
12 mg	3	(8 %)
8 mg	5	(13 %)
4 mg	3	(8 %)
2 mg	1	(3 %)
None	26	(67 %)

Difference between 24 hour subscale scores and the past seven day scores

In Table 3, paired t-test was conducted to determine the degree of systematic difference between the past 24 hours and the past seven days on FACT-G and FACT-Br subscale scores at baseline and one month follow-up. There was no statistically significant difference between the past seven day and past 24 hour subscale scores at both baseline and one month follow-up (p > 0.05). Consequently, the past 24 hour subscale scores were similar as the past seven days for each FACT-G and FACT-Br subscale.

Table 2. Correlation between FACT-G and FACT-Br subscale scores for the past seven days and past 24 hours at baseline and one month follow-up (n=40 patients)

FACT-G and FACT-Br at Post 7 Days	FACT-G and FACT-Br at Post 24 Hours	
	Baseline (n=40)	One month follow-up (n=40)
Physical Well-being Subscale Score (PWB)	0.98	0.95
Social/Family Well-being Subscale Score (SWB)	1.00	1.00
Emotional Well-being Subscale Score (EWB)	1.00	0.98
Functional Well-being Subscale Score (FWB)	0.99	0.99
FACT-G Total Score (FACT-G)	0.99	0.99
Brain Cancer Subscale (BrC)	1.00	1.00
FACT-Br Total Score (TOTAL)	1.00	1.00

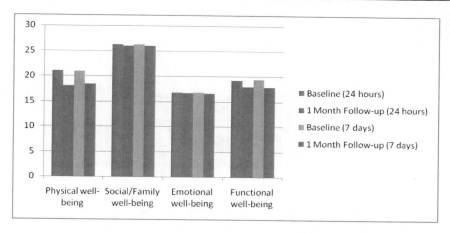

Figure 1. Mean FACT-G subscale scores for the past 24 hours and past seven days at baseline and one month follow-up (n=40 patients).

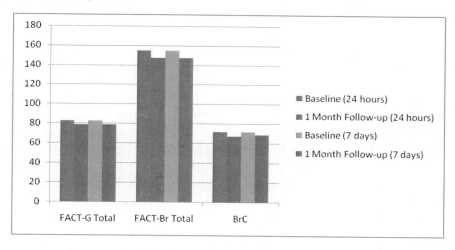

Figure 2. Mean FACT-G total, FACT-Br total, and BrC subscale scores for the past 24 hours and past seven days at baseline and one month follow-up (n=40 patients).

Table 3. Mean difference (95% CI) between 24 hours and 7 days subscale scores of the FACT-G and FACT-Br at baseline and one month follow-up (n=40 patients)

	24 hours mean (SD)	7 days mean (SD)	Mean difference (95% CI)	p-value
At baseline				
Physical Well-being Subscale Score	21.0 (5.3)	20.9 (5.6)	0.11 (-0.27, 0.49)	0.5608
Social/Family Well-being Subscale Score	26.3 (3.5)	26.3 (3.6)	0.03 (-0.03, 0.08)	0.3236
Emotional Well-being Subscale Score	16.8 (4.9)	16.8 (4.9)	0 (-0.01, 0.01)	0.9999
Functional Well-being Subscale Score	19.2 (6.2)	19.4 (6.3)	-0.18 (-0.49, 0.13)	0.2459
FACT-G Total Score	83.0 (15.8)	83.0 (16.2)	-0.05 (-0.68, 0.58)	0.8831
BrC Subscale Score	71.9 (13.3)	71.8 (13.4)	0.15 (-0.11, 0.41)	0.2487
FACT-Br Total Score	155.0 (27.4)	154.8 (28.1)	0.11 (-0.61, 0.84)	0.7587
At one month follow-up				
Physical Well-being Subscale Score	18.1 (7.2)	18.1 (7.0)	0 (-0.72, 0.72)	0.9999
Social/Family Well-being Subscale Score	26.1 (4.2)	26.1 (4.2)	0 (-0.01, 0.01)	0.9999
Emotional Well-being Subscale Score	16.7 (5.7)	16.6 (5.7)	0.13 (-0.21, 0.46)	0.4420
Functional Well-being Subscale Score	18.0 (7.1)	17.9 (7.0)	0.18 (-0.05, 0.41)	0.1282
FACT-G Total Score	79.2 (19.0)	78.9 (18.3)	0.31 (-0.55, 1.16)	0.4707
BrC Subscale Score	67.5 (19.0)	68.8 (17.3)	0.05 (-0.02, 0.13)	0.1600
FACT-Br Total Score	148.1 (34.5)	147.7 (34.1)	0.36 (-0.52, 1.23)	0.4115

Discussion

This is the first study to assess whether the FACT-Br (including the FACT-G) can be used to assess QOL in brain metastases patients based on the past 24 hours rather than the past seven days. QOL questionnaires commonly used in studies involving brain metastases patients, such as the FACT-Br and EORTC QLQ-BN20, were originally validated with a recall period of seven days. However, our study revealed that the 24 hour FACT-Br scores were strongly associated with the seven day subscale scores for patients. Consequently, this allows the opportunity for a recall period of 24 hours to be used for the FACT-G and FACT-Br in future studies when necessary.

A commonly used palliative QOL assessment tool with a short recall period is the Edmonton Symptom Assessment Scale (ESAS). The ESAS is a 10 item patient rated visual analogue scale that assesses current symptoms at the time of visit for palliative patients (11). Chang et al. conducted a validation study of the ESAS by administering this tool alongside the FACT-G and the Memorial Symptom Assessment Scale (MSAS). Both the FACT-G and MSAS are palliative QOL instruments with a recall period of seven days. After successfully completing the validation of the ESAS, the authors found some discrepancies in scores amongst the three instruments. For instance, the symptom prevalence measured appeared to be higher on the ESAS in comparison to the MSAS. The authors suggested a possible reason for this difference in scores could be attributed to the fact that the MSAS has a recall period of seven days, while the ESAS is considerably shorter (12). Although the authors did not proceed to further explain how the differences in recall period can affect the results, these results show a significance of using different recall periods in QOL assessment tools.

Some researchers have specifically investigated the choice of recall periods for QOL assessment tools. For instance, a literature review conducted by Stull et al. examined the optimal recall periods for patient reported outcomes. The authors found that the longer the time period between an event or experience and the rating of that experience, the more difficult and less accurate the event is recalled by the patient. Furthermore, the authors suggested that symptoms often fluctuate on a day-to-day basis, and as a result, longer recall periods may not capture these fluctuations in symptoms (13).

Norquist et al. examined the rationale behind selecting different recall periods. For instance, the authors suggested that a shorter recall period (immediate or daily recall) may be necessary for patients with memory deficits, daily variations in symptoms, and episodic symptoms. The authors also suggest longer recall periods (weekly recall or longer) may be necessary for patients with unnoticeable changes in symptoms over short time intervals (14). These studies provide a clear rationale for the use of the 24 hour recall period versus the seven day recall period for the FACT-Br and FACT-G.

Brain metastases patients with rapidly progressing disease, poor performance status, and neurocognitive decline, may benefit from QOL questionnaires with a shorter recall period in comparison to patients with stable disease, good performance status, and good neurocognitive status. A decline in memory function in patients can occur as a result of disease progression, or even in response to specific treatment regimens (9,10,15). For instance, a study conducted by Kondziolka et al. examined symptoms after combined WBRT and SRS in comparison to SRS alone. Overall, 72% of patients who received WBRT reported problems with short-term memory, and 33% reported problems with long-term memory. These problems were significantly reported more frequently in patients who received WBRT in comparison to patients who received SRS alone (16). Furthermore, a meta-analysis by Tsao et al. revealed similar findings and concluded that SRS alone results in fewer side effects and favourable neruocognitive outcomes in comparison to WBRT (17). Consequently, in addition to considering disease and neurocognitive factors, these studies show that the type of brain metastases specific treatment that the patient receives could also influence which recall period (24 hours versus seven days) of the FACT-G and FACT-Br that the patient may benefit more from.

The Overactive Bladder Questionnaire (OAB-q) is another QOL assessment tool used to assess various symptoms in patients with an overactive bladder condition. This questionnaire was originally validated with a fairly lengthy recall period of four weeks. However, Coyne et al. conducted a study very similar to ours, to validate the use of the questionnaire with a shorter recall period of one week. The authors suggested that a shorter recall period may be better suited based on the duration or frequency of symptoms, the type of symptoms being assessed, and the characteristics of the conditions or treatments being tested. Overall, the authors concluded that future studies can use the shorter or longer recall period of the OAB-q based on the needs of the study (18).

Similarly, the 24 hour or seven day recall periods of the FACT-G and FACT-Br can be selected based on the types of patients enrolled in the study, and/or the nature of the study. Not only will the 24 hour recall period benefit patients with a decline in neurocognitive function, but the 24 hour version of the FACT-G and FACT-Br can also be used in future studies that investigate changes in QOL of brain metastases patients on a daily basis. For instance, daily assessments may be helpful in studies examining immediate changes in QOL in response to specific treatments (i.e., WBRT). A shorter recall period in this case could help detect when certain symptoms occur and changes in symptoms that may fluctuate on a daily basis (i.e., fatigue, seizures, headaches, etc).

The use of the FACT-G and FACT-Br to assess QOL based on the past 24 hours was generally well received by patients; however, limitations still exist within this research design that could be improved for future efforts.

For instance, our patient sample consisted of patients with relatively good performance status, good neurocognitive status, and no inpatients. Consequently, our results showed that the seven day and 24 hour subscale scores were highly correlated. Patients with poorer performance status or neurocognitive function may have shown a greater difference in subscale scores for the past 24 hours in comparison to the past seven days.

Future studies could potentially explore the extended use of the FACT-G and FACT-Br (both the 24 hour and seven day recall periods) to detect changes in QOL beyond one month post treatment.

Conclusion

The assessment of QOL in patients with brain metastases continues to be an important aspect of palliative care in regards to assessing the overall disease state and efficacy of treatment. The use of the FACT-Br (supplemented by the FACT-G) is commonly used in clinical trials, and was originally validated to assess QOL in patients based on the past seven days.

Our study revealed that the past 24 hour subscale scores were significantly predictive of the past seven days for all FACT-G and FACT-Br subscales at baseline and one month follow-up. Thus, the FACT-G and FACT-Br can successfully be used to assess QOL based on the past 24 hours in brain metastases patients. Future clinical trials can use a 24 hour recall period for the FACT-G and FACT-Br in patients with poor neurocognitive and/or performance status, or for daily assessments based on the needs of the study.

Appendix I

Below is a list of statements that other people with your illness have said are important. **Please circle or tick one number per line to indicate your response as it applies to the *past 7 days (by circling) and 24 hours (by ticking over)***

FACT-Br VERSION 4

	ADDITIONAL CONCERNS	Not at all	A little bit	Some- what	Quite a bit	Very much
Br1	I am able to concentrate.	0	1	2	3	4
Br2	I have had seizures (convulsions).	0	1	2	3	4
Br3	I can remember new things.	0	1	2	3	4
Br4	I get frustrated that I cannot do things I used t.	0	1	2	3	4

ADDITIONAL CONCERNS	Not at all	A little bit	Some-what	Quite a bit	Very much
Br5 I am afraid of having a seizure (convulsion).	0	1	2	3	4
Br6 I have trouble with my eyesight.	0	1	2	3	4
Br7 I feel independent.	0	1	2	3	4
NTX6 I have trouble hearing.	0	1	2	3	4
Br8 I am able to find the right word(s) to say what I mean.	0	1	2	3	4
Br9 I have difficulty expressing my thoughts.	0	1	2	3	4
Br10 I am bothered by the change in my personality.	0	1	2	3	4
Br11 I am able to make decisions and take responsibility.	0	1	2	3	4
Br12 I am bothered by the drop in my contribution to the family.	0	1	2	3	4
Br13 I am able to put my thoughts together.	0	1	2	3	4
Br14 I need help in caring for myself (bathing, dressing, eating, etc.).	0	1	2	3	4
Br15 I am able to put my thoughts into action.	0	1	2	3	4
Br16 I am able to read like I used to.	0	1	2	3	4
Br17 I am able to write like I used to.	0	1	2	3	4
Br18 I am able to drive a vehicle (my car, truck, etc.).	0	1	2	3	4
Br19 I have trouble feeling sensations in my arms, hands, or legs.	0	1	2	3	4
Br20 I have weakness in my arms or legs.	0	1	2	3	4
Br21 I have trouble with coordination.	0	1	2	3	4
An10 I get headaches.	0	1	2	3	4

FACT-G VERSION 4

Below is a list of statements that other people with your illness have said are important.

Please circle or tick one number per line to indicate your response as it applies to the *past 7 days (by circling) and 24 hours (by ticking over).*

Please circle or tick one number per line to indicate your response as it applies to the *past 7 days (by circling) and 24 hours (by ticking over).*

EMOTIONAL WELL-BEING

	Not at all	A little bit	Some-what	Quite a bit	Very much
GE1 I feel sad	0	1	2	3	4
GE2 I am satisfied with how I am coping with my illness	0	1	2	3	4
GE3 I am losing hope in the fight against my illness	0	1	2	3	4
GE4 I feel nervous	0	1	2	3	4
GE5 I worry about dying	0	1	2	3	4
GE6 I worry that my condition will get worse	0	1	2	3	4

FUNCTIONAL WELL-BEING

		Not at all	A little bit	Some-what	Quitea bit	Very much
GF1	I am able to work (include work at home)	0	1	2	3	4
GF2	My work (include work at home) is fulfilling	0	1	2	3	4
GF3	I am able to enjoy life	0	1	2	3	4
GF4	I have accepted my illness	0	1	2	3	4
GF5	I am sleeping well	0	1	2	3	4
GF6	I am enjoying the things I usually do for fun	0	1	2	3	4
GF7	I am content with the quality of my life right now	0	1	2	3	4

Acknowledgments

We thank the generous support of the Bratty Family Fund, Michael and Karyn Goldstein Cancer Research Fund, Joseph and Silvana Melara Cancer Research Fund, and the Ofelia Cancer Research Fund.

Conflicts of interest: None.

References

[1] Serres S, Soto MS, Hamilton A, McAteer MA, Carbonell WS, Robson MD, et al. Molecular MRI enables early and sensitive detection of brain metastases. Proc Natl Acad Sci USA 2012;109(17):6674-9.

[2] Eichler AF, Loeffler JS. Multidisciplinary management of brain metastases. Oncologist 2007;12(7):884-98.

[3] Thomas SS, Dunbar EM. Modern multidisciplinary management of brain metastases. Curr Oncol Rep 2010;12(1):34-40.

[4] Posner JB. Management of central nervous system metastases. Semin Oncol 1977;4(1):81-91.

[5] Chang EL, Wefel JS, Maor MH, Hassenbusch SJ,3rd, Mahajan A, Lang FF, et al. A pilot study of neurocognitive function in patients with one to three new brain metastases initially treated with stereotactic radiosurgery alone. Neurosurgery 2007;60(2):277-83.

[6] Movsas B. Quality of life in oncology trials: a clinical guide. Semin Radiat Oncol 2003;13(3):235-47.

[7] Chen E, Cella D, Zeng L, Thavarajah N, Zhang L, Chang E, et al. Content validation of the FACT-Br with patients and health-care professionals to assess quality of life in patients with brain metastases. J Radiat Oncol 2012.

[8] Caissie A, Nguyen J, Chen E, Zhang L, Sahgal A, Clemons M, et al. Quality of life in patients with brain metastases using the EORTC QLQ-BN20+2 and QLQ-C15-PAL. Int J Radiat Oncol Biol Phys 2012;83(4):1238-45.

[9] Chang EL, Wefel JS, Hess KR, Allen PK, Lang FF, Kornguth DG, et al. Neurocognition in patients with brain metastases treated with radiosurgery or radiosurgery plus whole-brain irradiation: a randomised controlled trial. Lancet Oncology 2009;10(11):1037-44.

[10] Peacock KH, Lesser GJ. Current therapeutic approaches in patients with brain metastases. Curr Treat Options Oncol 2006;7(6):479-89.

[11] Nekolaichuk C, Watanabe S, Beaumont C. The Edmonton Symptom Assessment System: A 15-year retrospective review of validation studies (1991--2006). Palliat Med 2008;22(2):111-22.

[12]   Chang VT, Hwang SS, Feuerman M. Validation of the Edmonton Symptom Assessment Scale. Cancer 2000;88(9):2164-71.

[13]   Stull DE, Leidy NK, Parasuraman B, Chassany O. Optimal recall periods for patient-reported outcomes: challenges and potential solutions. Curr Med Res Opinion 2009;25(4):929-42.

[14]   Norquist JM, Girman C, Fehnel S, DeMuro-Mercon C, Santanello N. Choice of recall period for patient-reported outcome (PRO) measures: criteria for consideration. Qual Life Res 2012;21(6):1013-20.

[15]   Wong J, Hird A, Kirou-Mauro A, Napolskikh J, Chow E. Quality of life in brain metastases radiation trials: a literature review. Curr Oncol 2008;15(5):25-45.

[16]   Kondziolka D, Niranjan A, Flickinger JC, Lunsford LD. Radiosurgery with or without whole-brain radiotherapy for brain metastases: the patients' perspective regarding complications. Am J Clin Oncol 2005;28(2):173-9.

[17]   Tsao M, Wei X, Sahgal A. A meta-analysis evaluating stereotactic radiosurgery, whole-brain radiotherapy, or both for patients presenting with a limited number of brain metastases. Cancer 2011;118(9):2486-93.

[18]   Coyne KS, Gelhorn H, Thompson C, Kopp ZS, Guan Z. The psychometric validation of a 1-week recall period for the OAB-q. Int Urogynecol J 2011;22(12):1555-63.

In: Pain Management Yearbook 2013
Editor: Joav Merrick

ISBN: 978-1-63117-944-0
© 2014 Nova Science Publishers, Inc.

Chapter 29

Mindfulness training does not reduce inflammatory cytokine levels in chronic tension-type headache

Stuart Cathcart, PhD[*1], *Chris Della Vedova, PhD*[2],
Maarten Immink, PhD[3], *Michael Proeve, PhD*[4]
and John Hayball, PhD[2]

[1]Centre for Applied Psychology, Faculty of Health, University of Canberra
[2]School of Pharmacy and Medical Sciences, University of South Australia
[3]School of Health Sciences, University of South Australia
[4]School of Psychology, University of Adelaide, Australia

Abstract

To examine effects of mindfulness training on serum pro-inflammatory cytokine levels in chronic tension-type headache (CTH) sufferers. Method: Forty-three CTH sufferers participated in a randomized wait-list controlled trial of a mindfulness intervention for headache. Serum concentrations of cytokines IL1-β, IL-2, IL-6, IL-8, IL-12, IL-18, IFN-γ, MCP-1 and TNF-α were measured before and after treatment/wait-list control conditions. Results: Repeated Measures Analysis of Variance revealed that IL1-β, IL-6, IL-8, MCP-1 and TNF-α decreased from pre to post assessments in the treatment and wait-list groups, with no group or group x time effects. Conclusions: Mindfulness training compared to a wait-list control condition does not reduce serum cytokine levels in CTH sufferers.

Keywords: Mindfulness, headache, cytokines, randomized controlled trial

* Correspondence: Stuart Cathcart, PhD, Centre for Applied Psychology, University of Canberra, Bruce 2601, Australia. E-mail: stuart.cathcart@canberra.edu.au.

Introduction

Mindfulness training has been reported as beneficial for reducing symptoms in several chronic pain conditions, including headache (1,2). One potential mechanism for the therapeutic effects of mindfulness may be a reduction in pro-inflammatory cytokine (PIC) levels. Cytokines are regulatory proteins secreted by numerous cells including immune cells in the periphery and microglia in the Central Nervous System (CNS). Pro-inflammatory cytokines are involved in both stress and pain processing (3,4), and are increased in several chronic pain conditions, including headache (5,6). Mindfulness-based interventions have been shown to reduce PIC levels in healthy and clinical samples (7,8), however this has not been examined in CTH sufferers to date.

Elsewhere we reported elevated PIC levels in the present sample of CTH sufferers (9), and a reduction in headache activity following mindfulness intervention (10). The present study examines if the mindfulness intervention reduced PIC levels in that sample of CTH sufferers.

Methods

Participant information has been reported in detail elsewhere (9,10). Briefly, Fifty-eight volunteers satisfying diagnosis of CTH were recruited from the general population and completed pre-treatment measures. Forty-three participants completed post-treatment measures (N=24 treatment, N=19 wait-list). Volunteers were excluded if they reported any chronic pain other than CTH, satisfied other headache diagnoses including migraine or suspected Medication Overuse Headache, or had major medical or psychiatric diagnoses concurrent or in the past 12 months. The mean age of the total sample was 45.5 years (SD=13.8), 37% were male.

Measures

Blood samples (9mL) were collected via venepuncture by a phlebotomist nurse at the School of Psychology, University of South Australia. All participants had their blood taken between 9am and 11am, to control for circadian variation in cytokine levels. Samples were collected in ethylenediaminetetracetic acid (EDTA) and serum clotting tubes, and transported in biohazard containers to the Experimental Therapeutics Laboratory, Hanson Institute. The tubes were centrifuged at 2,500 x g for 10 minutes at room temperature, and the blood components (serum, plasma, buffy coat cells) were aliquoted separately (500μL) into labelled 1.8mL cryovials (Nunc, Roskilde, Denmark). The cryovials were placed into liquid nitrogen to snap freeze, and stored at -70oC before analysis.

Determination of cytokine levels

Cytokine levels in serum samples were analyzed using an established cytometric bead array kit (FlowCytomix; Bender MedSystems, Vienna, Austria) according to the manufacturers' instructions. The kit reagents were diluted 1:2 for each run, and all samples were run in duplicate. Standard curves for each cytokine were included in each run, and sample concentrations were calculated using FlowCytomix Pro software.

Intervention

The intervention was based on Mindfulness-Based Stress Reduction (MBSR) and Mindfulness Based Cognitive Therapy (MBCT), and is detailed elsewhere (10). Delivered by one of the authors (MI), the intervention involved six 1-hour group classes held twice per week for three weeks, and 30mins daily home practice. The program was developed by some of the authors (SC, MP, MI) who are psychologists (SC, MP) with formal training and teaching, practice, and research experience in mindfulness and/or meditation.

Three formal mindfulness meditation practices were taught: 1) body scan meditation, which involves focusing on each region of the body systemically from the foot to the head, and noticing the sensations that are present with openness and curiosity; 2) formal sitting meditation, focusing on mindfulness of breath and other experiences such as sounds and thoughts; 3) three-minute breathing space, which involves three sequential steps of a) focusing awareness of present internal experiences, b) focusing awareness on the breath, and c) expanding awareness to the body as a whole.

Home practice was supported by a written instruction manual and a compact disc containing audio-recorded instructions. The program also included other activities so that participants could practice applying concepts of mindfulness to activities of daily living, recognizing nourishing and draining activities, and documenting observations and reactions to pleasant and unpleasant events.

Procedures

The study was approved by the University of South Australia Human Research Ethics Committee. Following a screening interview and provision of written consent to participate, volunteers completed questionnaires and had blood drawn for cytokine analysis. Headache sufferers were then randomly assigned to either treatment or wait-list conditions. Post-treatment measures were recorded in all CTH participants in the week following completion of the intervention by the treatment group. The wait-list control group commenced mindfulness training the following week.

Results

Repeated Measures Analysis of Variance results (table 1) yielded significant Time effects indicating a decrease from pre to post assessments for IL1-β (F $(1,41) = 9.65$, p $< .01$, $\eta=.15$), IL-6 (F $(1,41) = 15.56$, p $< .01$, $\eta=.22$), IL-8 (F $(1,41) = 5.13$, p $< .04$, $\eta=.10$), MCP-1 (F $(1,41) = 10.66$, p $< .01$, $\eta=.17$) and TNF-α (F $(1,41) = 11.54$, p $< .01$, $\eta=.18$). Group and Group x Time effects were not significant for any measure (all p>.05).

Table 1. Cytokine levels before and after mindfulness intervention and wait-list control conditions in chronic tension-type headache sufferers

| Measure[1] | Mindfulness group N=24 | | | | Wait-list group N=19 | | | | Test value[2] | | |
| | Pre | | Post | | Pre | | Post | | Group effect | Time effect | G x T effect |
	Mean	SD	Mean	SD	Mean	SD	Mean	SD			
IL-1β	3.59	.53	2.57	1.95	3.56	.62	3.03	1.48	.42	9.65**	.98
IL-2	2.53	1.19	1.81	1.89	2.26	.50	2.17	1.10	.05	3.11	1.93
IL-6	15.22	1.95	10.09	7.59	14.77	1.97	12.12	5.66	.65	15.56**	1.57
IL-8	35.08	110.9	24.32	85.17	14.46	9.59	11.85	9.11	.62	5.13*	1.91
IL-12	1.74	.46	1.27	.98	1.70	.46	1.65	.88	1.27	3.63	2.28
IL-18	1.05	.93	.85	.95	.92	1.01	.70	.92	.48	1.43	.01
IFN-γ	1.66	.38	1.31	1.03	1.62	.48	1.63	.88	.91	1.44	1.57
MCP-1	223.76	99.68	159.38	151.11	278.10	153.70	230.79	203.74	2.81	10.66**	.25
TNF-α	6.40	.81	4.41	3.30	6.21	.83	5.31	2.56	.66	11.54**	1.67

[1.] Serum cytokine levels (mean fluorescent intensity) IL-1β; Interleukin 1-beta, IL-2; interleukin-2, IL-6; interleukin-6, IL-8; interleukin-8, IL-12; interleukin-12p70, IL-18; interleukin-18, IFN-γ; interferon-γ, MCP-1; Monocyte Chemoattractant Protein-1, TNF-α; Tumour Necrosis Factor-alpha.

[2.] Repeated measures analysis of variance F value, all df=1,41.

* p<.05, ** p<.01.

Discussion

To our knowledge, this is the first study to examine effects of mindfulness training on pro-inflammatory cytokines in CTH sufferers. The results indicate a pre to post treatment reduction in several of the PIC's examined, in both the treatment and wait-list groups, with no difference between groups. This indicates that mindfulness training compared to a wait-list control group does not reduce PIC levels in CTH sufferers. Elsewhere we have reported that the mindfulness training reduced headache activity in this sample of CTH sufferers (10). Although we did not presently examine relationships between headache activity and PIC's, the findings suggest the therapeutic effect of the intervention previously observed was not due to a reduction in PIC levels. The results also call in to question previous uncontrolled findings of effects of mindfulness training on cytokines (e.g., 8). The cause of the decrease in PICs in the treatment and wait-list groups is unclear. One possibility is non-specific effects common to both treatment and wait-list conditions (e.g., expectancy). Alternatively, the reduction in PIC levels may be coincidental.

Limitations to the present study include the brief nature of our intervention, the lack of an active control group, and the lack of longer-term follow-up. The lack of significant findings is unlikely due to low power associated with the small sample size, since time effects were observed and there were no trends indicating a group x time effect. The above limitations withstanding, the present results indicate that mindfulness training, elsewhere shown to reduce headache activity in this sample of CTH sufferers, does not reduce PIC levels in the same sample. Replication and extension of the present results would further understanding of the importance of PICs in, and the mechanisms of mindfulness intervention for, CTH.

Acknowledgments

The authors are grateful to Nicola Galatis and Margaret Mitchell for assistance in data collection. This research was funded in part by a Medical Advances without Animals Trust grant.

This study is registered with the Australian and New Zealand Clinical Trials Registry, number ACTRN12610001039077

References

[11] Morone NE, Greco CM, Weiner DK. Mindfulness meditation for the treatment of chronic low back pain in older adults: a randomized controlled pilot study. Pain 2008;134:310-9.

[12] Kabat-Zinn J, Lipworth L, Burney R. The clinical use of mindfulness meditation for the self-regulation of chronic pain. J Behav Med 1985;8:163-90.

[13] Chapman C, Tuckett R, Song C. Pain and stress in a systems perspective: Reciprocal neural, endocrine, and immune interactions. J Pain 2008;9(2):122-45.

[14] Marchand F, Perretti M and McMahon SB. Role of the immune system in chronic pain. Nat Rev Neurosci 2005;6:521-32.

[15] Bazzichi L, Rossi A, Massimetti G, Giannaccini G, Giuliano T, De Feo F, Ciapparelli A, Dell'Osso L, Bombardieri S. Cytokine patterns in fibromyalgia and their correlation with clinical manifestations. Clin Exp Rheumatol 2007;25:225–30.

[16] Koçer A, Koçer E, Memişoğullari R, Domaç FM, Yüksel H. Interleukin-6 levels in tension headache patients. Clin J Pain 2010;26(8):690-3.

[17] Koh KB, Lee Y, Beyn KM, Chu SH, Kim DM. Counter-stress effects of relaxation on proinflammatory and anti-inflammatory cytokines. Brain Behav Immun 2008;22(8):1130-7.

[18] Carlson LE, Speca M, Faris P et al. One year pre-post intervention follow-up of psychological, immune, endocrine and blood pressure outcomes of mindfulness-based stress reduction (MBSR) in breast and prostate cancer outpatients. Brain Behav Immun 2007 21(8):1038-49.

[19] Della-Vedova, C. Cathcart, S. Dohnalek, A., Immink, M. & Hayball, J. Peripheral interleukin-1 Beta and Interleukin-18 levels are elevated in Chronic Tension-Type Headache. Pain Res Manage, in press.

[20] Cathcart S, Galatis N, Immink M, Proeve M, Petkov J. Brief mindfulness-based meditation for chronic tension-type headache: A randomized controlled trial. Behav Cog Psychother, in press.

In: Pain Management Yearbook 2013
Editor: Joav Merrick

ISBN: 978-1-63117-944-0
© 2014 Nova Science Publishers, Inc.

Chapter 30

Avascular necrosis of the femoral head in metastatic breast cancer

Breanne Lechner, BSc(C)[1], Nemica Thavarajah, BSc(C)[1],
Linda Probyn, MD[2], Natalie Pulenzas, BSc(C)[1],
Lori Holden, MRTT[1], Natalie Lauzon, MRTT[1]
and Edward Chow, MBBS[1]*

[1]Rapid Response Radiotherapy Program, Department of Radiation Oncology, Odette
Cancer Centre, Sunnybrook Health Sciences Centre,
University of Toronto, Toronto, Ontario, Canada
[2]Department of Diagnostic Radiology, Sunnybrook Health Sciences Centre,
University of Toronto, Toronto, Ontario, Canada

Abstract

Avascular necrosis (AVN) of the femoral head is an acute condition that commonly presents as unilateral hip pain. Causes of AVN can be categorized as traumatic, non-traumatic and idiopathic. AVN has been described as a complication of many treatments commonly used in cancer patients including corticosteroid therapy, chemotherapy, and radiation. We present the case of a 70 year old patient with known breast cancer metastatic to bone and liver with the development of AVN of the femoral head.

Keywords: Metastatic breast cancer, avascular necrosis, radiation, chemotherapy

* Correspondence: Edward Chow, MBBS, MSc, PhD, FRCPC, Department of Radiation Oncology, Odette Cancer Centre, Sunnybrook Health Sciences Centre, 2075 Bayview Avenue, Toronto, Ontario, Canada M4N 3M5. E-mail: edward.chow@sunnybrook.ca

Introduction

Avascular necrosis (AVN) is defined as cellular death of bone components caused by a decrease or disruption of blood supply to the bone tissue of the affected area (1). AVN is most commonly encountered in the hip (2). AVN of the femoral head is an acute condition that commonly presents as unilateral hip pain (1). There are three main causes of AVN: traumatic, non-traumatic, and idiopathic (1). In idiopathic cases, the cause of the AVN is unknown. Traumatic causes of AVN include severe fracture and dislocation (1). Non-traumatic causes of AVN can include advanced diseases such as cancer. Other non-traumatic causes can include the use of corticosteroids, chemotherapy treatments, and irradiation of the area (3). These therapies associated with AVN risk are also common treatment options for patients with cancer. In this report, we present the case of a 70 year old advanced cancer patient with AVN of the femoral head.

Case report

A now 70 year old female was initially diagnosed with bilateral breast cancer in 1987 at the age of 45 years. The pathology of the disease has since been identified as ER/PR positive, HER-2/neu negative breast cancer. She initially underwent breast conservation surgery and post-operative breast radiation. She had local recurrence in 1996 and underwent re-excision. In March 2008, the patient had magnetic resonance imaging (MRI) of the spine that indicated metastatic disease at the L5 level with significant cauda equina syndrome involving L5-S1. Since that time, she has presented with several additional bony metastases particularly known to the sacral area in the pelvis and in the C4, T11, L4 and L5 vertebral bodies. There are also notable metastases identified in the liver as well.

In terms of systemic treatment, the patient was treated with Tamoxifen between 1997 and 2008, and was then switched to Letrozole for the duration of 2008 to March 2010. She then changed to Exemestane concurrently with Clodronate until February 2011. The patient received Faslodex intramuscular injections starting in April 2011. In efforts to treat progression of the disease, the patient was put on Capecitabine in October 2012 and continued until the present.

Radiotherapy treatment was also used to palliate pain due to extensive bone metastases. The patient was fist referred to the Rapid Response Radiotherapy Program (RRRP) at the Odette Cancer Centre in 2008. She received 20 Gy in five fractions to the lumbar and sacral spine in May 2008. In September of 2008, she received 20 Gy in ten fractions as a retreatment due to worsening pain. In March 2010, the patient received 20 Gy in five fractions to the right ilial region in the RRRP. The patient also was treated in March of 2011 with 20 Gy in five fractions to the T10 and L1 vertebral bodies in the RRRP.

The patient was referred again to the RRRP in June of 2012, presenting with a one year history of left groin pain that worsened upon walking. A bone scan from January 2012 showed new areas of bony metastases at L3, in the acetabulum, and the ischium. The scan also showed previously described loci at the left first rib posteriorly, the left eighth rib laterally, T7, T11, L4, L5, the right sacroiliac and the right medial iliac bone. In regards to her pain, radiographic images, computed tomography (CT) images, and a bone scan showed metastatic deposits in both the left femoral head as well as the acetabulum. Based on consultation with an orthopedic surgeon, the area was at a low risk for fracture and thus the patient proceeded with radiation therapy. The patient received a total of 30 Gy in ten fractions to the hip for palliation of pain and promotion of bone healing. In December of 2012, a CT scan of the pelvis demonstrated collapse of the anterior and superior articular surface within the left femoral head that extended over 2.5 cm of weight-bearing surface. Additionally, there was evidence of irregularity and bone remodeling. This abnormality showed a large area of sclerosis within the underlying femoral head. What was previously described as metastatic disease on prior CT scans and radiographic images has now been identified as advanced AVN of the femoral head by the radiologist reviewing the CT images.

Figures 1- 3 show the areas of AVN in the patient's hip. These images demonstrate from various views the area consistent with AVN of the left femoral head. As of January 2013, the patient was experiencing pain in her left hip, at the site of AVN. Despite receiving 3 mg of hydromorph contin twice daily with 1 mg for breakthrough pain, she was still experiencing significant pain. An orthopedic surgeon suggested the possibility of hip replacement surgery to better control the pain. Ultimately, the patient declined surgery and preferred to continue with hydromorph contin for pain management.

Discussion

The early diagnosis of AVN of the femoral head can be difficult as it often appears as areas of sclerosis and plain radiographs often appear normal in the initial stages (4). The symptoms of AVN are often nonspecific, and can thus be attributed to the progression of bone metastases in cancer patients (3). In this case, although the abnormality was noted in prior radiograph images of the affected area, it was previously considered to be metastatic disease. It was not until the AVN had become quite extensive that it was diagnosed as such by the radiologist examining the patient's CT images.

While AVN can begin as a painless bone abnormality, the bone can become profusely painful over time (1). Like in the presented case, when lower extremities such as the hip are affected it can often lead to difficulty walking and groin pain (1). This can be seriously problematic, especially for patients with advanced disease and other comorbidities.

AVN can usually be treated by joint replacement surgery (1) though in this particular case the patient decided not to pursue that option. Additional treatment options for AVN include treatment with bone strengthening agents, pain medications, and limiting the amount of weight bearing activity (1). In this case, the patient was actively taking the bisphosphonate Clodronate and developed AVN. There is much controversy in the literature in regards to bisphosphonate usage and AVN. Cases have been reported in which the use of bisphosphonates has been associated with the development of AVN, zoledronic acid in particular (5). Conversely, a systemic review of the literature by Cardozo et al. (6) has also demonstrated positive results in the use of various bisphosphonates to treat AVN.

In this case, the patient had also received both radiation to the affected area and was actively taking pain medications without adequate pain relief. Cases have also reported the development of AVN after irradiation (3). The risk of development of AVN is highest with conventional external beam radiation compared to other types of radiation therapy (3). Cases have also been reported of patients that received steroid treatment before radiation therapy and subsequently developed AVN (4).

Patients treated with long-term or high-dose steroid administration have been suggested to be at greater risk of developing AVN (6). Though steroid use is commonly accepted as a non-traumatic case of AVN, the processes by which this occurs are poorly understood (3). AVN in cancer patients has often been linked to the use of chemotherapy, in particular when associated with corticosteroid treatment, the femoral head being the site usually affected (6). Cases have been reported of patients developing AVN after use of steroids such as prednisone, prednisolone, and cyproterone acetate (3,4,7). In this case, the patient had been receiving Faslodex, a steroidal estrogen antagonist, as hormonal therapy and Capecitabine as chemotherapy at the time of development of AVN (8). Cases have also been documented in which patients receiving chemotherapy that did not include steroids had developed AVN (6).

Evidently, there are several possible factors that can contribute to the development of AVN. Further research investigating and identifying the causation of AVN in advanced cancer patients is needed to better understand what is the best method of treatment for patients with advanced cancer, and if these treatments could have negative consequences. Understanding the mechanisms of how various cancer treatments can interact and documenting cases of the reported outcomes of these interactions is important for patient care. Understanding potential risk factors may also contribute to earlier detection and identification of AVN. Minimizing potential complications with treatments and maximizing the benefit of treatments is the aim for all health professionals.

References

[1]   Summers, C. Avascular necrosis of the femoral head. Nurse Pract 2011;36(1):6-10.
[2]   Bose VC, Baruah BD. Resurfacing arthroplasty of the hip for avascular necrosis of the femoral head: A minimum follow-up of four years. J Bone Joint Surg Br 2010;92(7):922-8.
[3]   Chan E, Chan G, Ehrlich L, Huii P, Kreder H, Chu W, et al. When the tumour is not the culprit: Avascular necrosis of the hip in a patient with castration-resistant prostate cancer. Curr Oncol 2013;20(1):48-51.
[4]   Macdonald AG, Bissett JD. Avascular necrosis of the femoral head in patients with prostate cancer treated with cyproterone acetate and radiotherapy. Clin Oncol (R Coll Radiol) 2001;13(2):135-7.
[5]   Didden K, De Smet L, Vandenberghe L, Sciot R, Degreef I. Avascular necrosis of the proximal carpal row of the wrist. A possible complication of bisphosphonate administration. Chir Main 2012;31(6):355-7.
[6]   Harper PG, Trask C, Souhami RL. Avascular necrosis of bone caused by combination chemotherapy without corticosteroids. Br Med J (Clin Res Ed) 1984;288(6413):267-8.
[7]   Kosaka Y, Mitsumori M, Araki N, Yamauchi C, Nagata Y, Hiraoka M, et al. Avascular necrosis of bilateral femoral head as a result of long-term steroid administration for radiation pneumonitis after tangential irradiation of the breast. Int J Clin Oncol 2006;11(6):482-6.
[8]   Robertson JF. Faslodex (ICI 182, 780), a novel estrogen receptor downregulator--future possibilities in breast cancer. J Steroid Biochem Mol Biol 2001;79(1-5):209-12.

In: Pain Management Yearbook 2013
Editor: Joav Merrick

ISBN: 978-1-63117-944-0
© 2014 Nova Science Publishers, Inc.

Chapter 31

Intramedullary spinal cord metastasis from melanoma: A case report

Sean Gretz, Michael Poon, BSc(C), Gillian Bedard, BSc(C),
Julia Digiovanni, Marko Popovic, BHSc(C)
and Edward Chow, MBBS*
Rapid Response Radiotherapy Program, Department of Radiation Oncology,
Odette Cancer Centre, Sunnybrook Health Sciences Centre, University of Toronto,
Toronto, Ontario, Canada

Abstract

Rates of malignant melanoma have been increasing in frequency. Studies have shown that up to 46% of patients with melanoma will experience metastases to the central nervous system. Intramedullary tumors are metastases inside the spinal cord that cause symptoms by compressing the nerves of the spinal cord. These lesions may affect neighboring nerve roots, blood vessels or vertebra. Impingement of these tumors on the spinal cord can cause paralysis and can be potentially life-threatening. Surgery is typically the most effective way of treating intramedullary tumors. These tumors are often difficult to remove due to the high risk of spinal cord damage; however, much has been done in the way of improving the process of removing intramedullary tumors surgically. A study by Kwak et al. found that by utilizing a combined split-spinous laminectomy and quadrant tube retractor system allowed for minimal trauma to the surrounding tissue. In addition to surgery, radiotherapy is a viable option for patients who are ineligible for surgery. While radiation has been shown to be less effective than surgery, it is more effective than radiographic monitoring of the patient. Without radiotherapy, one does not expect to see neurological improvement in patients. In the following case, a 69 year old gentleman presented to clinic with a intramedullary tumor in the C2/C3 region. Treatment options including surgery, radiosurgery, and radiotherapy

* Corresponding author: Dr Edward Chow MBBS, MSc, PhD, FRCPC Department of Radiation Oncology, Odette Cancer Centre, Sunnybrook Health Sciences Centre, 2075 Bayview Avenue, Toronto, ON Canada. Email: Edward.Chow@sunnybrook.ca.

were limited for this patient. This case demonstrates the importance and difficulties of determining the most effective course of treatment for intramedullary tumors of the spine.

Keywords: Intramedullary metastasis, melanoma, palliative radiotherapy

Introduction

Rates of malignant melanoma have been increasing in frequency. This cutaneous carcinoma is very resistant to treatment and thus aggressive measures are commonly taken (1). Studies have shown that up to 46% of patients with melanoma will experience metastases to the central nervous system (CNS), with CNS metastases being diagnosed in 75% of patients at autopsy (2). These metastases present as a plethora of symptoms including: motor dysfunction, confusion, headache, and nerve disturbances. After metastases present, treatment intent becomes palliative and the prognosis declines. Therefore treatments focus upon lessening symptoms and palliating pain.

Intramedullary tumors can be observed in cancer patients who experience metastasis to the spinal cord (3). Intramedullary tumors grow inside the spinal cord and cause symptoms by compressing the nerves of the spinal cord. Symptoms include: non-mechanical back pain as well as loss of sensation or muscle weakness in the legs, arms or chest. In severe instances, paralysis or scoliosis may result. These tumors are often difficult to remove due to the high risk of spinal cord damage (3). In patients with intramedullary tumors, the goal of treatment is to restore or preserve neurological function, stabilize the spine, and alleviate pain. In general, surgery is the primary treatment option. Removal of the tumor followed by radiation and/or chemotherapy has shown promising results (3). However, for non-operable lesions, non-surgical treatment options include observation, chemotherapy and radiation therapy.

There are cases in which metastatic tumors are inherently radio-resistant (3). Melanoma is one such type of cancer that has high radio-resistance. The expected outcome from treatment depends greatly on the age and overall health of the patient. In the case of metastatic tumors, the goal is almost always palliative. At best, treatment may provide the patient with an improved quality of life and prolonged life expectancy. In this report, we present the case of a 69 year old gentleman who developed an intramedullary tumor in the cervical spine as a result of malignant melanoma.

Case Report

A 69 year old gentleman originally presented to our clinic in September 2011 with malignant melanoma that had metastasized to the bone, lung, mediastinum, and liver. He presented with an extramedullary, intradural tumor that was compressing the C2 to C3 vertebrae and causing severe stenosis at C5. The patient had a laminectomy, decompression and excision of the intradural mass in September 2011. Pathology from the surgery showed that the mass was metastatic melanoma. During the surgery, only 98% of the tumor was resected leaving a small rim of tumor attached to the spinal cord. This was done in order to avoid the risk of causing significant neurological deficits. The patient then underwent post-operative radiotherapy to a dose of 30 Gy in 10 fractions to the entire cervical spine. Systemic therapy was started afterwards and the patient was treated with Ipilimumab for one year.

In May 2013, the patient returned to clinic with a new onset of numbness and pain. The pain was experienced in the patient's neck and radiated down to his arm. In addition, the patient was experiencing numbness in his fingers as well as decreased temperature and impaired fine motor sensation in his hands. An MRI was conducted in May 2013, which showed a recurrent tumor centered on the left side of the upper cervical spinal cord at the C2/C3 level (Figure 1). The maximal axial diameter of this mass was found to be 0.9 cm x 1.2 cm at C2/C3 base level with cranial caudal extension for 2.5 cm.

Given the problematic location of the metastatic lesion, this case was discussed with a neurosurgeon to determine if further surgical resection would be possible. It was determined that surgery would not be possible, as the tumor deposit was intramedullary. Given the location of the tumor the patient was deemed ineligible for stereotactic body radiotherapy.

As the patient was experiencing severe pain, the role of palliative radiotherapy was discussed. The patient had previously received a radiotherapy dose of 30 Gy in 10 fractions to the cervical spine. Therefore, the potential retreatment dose of radiotherapy was limited as any treatment given would near maximum biological equivalent dose. Either the patient could elect for a higher radiation dose or he could opt for a single treatment with less tumor control potential. The patient was informed that it was not possible to eradicate the tumor and that the treatment intent was to palliate his current symptoms. In addition, the patient was informed that the efficacy of the treatment is unknown and unlikely to alleviate all symptoms. The patient was also informed about the side effects of the radiotherapy to that area, which include fatigue, dermatitis, mucositis, esophagitis, as well as a potential transient increase in pain (pain flare). After further discussion, the patient opted for a dose fractionation of 20 Gy in 8 fractions. Given the patient's understanding that further radiation would not be possible, he chose to accept the increased risk of radiation myelopathy in favor of increased tumor control.

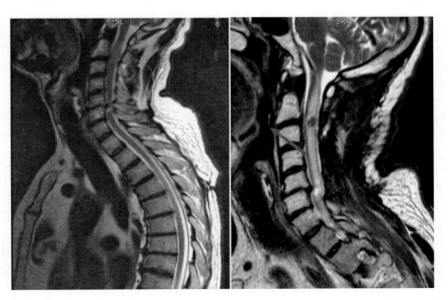

Figure 1. Recurrent intramedullary metastasis from melanoma centered on the left side of the upper cervical spinal cord at the C2/C3 level.

Discussion

Metastatic spread of tumors to the spinal cord potentially results in the development of intramedullary tumors (3). These tumors are highly dangerous due to their ability to grow within the spinal column and compress the spinal cord. In addition, these lesions may affect neighboring nerve roots, blood vessels or bones of the spine (3). Impingement of these tumors on the spinal cord can cause paralysis and potentially be life-threatening. Surgery is typically the most effective way of treating intramedullary tumors, with laminectomies being the most common surgical procedure for the removal of spinal cord tumors. However, as with all procedures, this surgery has its disadvantages, which primarily include: wide incisions, extensive muscle dissection and structural bone injury (4). These potential risks can render patients inoperable given the high likelihood of complication. The patient in the present case underwent a laminectomy when he first presented with extramedullary, intradural metastases, however for the recurrence, further surgery was not possible.

Kwak et al. (4) conducted a study in which 19 patients with intradural tumors measuring approximately 1.14 cm in size (0.8 cm-1.4 cm) were treated via a laminectomy. Eight patients received a combined split-spinous laminectomy and quadrant tube retractor system procedure, and eleven received a traditional total laminectomy. Pre-operative and post-operative evaluations consisted of pathological findings, surgical parameters, radiological findings, and functional examination. From this study, the investigators concluded that the combined split-spinous laminectomy and quadrant tube retractor system technique allowed for minimal trauma to the surrounding tissue (4). The data suggests that further development of these techniques could lead to an increase in surgical opportunities for patients who surgery was previously too dangerous. Perhaps with further development of these treatment techniques, patients who may today be deemed ineligible for a tradition laminectomy may one day be eligible for novel procedures like the combined split-spinous laminectomy and quadrant tube retractors system.

While surgery is not always an option for patients with intramedullary metastases, radiotherapy may be. While radiation has been shown to be less effective than surgery, it is more effective than radiographic monitoring of the patient. In a previous study, neurological improvements were seen in 33% of patients who underwent radiation treatment, as opposed to improvement rates of 58% in those patients who underwent surgery. Although rates of improvement are lower in patients who undergo radiation as compared to those with surgery, the results are far superior of patients treated palliatively. Without radiotherapy, no patients displayed neurological improvement (5).

Radiotherapy is a viable option for patients who are ineligible for surgery. However, the amount of radiation that can be safely delivered to the spinal cord is relatively low. In cases of recurrence, typically the patient cannot be treated with as large a dose as they were originally received. In the current case, the calculated biological equivalent dose for retreating the patient following a prior radiation dose of 30 Gy in 10 fractions was calculated to exceed the maximal dose tolerated in the spinal cord. When determining the optimal course of treatment, there is a tradeoff between symptom management and potential radiation myelopathy. Therefore, the patient was treated with a lower dose of 20 Gy in 8 treatments and told that no further radiation could be delivered after this retreatment. In the future, if the patient's disease progresses or reoccurs, unfortunately, they can only be medicated palliatively.

Conclusion

This case demonstrates the importance and difficulties of determining the most effective course of treatment for intramedullary tumors of the spine. Treatment options for this condition include surgery, radiosurgery, and radiotherapy. Due to the dangerous nature of intramedullary lesions, further development of surgical techniques is necessary. Future studies should seek to report the efficacy of radiotherapeutic retreatment of intramedullary lesions resulting from malignant metastases of melanoma. In addition, studies should seek to determine new treatments for patients with intramedullary metastases, especially for those patients who have a re-occurrence of their disease.

Acknowledgment

We thank the generous support of Bratty Family Fund, Michael and Karyn Goldstein Cancer Research Fund, Joseph and Silvana Melara Cancer Research Fund, and Ofelia Cancer Research Fund.

References

[1]   Rate WR, Solin LJ, Turrisi AT. Palliative radiotherapy for metastatic malignant melanoma: brain metastases, bone metastases, and spinal cord compression. Int J Radiat Oncol Biol Phys1988; 15(4):859-64.

[2]   Amer MH, Al-Sarraf M, Baker LH, Vaitkevicius VK. Malignant melanoma and central nervous system metastases. Incidence, diagnosis, treatment and survival. Cancer 1978; 42(2):660-8.

[3]   Sung WS, Sung MJ, Chan JH, Manion B, Song J, Dubey A, Erasmus A, Hunn A. Intramedullary spinal cord metastases: a 20-year institutional experience with comprehensive literature review. World Neurosurg 2012; 79(3):576-84.

[4]   Kwak YS, Kim KT, Cho DC, Kim YB. Minimally invasive removal of an intradural cervical tumor: Assessment of a combined split-spinous laminectomy and quadrant tube retractor system technique. J Korean Neurosurg Soc 2012; 52(4):427-31.

[5]   Poblete B, Kothbauer KF. Intramedullary spinal cord surgery. Monitoring the nervous system for anesthesiologists and other health care professionals. New York: Springer 2012:619-34.

In: Pain Management Yearbook 2013
Editor: Joav Merrick

ISBN: 978-1-63117-944-0
© 2014 Nova Science Publishers, Inc.

Chapter 32

Muscular metastases arising from squamous cell carcinoma of the lung

Nicholas Chiu, Leonard Chiu, Gillian Bedard, BSc(C),
Michael Poon, BSc(C), Marko Popovic, BHSc(C),
Erin Wong, BSc(C), Henry Lam and Edward Chow, MBBS *

Rapid Response Radiotherapy Program, Department of Radiation Oncology,
Odette Cancer Centre, Sunnybrook Health Sciences Centre, University of Toronto,
Toronto, Ontario, Canada

Abstract

Skeletal muscle metastases from lung cancer are a rare occurrence. Therefore, documentation of more cases of skeletal muscle metastases in the literature may be of use to health-care professionals in understanding the disease progression and consequent treatment procedure. The current report documents the case of a 66-year old woman with lung cancer who suffered from associated metastases including a metastatic tumor to the right rectus femoris. The patient underwent palliative radiation and is now deceased at the time of writing.

Keywords: Muscle metastases, lung cancer, radiation treatment

Introduction

Lung cancer is the leading cause of cancer-associated death around the world and is the second most commonly observed subcategory of cancer among both men and women (1). The

* Corresponding author: Edward Chow MBBS, MSc, PhD, FRCPC, Professor, Department of Radiation Oncology, Odette Cancer Centre, Sunnybrook Health Sciences Centre, 2075 Bayview Avenue, Toronto, ON Canada. E-mail: Edward.Chow@sunnybrook.ca.

first reported case of muscular metastasis was documented in 1854 by Wittich et al. and the first reported case of muscle metastases arising from a primary lung tumour was documented by Willis et al. (2). While lung cancer is quite regularly witnessed, skeletal muscle metastases from lung cancer are rare (1,3,4), and, as a result, the most effective strategy for treatment is not yet known (3). In addition, the typical prognosis for patients with skeletal metastases is poor (3). As more cases of skeletal muscle metastases are documented in the literature, procedures for treatment and their associated outcomes may be compared, thereby providing more information to aid health-care professionals in the deliberation process. In addition, an enhanced understanding of the mechanisms which yield resistance of skeletal muscle to metastases could aid in developing interventions for the prevention of metastatic disease (4). As such, it is of importance to document relevant cases of skeletal muscle metastases in the literature. The current report documents the case of a 66-year old woman with lung cancer who suffered from associated metastases including a metastatic tumor to the right rectus femoris that was confirmed to be squamous cell carcinoma.

Case Report

In 2013, a 66-year old female with a 50-pack-year smoking history and a chronic smoker's cough was admitted to the emergency department (ED) at Sunnybrook Health Sciences Centre after complaining of increasing dull and constant midline lower back pain over the span of two days. The patient described the pain as non-radiating and reported similar pain in both her hips. The back pain began 4 months ago, a time period during which the patient lost approximately 15 pounds and experienced associated fevers, chills, and sweats. In addition, the patient experienced muscle spasms in her back as well as developing weakness in her left leg over the past 2 weeks. Prior to admission to the emergency ward, the patient underwent a one-week span of nausea, vomiting, and polyuria. Upon the discovery of chest pain, the patient consulted her family physician 3-4 weeks prior to her admittance to the ED, and subsequent chest x-ray and CT scans confirmed the presence of an abnormal mass in her right lung. The patient was admitted to the emergency ward on April 13, five days prior to her scheduled outpatient biopsy.

In the ED, the patient was found to be hypercalcemic, for which she was treated with Pamidronate. Further investigations revealed extensive metastatic squamous cell carcinoma originating from the lung and involving the bones, liver, left adrenal gland, and the right rectus femoris muscle (Figure 1)

Specifically, a CT scan of the chest detected a primary bronchogenic carcinoma with enlarged mediastinal and hilar lymph nodes in the right lower lobe of the lungs. Bilateral pleural effusions were also observed and bone metastases were detected involving the manubrium, thoracic spine, and ribs with bilateral fractures. A CT scan of the abdomen and pelvis showed multiple bilobar liver metastases—the largest of which measured 3 cm, progressing in size from an earlier CT scan performed 12 days previous. The left adrenal metastatic tumor measured 1.2 cm in size and further bone metastases were seen involving the right iliac and sacroiliac joint as well as the T12 and L3 vertebrae with pathological fractures in both locations. A biopsy of the right rectus femoris metastasis confirmed the presence of squamous cell carcinoma. A CT scan of the head showed no evidence of metastatic growth.

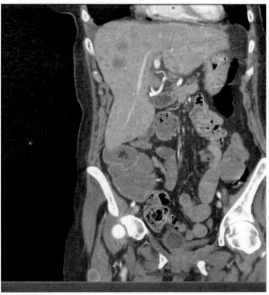

Figure 1. Right rectus femoris enhancing metastasis (arrow shown in red).

During her admission as an inpatient to the Medical Oncology Service, Palliative Care was involved with pain management as well as management of her constipation and nausea. While she continued to maintain good ECOG performance status, she suffered from delirium—a complication that she improved only gradually from. The patient was prescribed systemic therapy consisting of platinum-based chemotherapy to be started as an outpatient and was referred to the Department of Radiation Oncology for palliative radiation. An MRI of spine was done to rule out spinal cord compression and a repeat bone scan showed widespread metastases with an uptake in the midshaft of the right femur. The patient was treated with palliative radiation for her painful bone metastasis where she received a single 8 Gy to the thoracic and lumbar spine, the pubic symphysis, and the right pelvic bone for palliation and pain control. Unfortunately, the patient is now deceased at the time of writing.

Discussion

Metastases from lung cancer are known to commonly involve the liver, adrenal glands, bone, and brain (1,5). All such metastatic sites, except metastases to the brain, were observed in this patient. As skeletal muscle metastases are rarely the only clinical manifestation of lung cancer (3), it is frequently the case that muscle metastases are only detected after the primary lung abnormality has been diagnosed and the tumor has metastasized via hematogenous spread or through the lymphatic system (1,3).

Again, such trends were observed in the 66-year-old patient. In particular, the presence of metastatic growth in the right rectus femoris was discovered only after the patient's primary lung cancer site as well as various multiple metastatic sites, including the liver, had been discovered. As such, the patient had already advanced to a terminal stage of cancer by the time the metastatic growth to her skeletal muscle was identified.

Late-stage diagnosis of skeletal muscle metastases is not uncommon, as various studies have noted the difficulty in establishing a diagnosis of skeletal muscle metastases due to the lack of symptoms it causes (6-8). In fact, skeletal muscle metastases are often not detected unless the presence of a tumor is evident (6-8), as was the case in the current report. Unfortunately, while various studies have identified CT scanning to be an effective means of evaluating the extent of skeletal muscle tumors (6,9), identifying malignant growth via image analysis alone is difficult (6). Moreover, once diagnosed, most patients suffering from skeletal muscle metastasis arising from lung carcinoma die within a year of diagnosis (6,10). Due to this poor prognosis, earlier intervention and prevention is of necessity.

Although patients experiencing metastatic growth in the skeletal muscles are often terminal (6,11), not all such patients fall into this category. A study done in 2009 by Kulahci et al. describes a case in which a 70-year old patient experienced metastatic growth in the left rectus femoris from laryngeal squamous cell carcinoma and who successful underwent surgical excision of the metastases (12).

Twenty-one months after the removal of the metastatic growth, the patient showed no signs of distant muscular recurrence. The patient, however, passed away two years later from brain and suprarenal metastases. Kulahci et al. subsequently recommended surgical removal as a possible treatment procedure in the case of an isolated muscular metastasis, especially if there has been locoregional control of the tumor. They do note, however, that treatment options for skeletal muscle metastases rarely alter the survival outcome (12).

The case reported by Kulahci et al. reported a different primary site than the current case, however, and we note that results from such a case may not be comparable, especially since the current case involves a stage IV terminal patient and extensive metastatic disease was not documented by Kulahci et al. Nevertheless, we recommend that case reports of treatment procedures for metastatic growth in skeletal muscles be done to identify effective treatment options. Perhaps in doing so, optimal treatment procedures in dealing with skeletal muscle metastasis for patients experiencing different stages of disease progression may be identified.

Conclusion

Documentation of more cases of skeletal muscle metastases may be of use to health care professionals in understanding the disease progression of such rare metastatic occurrences. We recommend that further studies of treatment procedures for metastatic growth in skeletal muscles be done in order to identify optimal treatment procedures for patients of various stages of disease progression. Finally, as more studies of relevant cases are documented in the literature, comparisons in treatment procedures should be made to identify more effective treatments for the disease.

References

[1]   Giugliano FM, Alberti D, Guida G, De Palma G, Ladanza L, Mormile M, Cammarota F, Montanino A, Fulciniti F, Ravo V, Muto P. Non small-cell lung cancer with metastasis to thigh muscle and mandible: Two case reports. J Med Case Rep 2013; 7(98):1-5.

[2]   Daniel P, Ahmad SN, Nicolas V, Patrice G, Josiane O, Michel P, Jerome M. Skeletal muscle metastasis from non-small cell lung cancer. J Thorac Oncol 2009; 4(10): 1236-41.

[3]   Di Giorgio A, Sammartino P, Cardini CL, Al Mansour M, Accarpio F, Sibio S, Di Seri M: Lung cancer and skeletal muscle metastases. Ann Thorac Surg 2004; 78:709-11.

[4]   Sridhar KS, Rao RK, Kunhardt B. Skeletal muscle metastases from lung cancer. Cancer 2006; 59(8):1530-3.

[5]   Molina JR, Yang P, Cassivi SD, Schild SE, Adjei AA: Non-small cell lung cancer: epidemiology, risk factors, treatment, and survivorship. Mayo Clin Proc 2008; 83:584-94.

[6]   Hasegawa S, Sakurai Y, Imazu H, Matsubara T, Ochiai H, Funabiki T, Suzuki K, Mizoguchi Y, Kuroda M, Kasahara M. Metastasis to the forearm skeletal muscle from an adenocarcinoma of the colon: Report of a case. Surg Today 2000; 30:1118-23.

[7]   Pearson CM. Incidence and type of pathologic alterations observed in muscle in a routine autopsy survey. Neurology 1959; 9(11):757-66.

[8]   Wilson J, Korobkin M, Genant H, Bovill E. Computed tomography of musculoskeletal disorders. Am J Roentgenol 1978; 131(1):55-61.

[9]   Heelan W, Watson R, Smith J. Computed tomography of lower extremity tumors. Am J Roentgenol 1979; 132:933-7.

[10] Tsunezuka Y, Saito H, Masuda S. A case of adenosquamous cell carcinoma of the lung which was founded by metastasis to the skeletal muscle. Jpn J Lung Cancer 1994; 34:411-6.

[11] Willis RA. The spread of tumours in the human body. Butterworth 1952; 3:284-5.

[12] Kulahci Y, Zor F, Onguru O, Bozkurt M, Duman H. Distant muscular (rectus femoris) metastasis from laryngeal squamous cell carcinoma. J Laryngol Otol 2009; 123:1381-3.

In: Pain Management Yearbook 2013
Editor: Joav Merrick

ISBN: 978-1-63117-944-0
© 2014 Nova Science Publishers, Inc.

Chapter 33

Extrapulmonary tuberculosis mimicking widespread metastatic disease: A case report

*Leila Makhani, Kristopher Dennis, Janet Nguyen, Florencia Jon and Elizabeth Barnes, MD**

Rapid Response Radiotherapy Program, Department of Radiation Oncology, Odette Cancer Centre, Sunnybrook Health Sciences Centre, University of Toronto, Toronto, Ontario, Canada

Abstract

Tuberculosis (TB) can mimic malignant disease as the radiological appearance is non-specific and often resembles tumerous lesions. This report describes the case of a 52-year old woman who presented with spinal cord compression, as well as clinical and radiological signs consistent with metastatic hepatic and pulmonary disease. She was treated with emergent vertebral decompression surgery and histological reports from the operative specimen revealed infection with Mycobacterium tuberculosis. Her diagnosis was eventually confirmed to be widespread disseminated TB. This report highlights the importance of pathological confirmation of presumed malignancy seen on imaging, as well as the inclusion of TB in the differential diagnosis of suspected tumerous lesions.

Keywords: tuberculosis, metastatic disease, differential diagnosis

---

* Corresponding author: Elizabeth Barnes, MD, Department of Radiation Oncology, Odette Cancer Centre, Sunnybrook Health Sciences Centre, University of Toronto, 2075 Bayview Ave, Toronto, Ontario, Canada M4N 3M5. Email: toni.barnes@sunnybrook.ca.

Introduction

An understanding of the various clinical manifestations of tuberculosis (TB) is important for its effective diagnosis and treatment. It is estimated that nearly one third of the world's population is infected with TB (1) and although it is more prevalent in sub-Saharan Africa, India and China, TB still prevails in the west. The United States, Western Europe and Canada encounter approximately 25 cases per 100,000 inhabitants per year (2). Moreover, the recent ease of global travel enables the carriage of Mycobacterium tuberculosis species across continents.

Although M. tuberculosis largely infects the lungs, extrapulmonary manifestation, which is more difficult to diagnose, can also occur (3,4). Tuberculosis has been known to mimic various metastatic conditions, including lung, pancreatic and ovarian carcinomas, and liver metastases (3,5-7). In the majority of these cases, patients were initially diagnosed with neoplastic disease based on radiological findings. However, subsequent tissue biopsies revealed infection with M. tuberculosis, emphasizing the importance and necessity of histological investigation. A delay in the detection and treatment of TB can lead to fatal consequences of unmitigated infection as well as the sequelae of inappropriately administered therapies for other presumed underlying disease processes (8). This highlights the crucial role of pathology in providing an accurate and timely diagnosis.

Herein we report an interesting case of disseminated TB mimicking widespread metastatic disease of unknown origin.

Case report

A 52-year old woman originally from the Philippines, having lived in Canada for 2 years, presented with a 3-month history of pain in the right scapular region. This led to a series of investigations beginning with routine blood work, which revealed incidental elevated liver enzymes. An ultrasound of her liver showed a mass in the hilum, which prompted a contrast enhanced computed tomography (CT) scan of the abdomen and pelvis. The CT scan uncovered multiple hepatic lesions, the largest measuring an aggregate 7.4 by 3.3 cm at the portal confluence and also causing intrahepatic bile duct dilatation due to mass effect. The differential diagnosis included liver metastases, multifocal cholangiocarcinoma and though less likely, a hepatoma. She was therefore referred to surgical oncology for consideration of liver resection.

Staging investigations were performed, including a CT scan of the chest that demonstrated what was believed to be multiple bilateral metastatic pulmonary nodules as well as a sizeable left pleural mass measuring 7.6 by 1.8 cm. In addition, the CT scan showed hilar and mediastinal adenopathy. A partially obscured pathological fracture involving C7 prompted a dedicated CT scan of the cervical spine, which confirmed the pathological fracture at C7 and demonstrated considerable height loss and associated soft tissue protrusion posteriorly. The resulting spinal canal narrowing of approximately 50% contributed to spinal cord compression and spinal instability. The patient was therefore immediately fitted with a cervical collar and rushed to the Emergency Department and referred to Neurosurgery for stabilization of her cervical spine.

At this moment in time, the patient was strongly believed to have widespread metastatic disease of unknown origin and was introduced to the radiation oncology team. The care plan included immediate surgery for decompression of the spinal cord which would also yield a tissue diagnosis. The patient would then be referred for palliative treatments in the form of chemotherapy and postoperative radiation therapy.

After contrast enhanced magnetic resonance imaging (MRI) of the cervical, thoracic and lumbar spine that confirmed the findings seen on CT (See Figure 1), the patient underwent C7 vertebrectomy, and excision of a 5 cm epidural lesion, believed to be tumour tissue. A donor bone allograft was inserted between C6 and T1 and was reinforced with a cervical plate. The patient remained stable throughout surgery and a final X-ray confirmed good positioning of the reinforcements.

Interestingly, the pathological diagnosis of the C7 specimen was necrotizing granulomatous inflammation with acid fast bacilli, consistent with Mycobacterium tuberculosis. Soon after, a CT guided biopsy of the lesion in the left lung confirmed caseating granulomata and the presence of acid fast bacilli, once again consistent with Mycobacterium tuberculosis. Pleural fluid was isolated and cultured for sensitivity. No resistance was indicated and the patient was started on ethambutol (800 mg PO daily), isoniazide (300 mg PO daily), pyrazinamide (500 mg twice daily) and rifampicin (300 mg, twice daily) and referred to a dedicated TB clinic for continued care and monitoring.

Discussion

The clinical and radiographic features of TB can mimic many diseases. TB remains a problem worldwide and should be included in the differential diagnosis for cases of presumed malignancy. Similar cases to that outlined here have been reported, in which TB was mistaken for metastatic disease and subsequently mistreated until tissue diagnosis revealed infection with M. tuberculosis.

Ringshausen et al. (8) described a fatal case of spinal TB in a 67-year old Caucasian man, misdiagnosed as metastatic lung cancer. Imaging of the chest and spine showed a compression fracture and a solitary pulmonary lesion. The initial tissue biopsy of the pulmonary lesion was unsuccessful in providing a specific diagnosis, and the patient was treated with three weeks of palliative radiotherapy to the thoracic spine. Following, the tissue sample obtained from the spinal decompression surgery revealed non-specific chronic inflammation and granulation. The patient's general condition deteriorated rapidly over the next three months, after which the diagnosis of TB was made with polymerase chain reaction (PCR) analysis of the surgically resected tissue (8).

Another similar case was a 51-year old woman provisionally diagnosed with a pancreatic tumour. Further imaging and endoscopic retrograde cholangio-pancreatography (ERCP) suggested serous cystadenoma of the pancreas. Pancreatic TB was only discovered after the mass was surgically removed at the request of the patient and sent for further histological testing (3). Three other similar cases are described, in which the patients were initially diagnosed with pancreatic carcinoma until histological analysis revealed infection with M. tuberculosis (9).

Tuberculosis can present in multiple ways, and hence, its misdiagnosis is not surprising. The lesson to be learnt from these cases is the crucial role that tissue analysis plays in the timely diagnosis and treatment of TB. Despite today's advanced imaging techniques, tissue biopsy remains the gold standard in confirming or refuting a provisional diagnosis made on the basis of radiological findings. Although there are multiple ways to obtain a tissue sample, some centres may be hesitant to perform fine needle aspiration in the case of suspected malignancy, due to the risk of tumour seeding along the needle track (7). It is reassuring to note that in the case of suspected spinal TB, CT-guided percutaneous biopsy of the vertebral body is known to be a safe method of diagnosing spinal lesions (10,11).

In our case, although post-operative radiation to the cervical spine would not have been life-threatening to the patient, it could have induced focal neurological symptoms, pain flare, fatigue, skin irritation and odynophagia, all of which would have been unnecessarily imposed on the patient. Indeed, patients receiving inappropriate treatment for missed TB are subject to the sequelae of treatment, as well as the symptoms of untreated infection. Our patient could have progressed locally and systemically and posed an infectious risk to those around her if she had remained undiagnosed.

In the face of complex cases of presumed malignancy, pathologic confirmation of disease (cancer, tuberculosis or otherwise) has a pivotal role in correct diagnosis and treatment. It is important to employ a higher index of suspicion for the diagnosis of TB, especially in patients who come from countries where the disease is endemic. Moreover, long-term TB treatment and monitoring may help to ensure disease control and reduce drug resistance.

Acknowledgments

The authors declare no conflicts of interest related to this manuscript

References

[1]   Lonnroth K, Raviglione M. Global epidemiology of tuberculosis: prospects for control. Semin Respir Crit Care Med 2008; 29(5):481-91.

[2]   WHO. Global Tuberculosis Control. Geneva: World Health Organization 2008.

[3]   Hong SG, Kim JS, Joo MK, Lee KG, Kim KH, Oh CR, et al. Pancreatic tuberculosis masquerading as pancreatic serous cystadenoma. World J Gastroenterol 2009;15(8):1010-3.

[4]   Aisenberg GM, Jacobson K, Chemaly RF, Rolston KV, Raad, II, Safdar A. Extrapulmonary tuberculosis active infection misdiagnosed as cancer: Mycobacterium tuberculosis disease in patients at a Comprehensive Cancer Center (2001-2005). Cancer 2005;104(12):2882-7.

[5]   Landen S, Ballet T, Kessler R, Badic B, Costache M, Dobos S, et al. Tuberculosis diagnosed after major hepatectomy for suspected malignancy. ActaChirBelg 2010;110(2):221-4.

[6]   Dursun P, Ersoz S, Gultekin M, Aksan G, Yuce K, Ayhan A. Disseminated peritoneal tuberculosis mimicking advanced-stage endodermal sinus tumor: a case report. Int J Gynecol Cancer 2006;16(Suppl 1):303-7.

[7]   Landen S, Ballet T, Bollars P, Badic B, Herman D, Delugeau V. Liver tuberculosis mistaken for malignancy. The role of needle biopsy. Acta Gastroenterol Belg 2010;73(2):278-9.

[8]   Ringshausen FC, Tannapfel A, Nicolas V, Weber A, Duchna HW, Schultze-Werninghaus G, et al. A fatal case of spinal tuberculosis mistaken for metastatic lung cancer: recalling ancient Pott's disease. Ann Clin Microbiol Antimicrob 2009;8:32.

[9]   Tan KK, Chen K, Liau KH, Ho CK. Pancreatic tuberculosis mimicking pancreatic carcinoma: series of three cases. Eur J Gastroenterol Hepatol 2009;21(11):1317-9.

[10]   Heyer CM, Al-Hadari A, Mueller KM, Stachon A, Nicolas V. Effectiveness of CT-guided percutaneous biopsies of the spine: an analysis of 202 examinations. AcadRadiol 2008;15(7):901-11.

[11]   Pertuiset E, Beaudreuil J, Liote F, Horusitzky A, Kemiche F, Richette P, et al. Spinal tuberculosis in adults. A study of 103 cases in a developed country, 1980-1994. Medicine 1999;78(5):309-20.

[12]   Tan KK, Chen K, Liau KH, Ho CK. Pancreatic tuberculosis mimicking pancreatic carcinoma: series of three cases. Eur J Gastroenterol Hepatol 2009;21(11):1317-9.

[13]   Heyer CM, Al-Hadari A, Mueller KM, Stachon A, Nicolas V. Effectiveness of CT-guided percutaneous biopsies of the spine: an analysis of 202 examinations. AcadRadiol 2008;15(7):901-11.

[14]   Pertuiset E, Beaudreuil J, Liote F, Horusitzky A, Kemiche F, Richette P, et al. Spinal tuberculosis in adults. A study of 103 cases in a developed country, 1980-1994. Medicine 1999;78(5):309-20.

In: Pain Management Yearbook 2013
Editor: Joav Merrick

ISBN: 978-1-63117-944-0
© 2014 Nova Science Publishers, Inc.

Chapter 34

Opioid-induced hyperalgesia and monotherapy intrathecal ziconotide: Experience with four cases

Mary Jean Walker[*] **and Lynn R Webster**

University of Utah, Salt Lake City, Utah and Lifetree Clinical Research,
Salt Lake City, Utah, United States of America

Abstract

Opioid-induced hyperalgesia (OIH) is reported to be a state of increased pain due to systemic and intrathecal (IT) opioid therapy. *Objective*: To determine the association with delivery of IT Ziconotide as monotherapy, and the reduction of OIH symptoms. Methods: A literature search of OIH presentation and symptoms assisted in the identification of patients who may qualify for the diagnosis. Four patients were identified who met the qualifications for OIH by examination, symptoms, and history. The patients were weaned off opioid therapy and started on IT ziconotide monotherapy with a dose range of 2.4 to 14 μg per day. The mean treatment duration was 11.25 months. Primary efficacy measures were the percent decrease in opioid usage and the mean decrease in pain intensity scores. *Results:* Patients were male, aged 48-66 years. Prior to initiation of ziconotide therapy, mean duration of severe chronic pain was 27.75 years, mean pain intensity score was 8/10 measured via numeric rating scale, and mean oral opioid dose was 408 oral morphine equivalents in addition to IT therapies. Ziconotide monotherapy reduced pain scores to a mean of 5.5/10, representing a 32% reduction from baseline. Two patients discontinued opioids, 1 patient was rotated off traditional opioids to 24 mg buprenorphine/naloxone, and one patient decreased oral morphine equivalents from 320 mg to 56 mg of oral hydromorphone per day, (224 morphine equivalents). *Conclusion:* Ziconotide monotherapy provided improved pain control accompanied by discontinued or substantially lowered opioid doses in this case series of patients with suspected OIH.

---

[*] Corresponding author: Mary Jean Walker, MSN, APRNDNP, Park City Spine and Pain. Park City, UT 84060, United States. Email: Jean.Walker2@imail.org.

Keywords: Pain, chronic pain, opioid

Introduction

Lack of efficacy in long-term opioid therapy is commonly seen in clinical practice and can result from pharmacologic opioid tolerance, opioid-induced abnormal pain sensitivity, or disease progression (1). Frequent solutions to this problem include opioid rotation, reduction of the daily dose, or detoxification. Opioid-induced hyperalgesia (OIH), a topic of widespread discussion and research in recent years, is now considered a primary differential diagnosis when loss of efficacy occurs in patients undergoing long-standing treatment with high-dose opioids. Chu et al. (2) defined OIH as a state of nociceptive sensitization caused by exposure to opioids and summarized 15 case reports documenting OIH in patients on high dose opioids. Opioid-induced abnormal pain sensitivity has much in common with the cellular mechanisms of neuropathic pain (3, 4). OIH has been observed in patients treated for pain. It has also been observed in patients being treated for pain who demonstrate addiction behaviors. (5) OIH occurs with both systemic and intrathecal (IT) use of opioid medications. Presentation of OIH can differ in origin and quality and may extend beyond the distribution of pre-existing pain.

The practitioner is often unable to distinguish between OIH and development of tolerance. The tapering of opioids is often fraught with challenges and sometimes, decreases in patient functionality. As practitioners attempt to decrease IT opioids in order to reduce hyperalgesia, we are left with the search for alternatives to improve the quality of life of our patients. Ziconotide offers a non-opioid alternative for management of chronic pain and is hypothesized to reduce OIH and tolerance to opioids.

Ziconotide, previously called SNX-111, is an IT analgesic approved by the FDA in December 2004 for the management of severe chronic pain not relieved by systemic analgesia, adjunctive therapies, or IT morphine in patients who are appropriate candidates for IT therapy (6). Ziconotide is the first non-opioid, IT-administered, neuronal-type calcium channel blocker approved in the United States (7). Developed from the venom of the Conus magus sea snail, the molecule is a synthetic version of the omega-conotoxin MVIIA. Ziconotide is a peptide with a large molecule compared with non-peptide drugs. Highly hydrophilic, it moves slowly from the cerebrospinal fluid through the parenchyma to its target site in the dorsal horn of the spinal cord. The onset of pain relief after initiation of the drug may be delayed by 2 to 4 hours. Maximum effects may develop after 8 to 12 hours (8).

Ziconotide is an N-type voltage-gated calcium channel blocker, which mediates normal sensory neuron excitability and neurotransmitter release (9). Blocking calcium influx into the nerve terminals reduces the release of pain-relevant neurotransmitters such as glutamate and neuropeptides from the primary afferent nerve terminals into the synaptic cleft (8).

The 2007 Polyanalgesic Consensus panel has approved ziconotide as a first-line drug for use in IT therapy (10). With the advent of this major step forward, interest has increased in the use and the mechanisms of action of this novel drug.

Many animal studies and animal models of pain using ziconotide showed strong anti-nociceptive effects (11, 12). The initial animal studies reported that IT ziconotide was at least

10 times more potent than IT morphine (13). The efficacy data in humans are less robust and based on a limited number of randomized, double-blind, placebo-controlled trials (11, 12).

In a case series report, ziconotide demonstrated benefit in patients with complex regional pain syndrome, pointing to a possible role in reducing the symptoms of OIH and reversing central sensitization (14). As an N-type calcium channel antagonist, ziconotide has been shown to block nerve injury-induced tactile allodynia in animal models (15).

The effect of ziconotide on OIH has not been studied in clinical trials; however, pharmacokinetic evidence is strong that ziconotide could help reverse the paradoxical sensitization and continue to reduce pain as opioids are discontinued. Clinical observations by practitioners who provide pain management support this hypothesis.

This brief retrospective case series investigates the ability of ziconotide to reverse or reduce OIH and to unwind central sensitization in patients with chronic pain. The current study is meant to lay a foundation for further research.

Literature review and search strategy

A literature review was performed by searching Pub Med, CINAHL, and GOOGLE Scholar for the terms ziconotide, opioid-induced hypersensitivity, SNX-111, and intrathecal pain therapy. Publications from the past seven years were preferentially selected. Also, publications for historical purposes were included. The pharmacological research presented in the early years of the development of ziconotide suggested that it could be beneficial in OIH. Therefore several animal studies and early pharmacological reports were included in the literature search.

Methods

Four patients were identified between 2007 and 2010 with suspected OIH, based on the following criteria: High-dose systemic and IT opioids, high levels of pain extending beyond the primary pain complaint as measured by a mean score greater than 5 and low functional ability as measured by a score greater than 50 on the Brief Pain Inventory. Medical records were reviewed for demographic information and medical histories. The clinical presentation of these four patients warranted a reassessment of their treatment plans. In these patients, the decision was made to trial ziconotide in their IT pumps.

The patients were weaned completely off their IT opioid regimens at variable rates prior to trialing with ziconotide via IT pump in a continuous infusion. No greater than a 20% reduction in any medication in the IT regimens was allowed at one time, and adjustments occurred no more often than weekly.

Ziconotide dose was titrated by 0.25 µg to 0.5 µg per day (16) every 2 weeks or every month as necessary. Lower incremental adjustments were made due to early clinical response in therapy and dose stabilization. Concurrent use of oral morphine equivalents was recorded upon initiation of ziconotide and with each therapeutic response reported to ziconotide.

Numeric Pain Rating Scale (NPRS), IT doses of opioids, systemic doses of opioids and other concomitant drugs, physical examination results, functional and quality of life changes, adverse events, and patient perspectives on treatment were evaluated. The NPRS for measurement of pain intensity was a 0 to 10 scale with 0 equaling no pain and 10 indicating the worst pain experienced. The NPRS is widely used and accepted within the pain management community as a valid and reliable tool (17). The primary efficacy measures were the percent decrease in opioid usage and the mean decrease in pain intensity scores. Secondary efficacy measures were the improvement in quality of life and functionality, measured by patient report and a Brief Pain Inventory quality-of-life 10-point scale administered at each visit (18). Safety was assessed by adverse event reports. All results were summarized descriptively.

Results

The patients were male, ages 48, 50, 55, and 66 years (see table 1). The mean duration of severe chronic back pain was 27.75 years. Each of the patients had exhausted multiple therapeutic options and multiple IT therapies prior to being weaned and placed on ziconotide monotherapy. The mean oral opioid dose was 408 oral morphine equivalents in addition to IT therapies, and the mean NPRS score was 8/10 (see figure 1) (18).

Table 1. Decrease in oral opioids expressed in morphine equivalents

Patient	Prior to treatment	After treatment	Percent decrease	Mean duration
M1 50 yrs	120mg	0mg	100	18 mo
M2 48 yrs	929mg	312mg	66	12mo
M3 66 yrs	623mg	0mg	100	10mo
M4 55 yrs	320mg	184mg	42.5	9mo

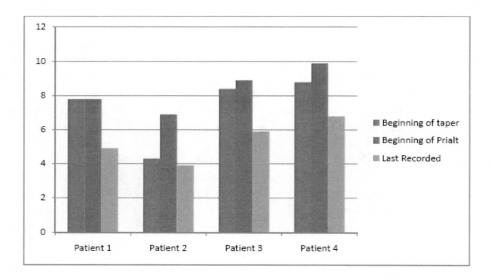

Figure 1. Average NPRS scores.

Mean treatment duration of ziconotide monotherapy was 11.25 months with a dose range of 2.4 µg to 14 µg per day. The mean NPRS report of 5.5/10 with ziconotide monotherapy represented a 32% reduction from baseline pain scores. Two patients are opioid free. One patient was rotated to 40 mg buprenorphine/naloxone, and 1 patient decreased his oral morphine equivalents from 320 mg to 56 mg of oral hydromorphone (see table 1) (19).

Case reports

Case study 1

This patient is a 50-year-old Caucasian male with chronic back pain due to an injury in 1983. He had two failed spine fusion procedures and several discectomies. He had lost 30 to 40 pounds due to nausea and the inability to eat. The nausea and anorexia were attributed to his chronic pain. He was unable to walk long distances and was bedridden due to his pain. He reported hyperalgesia in his lower extremities, and could not bear to have the sheets on his legs while sleeping. His medications prior to initiation of ziconotide therapy included diazepam, hydrocodone, hydromorphone, celecoxib, clonidine, morphine sulfate, methylnaltrexone, testosterone gel, promethazine, lanzoprazole, and lubiprostone. His oral morphine equivalents were 120 mg per day.

His morphine IT dose was 13.5 mg per day with clonidine 58.5 µg per day, hydromorphone 1.75 mg per day, and bupivacaine 3.75 milligrams per day.

He experienced several adverse effects related to his therapy prior to administering IT ziconotide. These included hypogonadism, nausea, and vomiting, sexual dysfunction, sleep apnea, and gastroparesis. He also experienced chronic obstructive pulmonary disease, unrelated to his opioid therapy.

The patient was weaned off IT medications over a 10-month period. He was seen monthly for a reduction in his IT pump rate. The average reduction per visit was 1 mg of morphine. Ziconotide using the 25 µg/ml vial was initiated at 1.2 µg per day IT until he reached a therapeutic level at 3.5 µg per day. He responded well at initiation and continued to improve at each titration.

He was followed for 18 months, and at his last evaluation, he was able to discontinue all oral pain medications and to walk 100 feet without assistance. He was no longer bedridden, able to walk his dog and drive his wife out to dinner. The patient reported an improvement in all aspects of his quality of life. At his last follow-up, he reported no increases in NPRS scores and no changes in his ziconotide dose of 3.5 ug per day.

He reported no adverse effects with ziconotide therapy. Following the titration and stabilization of his dose, he remained on only 2 of his previous drugs: diazepam and celecoxib.

Case study 2

This patient is a 48-year-old white male with chronic back pain due to an injury in 1991. He underwent a lumbar spine fusion from L4-S1 with 2 rods, 6 screws, and a discectomy. He was unable to sit or stand for long periods and had difficulty sleeping because of the pain. He had a history of three separate incidences of "driving under the influence" (DUI) charges against him due to medication overuse and misuse. His family relationships were strained due to his dysfunction.

His oral medication prior to initiation of ziconotide therapy included the following: fentanyl transmucosal lozenges, oxycodone extended-release, clonazepam, carisprodol, fentanyl transdermal, quetiapine, diazepam, alprazolam, morphine, oxycodone/ acetaminophen, hydromorphone, zolpidem, and trazodone. His total morphine equivalents were 929 mg per day. The adverse effects reported with this therapy included xerostomia, nausea, vomiting, muscle cramping, sedation, hypogonadism, and rhinitis.

His IT therapy prior to initiation of ziconotide included the following: clonidine 82.5 μg per day, hydromorphone 0.27 mg per day, fentanyl 5.5 mg per day, sufentanil 88 μg per day, and baclofen 275 μg per day. He was weaned off of his IT pump medications over 1.25 months with biweekly reductions of 20%. His pump was explanted due to an infection from a revised pump procedure 3 months prior to the initiation of ziconotide. During the period between explantation and implantation of his new pump, he was maintained on oral medications. After the resolution of the infection and implantation of a new pump, he was initiated on ziconotide using the 25 μg/ml vial at 1.2 μg per day. He responded to the ziconotide therapy after 3 weeks. He was maintained on 2.4 μg per day and reported this to be a therapeutic dose. He was able to work full time, ride a bike, and stated that he felt better than he had in 17 years. He was able to reestablish a relationship with his family. He reported no adverse effects with his ziconotide therapy.

He was evaluated at 12 months and reported ongoing and continued quality of life, low pain scores, and no changes in his ziconotide dose. His oral medications at follow-up included buprenorphine/naloxone, tizanidine, and quetiapine.

Case study 3

A 66-year-old white male had sustained multiple lower back injuries and reported a history of pain for more than 20 years. Multiple cervical root lesions were present. He also had lumbosacral arthritis, degenerative disc disease in the cervical spine, and a history of lumbar spine fusion with failed postoperative results. He was unable to sit or stand for long periods. Severe muscle spasms occurred frequently throughout the day and were debilitating for him. He was unable to work and was extremely limited in his daily activities. Pain also disrupted his sleep. His oral medications prior to initiation of ziconotide therapy included the following: oxycodone extended-release, fentanyl transdermal, diazepam, baclofen, alprazolam, clonazepam, zolpidem, hydromorphone, eszopiclone, eletriptan, frovatriptan, promethazine, celecoxib, and acetaminophen/caffeine. His oral morphine equivalents were 623 mg per day. His reported adverse effects included the following: headaches, urinary retention, xerostomia, vomiting, syncope, hypotension, insomnia, constipation, and gastroparesis. His IT therapy included the following: clonidine 133 μg per day, hydromorphone 17 mg per day, sufentanil 7 μg per day, baclofen 400 μg per day, bupivacaine 5.3 mg per day. He was weaned off the IT medications over a 4.5-month period as follows: a 20% reduction during the first month, followed by every week for 2 months, followed by every other day until his dose was sufficiently low to remove the IT medications. Ziconotide monotherapy was initiated with the

25 µg/ml vial. His starting dose was 1.2 µg per day. He reported a positive response to therapy at the initiation of therapy. He reached an adequate therapeutic dose at 2.2 µg per day. He had a personal therapeutic monitor which allowed him a 0.25 µg bolus each day. He reported urinary retention, confusion, mental status changes, syncope, nausea and vomiting with monotherapy IT ziconotide. The adverse effects were self-limiting and resolved with dose reductions. He reported ongoing problems with insomnia but was able to improve his activity level and help with activities around the house. He stated that "the ziconotide and buprenorphine/naloxone combination saved my life."

He was able to eliminate all oral and IT opioids, remaining on naproxen for pain and eszopiclone for insomnia. He was evaluated at 10 months and was on ziconotide at the time of review.

Case study 4

A 55-year-old white male reported chronic back pain due to a work-related injury in 1994. He underwent a lumbar spine fusion, but his pain never resolved. He had been treated with a spinal cord stimulator, which had failed. He reported that he was unable to complete even simple household duties and self-care and spent most of every day in bed. His sleep was disrupted due to the pain. His medications prior to initiation of ziconotide monotherapy included the following: morphine sulfate, fentanyl, tapentadol, pregabalin, naproxen, lamotrigine, lidocaine transdermal, trazodone, clonazepam, celecoxib, and tizanidine. His morphine equivalents were 320 mg per day. He complained of dyspepsia, depression, constipation, and dysphagia.

His IT pump was programmed to deliver clonidine 200 µg per day, fentanyl 300 µg per day, hydromorphone 41.9 mg per day, and bupivacaine 9.6 mg per day. He was weaned off his IT pump medications over a 5-month period. He was able to tolerate a 20% reduction each month. After tapering and removing the IT medications, he was initiated on ziconotide using the 25 µg/ml vial to be delivered at 1.2 µg per day. He was titrated to a therapeutic effect of 14 µg per day. He reported a response to therapy at 5 weeks. He reported his back pain was decreasing, he was no longer bedridden, and he was able to walk faster and complete household duties. He was able to do minimal work in the yard, go fishing, and take care of his personal needs . He appeared at the clinic groomed, which was a change in his presentation prior to ziconotide therapy.

He was evaluated at 9 months and was tolerating his ziconotide therapy without significant difficulty. His continued oral medications included hydromorphone 56 mg per day, duloxetine, and diclofenac transdermal patches.

Discussion

The patients in this case series presented with symptoms consistent with OIH. Hyperalgesia is primarily a clinical diagnosis; therefore, the diagnosis is arbitrary. The fact that the patients improved in function, had a reduction in pain, and were on little to no opioids following the treatment, is a strong indicator that OIH was the cause of their excessive pain, and unresponsiveness to opioid therapy.

The NPRS pain scores rose initially when weaning patients off their pre-ziconotide IT therapy regimens. Patients were monitored closely for signs and symptoms of withdrawal and treated appropriately. Patients tolerated weaning off their IT regimens with variable rates due to individual patient circumstances. Some patients were unable to return to the clinic more often than once a month because of travel restrictions. A dose reduction of ≤20% of any component in the IT regimens was the standard. No reductions took place more often than once a week unless there was an emergency situation. Patient No. 2 developed an infection in his IT pump pocket, necessitating an escalation in the weaning schedule to twice a week.

When the clinical response and therapeutic window to ziconotide was achieved, all of the patients were able to significantly reduce or discontinue oral and systemic opioids and non-opioid drugs. This dose reduction was voluntary by the patients because symptoms no longer were present that necessitated drug use, and the patients no longer wanted to be on opioids as part of their pain management treatment.

Initial clinical trials with fast titration of ziconotide were associated with serious adverse events, primarily cognitive. Subsequently, the FDA approved ziconotide for a slow titration rate, not to exceed 2.4 μg per day. The drug is initiated at a low dose and titrated slowly over several months. The most frequently reported adverse events (>25%) in clinical trials of 1254 patients (662 patient years) with slow titration of ziconotide were dizziness, nausea, confusion, and nystagmus. (Pharma, 2010). Ataxia was reported in 14% of the study group, and hallucinations in 2%, which resolved with tapering or discontinuing the dose.

This series of patients had a clinical response very early in titration of ziconotide and reported no or few adverse events, which were managed by downward titration. As the ziconotide dose was tapered and the adverse effects diminished, the therapeutic window was identified. Once stabilized on a dose, the patients generally did not require changes in their dose. The patients described in this case report had a 20% to 40% reduction in NPRS scores. All had clinically significant increases in their functionality over their previous regimens. This outcome was clinically stable over the duration of the measurement period.

Conclusion

Monotherapy of a continuous infusion of IT ziconotide may prove to be an excellent option for treatment of OIH. All patients displayed moderate improvement in their NPRS scores and quality of life. Three of the four patients did not report any adverse events from ziconotide therapy. Patient No. 3 had cognitive adverse effects that resolved upon a decrease in the rate of administration. Although these patients showed improvement with IT ziconotide, further studies are needed to determine the full effects of ziconotide on OIH.

Acknowledgments

We wish to express our sincere appreciation for the assistance of KeriKasun, PharmD of Jazz Pharmaceuticals for her assistance in reviewing this manuscript.

References

[1] Ballantyne JC, Mao J. Opioid therapy for chronic pain. New Engl J Med 2003;349(20):1943-53.

[2] Chu LF, Angst MS, Clark D. Opioid-induced hyperalgesia in humans: Molecular mechanisms and clinical considerations. Clin Journal Pain 2008; 24(6):479-96.

[3] Mao J, Price DD, Mayer DJ. Thermal hyperalgesia in association with the development of morphine tolerance in rats: roles of excitatory amino acid receptors and protein kinase. C J Neurosci 1994; 14(4):2301-12.

[4] Mao J, Price DD, Mayer DJ. Mechanisms of hyperalgesia and morphine tolerance: a current view of their possible interactions. Pain 1995; 62(3): 259-74.

[5] Compton MA. Cold-pressor pain tolerance in opiate and cocaine abusers: correlates of drug type and use status. J Pain Symptom Manage 1994; 9(7):462-73.

[6] Lynch SS, Cheng CM, Yee JL. Intrathecal ziconotide for refractory chronic pain. Ann Pharmacother 2006; 40(7-8):1293-1300.

[7] AzurPharma. Prialt package insert. 2010; Accessed 2011 Jul 28.URL: http://www.azurpharma.com/pdf/prialt/PRLTp-10-01-R6%20Cropped%20for% 20Web.pdf.

[8] Schmidtko A, et al. Ziconotide for treatment of severe chronic pain. Lancet 2010; 375(9725):1569-77.

[9] Perret D, Luo ZD. Targeting voltage-gated calcium channels for neuropathic pain management. Neurotherapeutics 2009; 6(4):679-92.

[10] Deer T, et al. Polyanalgesic consensus conference 2007; Recommendations for the management of pain by intrathecal (intraspinal) drug delivery: report of an interdisciplinary expert panel. Neuromodulation 2007; 10(4):300-28.

[11] Wallace MS. Ziconotide: a new nonopioid intrathecal analgesic for the treatment of chronic pain. Expert Rev Neurother 2006; 6(10):1423-8.

[12] Bowersox SS, Luther R. Pharmacotherapeutic potential of omega-conotoxin MVIIA (SNX-111), an N-type neuronal calcium channel blocker found in the venom of Conus magus. Toxicon 1998; 36(11): 1651-8.

[13] Vanegas H, Schaible H. Effects of antagonists to high-threshold calcium channels upon spinal mechanisms of pain, hyperalgesia and allodynia. Pain 2000; 85(1-2):9-18.

[14] Kapural L, et al. Intrathecal ziconotide for complex regional pain syndrome: Seven Case Reports. Pain Pract 2009; 9(4):296-303.

[15] Chaplan SR, Pogrel JW, Yaksh TL. Role of voltage-dependent calcium channel subtypes in experimental tactile allodynia. J Pharmacol Exp Ther 1994; 269(3):1117-23.

[16] Burton AW, et al. Considerations and methodology for trialing ziconotide. Pain Physician 2010;13(1):23-33.

[17] Madigan Army Medical Center, Clinical practice guidelines: provider tools 2010. Accessed 2011 Jul 10. URLhttp://www.mamc.amedd.army.mil/clinical/standards/ pain_pro.htm

[18] Partners against pain, Pain treatment topics, pain and disability assessment tools 2010. Accessed 2011 Jul 12. URL:http://www.mamc.amedd.army.mil/clinical/ standards/ pain_pro.htm

[19] Yassen A, et al. Animal-to-human extrapolation of the pharmacokinetic and pharmacodynamic properties of buprenorphine. Clin Pharmacokinet 2007; 46(5):433-47.

[20] Cowan A, Lewis JW, Macfarlane IR. Agonist and antagonist properties of buprenorphine, a new antinociceptive agent. Br J Pharmacol 1977; 60(4):537-45.

In: Pain Management Yearbook 2013
Editor: Joav Merrick

ISBN: 978-1-63117-944-0
© 2014 Nova Science Publishers, Inc.

Chapter 35

Instruments to measure acute pain: An integrative review

*Dru Riddle**

School of Nurse Anesthesia, Texas Christian University,
Fort Worth, Texas, United States of America

Abstract

Acute pain impacts approximately 45% of the world's population and is a cause of delayed discharge and increased cost to the healthcare system. If not appropriately treated, acute pain can transition into chronic pain resulting in long-term complications. The objective of this integrative review is to synthesize and describe the current instruments used to measure acute pain.

Methods: A systematic three-stage search strategy was used to review the literature.

Results: A total of 1,754 manuscripts were identified with eight meeting all inclusion criteria. Many of the instruments report various aspects of psychometrics but only five reported reliability, validity, and address feasibility.

Conclusions: Caution should be exercised when using the currently available instruments to measure acute pain. Since treatment decisions are often based solely on the pain measurement instrument, it is important to ensure the chosen instrument is both reliable and valid.

Keywords: Acute pain, instrument, review, psychometrics, integrative review

---

* Corresponding author: Dru Riddle, DNP, CRNA, Assistant Professor of Professional Practice, Texas Christian University, School of Nurse Anesthesia, TCU Box 298626, Fort Worth, Texas 76129, United States. Email: d.riddle@tcu.edu or druriddle@me.com.

Introduction

Pain, as a concept, is an unpleasant or unwanted feeling often brought on by an injury or illness (1). It is estimated that approximately 50% of the American population suffers from some form of acute or chronic pain (2). Within the past few years, there has been a push internationally to think of pain as the "Fifth Vital Sign" signifying its importance to both the patient and healthcare provider (3). Physiological implications of pain include: increased catecholamine release, changes in intrinsic cortisol levels, and delayed wound healing as well as psychological problems like depression and anxiety (4,5).

Pain is typically considered subjective, can be defined by the person experiencing it and can be described in multiple different ways. Theoretically, pain is defined as an aversive, uncomfortable, and unwanted sensation (6). To operationally define pain a score or rating on a particular measurement scale is often used. Given the heterogeneity of individual pain perceptions, the measurement of pain as a construct has been labeled difficult to accurately measure (7).

There are several defined types of pain including acute, chronic, and neuropathic pain. The focus of this review is to critically review the clinically used instruments that are aimed or focus on measuring acute pain. Acute pain is often defined as the normal physiologic response to adverse physical stimulus such as trauma, surgery, and acute illness (8). The patient's self-reported pain score often predicates treatment of acute pain and there are several instruments in use clinically that purport to measure pain. The purpose of this integrative literature review is to synthesize the best available evidence related to quantitative instruments used to measure acute pain.

Theoretical framework

Currently, several theories informing the study and pathophysiology of pain. As proposed originally by Melzack and Wall, the gate control theory of pain proposes that there is a natural physiologic factor (gate) that modulates pain impulses within the spinal cord (9). When a noxious impulse is perceived, large nerve fibers inhibit the transmission of some of the stimulus to the brain through afferent nerve tracts. The gate, or large nerve fibers, is effectively closed at this point and stimulation of the dorsal horn neurons of the spinal cord does not occur and the perception of pain is decreased (10).

The gating mechanism is influenced by nerve transmission descending from the brain and this mechanism is thought to explain some aspects of normal physiologic functioning in the face of pain (9). Factors influencing the gating mechanism include the amount of activity of pain fibers, the presence of analgesic medications, and emotional factors such as depression and mood (11). Although the gate control theory of pain does not explain everything regarding pain, an in-depth study of this framework does explain why various medications and treatment modalities are effective in controlling pain. Within the current literature, the gate control theory of pain is one of the accepted frameworks.

Search strategy

Using a three-step search strategy, the literature was queried to find relevant and related studies. Consultation with a health science reference librarian was utilized to hone and refine the search terms and databases. In the first step of the search, the key words "measurement" and "pain" were used in the Cumulative Index to Nursing and Allied Health Literature (CINAHL) and MEDLINE databases to ascertain relevant articles and additional key words related to the concept of interest. In the next step of the search strategy, all identified key words including acute pain, measurement, instrument, and self-report were utilized across CINAHL, MEDLINE, PUBMED, and PsychINFO databases. In the third step of the search, the reference list of all articles meeting inclusion criteria was searched for additional manuscripts. Figure 1 represents the search strategy and articles found with each step. Of note, one article was not found using a database search; instead the article was shared by a colleague and is included as it meets inclusion criteria (12). Overall, eight articles were utilized in this integrative review and table 1 represents the relevant findings from those articles.

For the purposes of this literature review, the focus was on instruments that are self-reported measures of acute pain levels. Instruments that are designed for use in sedated or cognitively impaired individuals were excluded. Additionally, as the focus of this review was the adult population, studies related to instruments for use specifically in children were also excluded. Lastly, only instruments that were available in the English language were examined. There are several studies that address the psychometric evaluation of instruments for application in other languages; these studies were excluded, as no translational services are available. There was no date-limit set for this literature search.

Results

Each of the eight studies included in this literature review represents a self-reported method of measurement of acute pain. Seven of the eight studies were conducted in the United States and one was conducted in England.

Overall, the quality of the studies was fair with medium to low-level evidence informing these results (13). The combination of these eight studies represents 1,278 total study participants. Only two of the eight studies reported a theoretical framework for their study design (14,15). Three of the eight studies reported information on a newly developed scale aimed at measuring acute pain (12,14,16). The remaining five studies examined psychometric properties of existing instruments with new applications or revised designs. Specific psychometric properties of the eight included studies are reported in table 1.

Reliability

Seven of the eight studies report some measure of reliability. In pain management research, reliability is commonly measured in reliability coefficients, which is a measure of stability and consistency over time (17). This is commonly reported as Cronbach's alpha. Six of the eight studies report reliability in terms of internal consistency with Cronbach's alpha scores. Consistently, the measures of internal consistency as represented by Cronbach's alpha are high (>0.95) across all six studies. The Visual Analog for Pain study used Interclass Correlation Coefficient (ICC) scores between one-minute measurements and the McGill Pain Questionnaire study performed three confirmatory factor analysis models to test for reliability (18,19).

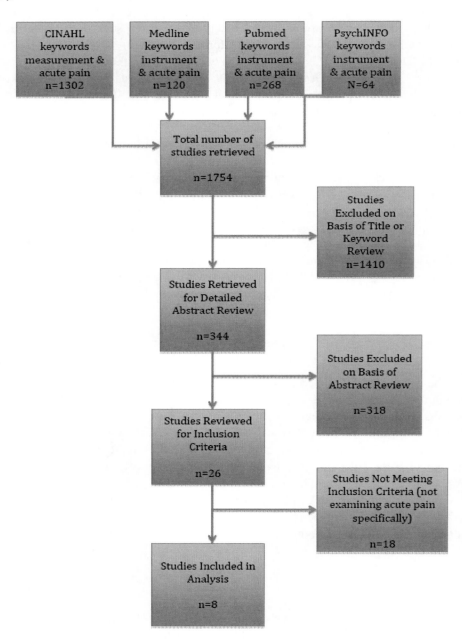

Figure 1. Search results.

Table 1. Data extraction and psychometric properties

Instrument Reference	Framework	Sample Subjects	Instrument Description and Scoring	Reliability	Validity	Feasibility	Level of Evidence[13]
Brief Pain Inventory Revised (BPI-R):(25)	Not reported	Adult surgical cancer patients at two VA hospitals in the US, n= 388	23-item self-report with response categories of 0-10 ordinal scale; higher number indicating more intense pain; 15 minutes to complete	Cronbach's alpha = 0.95 for medical patients Cronbach's alpha = 0.97 for surgical patients	Calculated by comparing BPI with VAS; Pearson correlation coefficients= 0.70 for medical patients; 0.60 for surgical patients	Reasonable, only 15 minutes to complete the 23-items; free instrument to use	2b
Brief Pain Inventory (BPI): (17)	Not reported	Adults with bone metastases receiving palliative radiotherapy for acute bone pain, n=45	11-item questionnaire with response categories 0-10 ordinal scale with 0 = no pain and 10 = worst pain possible including one question asking for list of medications	Cronbach's alpha = 0.950 for worst pain scores; 0.939 for average pain scores; and 0.939 for current pain scores	Reported as having strong validity with high correlation coefficients	Short, 11 item questionnaire applicable to metastatic cancer patient with acute bone pain	2b
PAULA the PAIN-METER (PAULA): (22)	Not reported	Adult patients in the post-anesthesia care unit having undergone surgery, n=65	Sliding ruler designed to be moved by the patient corresponding to level of perceived pain with response categories of 5 colored faces representing pain intensity	Internal consistency Cronbach's alpha =0.98	Not reported	Simple, slide rule design but only measures one aspect of pain. One-item instrument might be at risk for poor content validity.	2b

Table 1. (Continued)

Instrument Reference	Framework	Sample Subjects	Instrument Description and Scoring	Reliability	Validity	Feasibility	Level of Evidence[13]
Continuous Pain Score Meter (CPSM): [14]	Bio-feedback	Healthy adult volunteers, mean age 30, n=32	Electronic instrument that measures continuously the movement of a slider connected to a computer with a continuous range response varying from 0-10	Test-re-test reliability reported as "excellent" but no statistics were given	Considered valid by authors, no discussion of testing for validity	Required a sophisticated computer software and hardware assembly; no validity reported	2b
Multidimensional Affect and Pain Survey (MAPS): [15]	Frequency pattern of correlations	Oncology patients at one major medical center with various types of cancer, n=81	101 item instrument describing pain and pain symptoms and patient rate agreement with descriptor on a 0-5 point scale; 0= none at all, 5=very much so	Not reported	Factor analysis using pattern analysis approach	101 questions is a significant burden on the respondent; over 70 minutes was required to complete the instrument; difficult to score	2b
Defense and Veterans Pain Rating Scale (DVPRS): [12]	Not reported	Military members (active duty or retired); n=350	5-item VAS plus PFS with response categories 0-10 with 0=none and 10=worst combined with 4 supplemental questions with response categories 0-10 indicating degree of agreement with the statement	Internal consistency reliability Cronbach's alpha =0.902	Principal component factor analysis for construct validity factor loadings >0.82	8-9th grade reading level; easy to administer and quick to answer, little burden on the participants, unknown about availability outside the military population; useful in clinical research	1b

Instrument Reference	Framework	Sample Subjects	Instrument Description and Scoring	Reliability	Validity	Feasibility	Level of Evidence(13)
Visual Analog Scale for Pain (VAS): (18)		Adult patients in the emergency room of two facilities, n=96	1-item scale with response categories continuous along a 100mm line representing a continuum of pain levels; one end "least possible pain" other end "worst possible pain"	ICC were used with 0.97 ICCs between 1-minute measurements	Convergent validity when correlated with NPS 0.95	Simple, 1-item scale, usable for those not able to read, universal in language, widely used; useful in clinical research	1b
McGill Pain Questionnaire (MPQ): (19)	Not reported	Adult patients participating in larger RCT in VA medical system; n=221	22-item pain descriptors including 4 summary scales assessing continuous, intermittent, descriptors, and affect with a 0-10 rating scale; 0=none, 1=worst possible	3 confirmatory factor analysis models used; reliability for 3 models are r=0.98; r=0.88; r=0.86	Convergent validity as compared to itself r=0.74; discriminant validity reported as "excellent" but without statistics	Widely used instrument that requires only 10 minutes to complete; comprehensive examination of pain; limited to English speaking/reading patients	1b

Validity

Seven of the eight studies report validity results with varying methods for calculating and reporting validity. Two studies reported strong validity but did not provide psychometric calculations to support this statement. The remaining five studies reported validity primarily using factors analysis and are reporting convergent validity. Where reported, various validity scores are strong but often-exact statistical measures are not specifically reported in the manuscript.

Discussion

This integrative review found eight unique scales that measure acute pain. Previous reviews on pain instruments have been broad in scope and have not examined pain instruments related specifically to acute pain; therefore, the included eight studies represent only those instruments for which studies have examined psychometric properties for measurement of acute pain. According to this literature review, the McGill Pain Questionnaire and the Visual Analog Scale for Pain are the two most commonly used pain instruments in the clinical setting (20).

Strong reliability scores have been reported in most of the included studies; psychometric scoring for validity is sparse. There are many studies that indicated the instrument is valid but did not provide supporting evidence to the reader. As pain is a subjective concept necessitating patient reported scores for quantification, the lack of consistent validity scores raises concerns. As validity of a scale is foundationally a measure of how well the instrument measures what it purports to measure, it is possible that those instruments with no validity scores are not actually measuring pain but some other construct.

Although reliability was shown to be strong across the entire included instruments, the lack of consistent reporting of validity raises concern. This is especially important when considering clinical implications of pain management. As a subjective concept, pain can only be measured indirectly by asking the patient about his or her pain levels. To measure pain, it is necessary to use an instrument to quantify the pain level, which is individualized. Treatment decisions and patient care are planned based on the reported pain levels. If an instrument is used that does not have adequate validity, there is a danger of reporting a score that is not a true representation of the construct being measured. In this situation, potent and lethal medications could be administered and inappropriate discharge planning, or incorrect pain management procedures could be performed based on an erroneous pain score.

Additionally, many studies have shown that pain is far more complex than what is represented by a single score (5,21). In measuring pain, this balance between a simple, quick, and useful instrument and an instrument that is comprehensive enough to measure the multiple facets of pain is difficult. This balance can be seen in this review by examining 1-item instruments, like the PAULA scale, as compared to an instrument like the MAPS scale that includes 101-items and requires considerable time to complete (15,22). The key to finding an appropriate and useful instrument to measure pain is finding an instrument that is comprehensive enough to capture all of the facets of pain, short enough not to be burdensome to the patient, and has applicability to a wide range of the population.

One additional consideration that is not addressed in any of the studies is the phenomenon of sedation related to pain treatment. Frequently, acute pain is treated with medication that can cause sedation; sometimes this sedation can be profound. None of the studies examined the feasibility of using the instrument with a patient who is being actively treated for acute pain episodes. This raises concerns regarding the reliability of the instrument across the spectrum of an episode of acute pain. A clinical example is the patient in the immediate post-operative period receiving opioid analgesics for acute surgical pain. Although important to measure pain in this particular population, reliability of the various available instruments has not been established in the face of a sedated patient.

Further research aimed at establishing validity of the various instrument used to measure acute pain is warranted. When clinical treatment decisions are based largely on scores obtained from pain instruments, it is of paramount importance to ensure the instruments are indeed measuring the construct of pain and not some other construct. This is critically important given the untoward side effects of the most commonly used treatment for acute pain: opioid analgesics (23). The side effect profile of opioid analgesics can range from bothersome pruritus and constipation to severe respiratory depression and respiratory arrest (24). Given the significant and dangerous side effects of the treatment of acute pain, it is essential that the instruments used to measure the construct on which treatment is based be reliable and valid for that construct.

Conclusion

There are several instruments available to measure the construct of pain. Of the eight reviewed instruments, only five have reliability and validity that would warrant clinical applicability. It is useful to have a varying and wide array of instruments that will fit with various populations. It is incumbent on the person administering the instrument, however, to make sure that it is reliable, valid, and applicable to the population in question. Fortunately, several instruments with excellent validity and reliability are feasible to use in measuring pain.

Acknowledgment

The author did not receive funding or sponsorship for this work. The author wishes to express his gratitude to Drs. Carolyn Jenkins and Mat Gregoski for their leadership and expert feedback and critique of this manuscript.

References

[1]   Beard DJ, Aldington D. Chronic pain after trauma. Trauma 2012; 14(1):57-66.
[2]   Bunten H, Liang W, Pounder D, Senevirante C, Osselton D. Interindividual variability in the prevalence of OPRM1 and CYP2B6 gene variations may identify drug-susceptible populations. J Analytical Toxicol 2011; 35:431-7.

[3]   Lanser P, Gesell S. Pain management: the fifth vital sign. Healthcare Benchmarks 2001;8(6):68.

[4]   Burton AW, Fine PG, Passik SD. Transformation of acute cancer pain to chronic cancer pain syndromes. Support Oncol 2012; 10(3):89-94.

[5]   Kavelaars A, Eijkelkamp N, Willemen HLDM, Wang H, Carbajal AG, Heijnen CJ. Microglial GRK2: A novel regulator of transition from acute to chronic pain. Brain Behav Immun 2011; 25(6):1055-60.

[6]   Childress SB, Stromness AR. Improving pain management at the end of life in the home care environment. Home Health Care Manage Pract 2003; 15(3):203-6.

[7]   Huskisson E. Measurement of pain. Lancet 1974; 304(7889):1127-31.

[8]   Carr DB, Goudas LC. Acute pain. Lancet 1999; 353(9169):2051-8.

[9]   Moayedi M, Davis KD. Theories of pain: from specificity to gate control. J Neurophysiol 2013; 109(1):5-12.

[10]   Dickenson AH. Editorial I Gate Control Theory of pain stands the test of time. Br J Anaesth 2002; 88(6):755-7.

[11]   Cryosoothe. Education, 2011. URL: http://www.cryosoothe.ca/education.

[12]   Buckenmaier CC, Galloway KT, Polomano RC, McDuffie M, Kwon N, Gallagher RM. Preliminary validation of the defense and veterans pain rating scale (DVPRS) in a military population. Pain Med 2013; 14(1):110-23.

[13]   Medicine OCfE-B. Levels of evidence, 2009. URL: http://www.cebm.net/?O=1025.

[14]   Boormans EM, van Kesteren PJ, Perez RS, Brölmann HA, Zuurmond WW. Reliability of a continuous pain score meter: real time pain measurement. Pain Pract 2009; 9(2):100-4.

[15]   Knotkova H, Clark WC, Keohan ML, Kuhl JP, Winer RT, Wharton RN. Validation of the Multidimensional Affect and Pain Survey (MAPS). J Pain. 2006; 7(3):161-9.

[16]   Machata A, Kabon B, Willschke H, Fässler K, Gustorff B, Marhofer P, et al. A new instrument for pain assessment in the immediate postoperative period. Anaesthesia 2009; 64(4):392-8.

[17]   Harris K, Zhang L, Chow E. Reliability of the Brief Pain Inventory (BPI) in patients with bone metastases. J Cancer Pain Sympt Palliat 2006; 2(2):3-15.

[18]   Bijur PE, Silver W, Gallagher EJ. Reliability of the visual analog scale for measurement of acute pain. Acad Emerg Med 2001; 8(12):1153-7.

[19]   Lovejoy TI, Turk DC, Morasco BJ. Evaluation of the psychometric properties of the revised short-form McGill Pain Questionnaire. J Pain 2012; 13(12):1250-7.

[20]   Kahl C, Cleland JA. Visual analogue scale, numeric pain rating scale and the McGill Pain Questionnaire: an overview of psychometric properties. Phys Ther Rev 2005; 10(2):123-8.

[21]   Jannetto PB, Pharmacogenomic considerations in the opioid management of pain. Genome Med 2010; 2(66):1-4.

[22]   Machata AM, Kabon B, Willschke H, Fässler K, Gustorff B, Marhofer P, et al. A new instrument for pain assessment in the immediate postoperative period. Anaesthesia 2009; 64(4):392-8.

[23]   Chou WY, Yang LC, Lu HF, Ko JY, Wang CH, Lin SH, et al. Association of mu-opioid receptor gene polymorphism (A118G) with variations in morphine consumption for analgesia after total knee arthroplasty. Acta Anaesth Scand 2006; 50(7):787-92.

[24]   Kolesnikov Y, Gabovits B, Levin A, Voiko E, Veske A. Combined catechol-O-methyltransferase and mu-opioid receptor gene polymorphisms affect morphine postoperative analgesia and central side effects. Anesth Analg 2011; 112(2):448-53.

[25]   Tittle MB, McMillan SC, Hagan S. Validating the brief pain inventory for use with surgical patients with cancer. Oncol Nurs Forum 2003; 30(2 part 1):325-30.

In: Pain Management Yearbook 2013
Editor: Joav Merrick

ISBN: 978-1-63117-944-0
© 2014 Nova Science Publishers, Inc.

Chapter 36

Pain management in endodontics

*Skanda Ramesh and Prasanna Neelakantan**

Undergraduate Clinic 6, Saveetha Dental College and Hospitals,
Saveetha University, Chennai, India

Abstract

Endodontic treatment is characterized by pain pre-operatively and sometimes post operatively as well. Understanding the mechanisms of pain involved in pulpo-periapical pathoses and root canal treatment are imperative to achieve optimal pain control and patient comfort. Preoperative pain control is achieved via local anaesthesia, anaesthetic premedication with analgesics, inter-appointment analgesics and post-operative analgesics. Dentists must have a clear idea of the medications of choice, their dosage, indications, contraindications and adverse effects. This review serves to address the pharmacological methods of pain control in root canal treatment.

Keywords: Analgesics, pain, antibiotics, steroids, local anaesthesia, endodontics

Introduction

In endodontics (a specialty that deals with the diseases of dental pulp and periradicular tissues), the importance of drug administration can be explained by three phases: pre-operative, intra-operative and post-operative. Allodynia refers to an exaggerated pain sensitivity in response to neutral or relatively innocuous stimuli, which results from previous exposures to painful stimuli (1), and hyperalgesia is defined as exacerbation of pain when a non-painful stimulus is applied(1).

---

* Correspondening author: Prasanna Neelakantan, MDS, 1500, 16th Main Road, Anna Nagar West, Chennai 600040, Tamil Nadu, India. E-mail: prasanna_neelakantan@yahoo.com.

Pre-operative pain management involves administration of local anaesthesia and prophylactic medication. Some patients report with a hot pulp (dental pulp that does not respond to local anaesthesia), wherein premedication with specific NSAIDs may be required. The process of root canal treatment involves gaining access to the pulp chamber, removal (extirpation) of the pulp, preparation and disinfection of the root canal system and sealing of the root canal space. Inter-appointment medication is given either as locally delivered chemicals (intracanal medicaments, which could be antiseptics or antibiotics), concomitant with systemic administration (oral route). Post-operative endodontics involves adequate pain management using analgesics. The use of steroids and antibiotics should be viewed cautiously in endodontics and justified as per cost-benefit analysis. This review discusses the pharmacological approach to pain management in endodontics, including local anaethesia, pre-anaesthetic analgesics, pre-operative and post-operative medication and pain relief via medicaments locally delivered within the root canal. The role of antibiotics in endodontics has also been critically discussed.

Pre-operative pain management

The objective of preoperative pain management is to offset the pain during treatment. This also enhances patient comfort to application of rubber dam, which is mandatory for endodontic procedures. Pain control before endodontic treatment is achieved using local anaesthetics (LA). Local anesthesia is induced when propagation of action potentials is prevented, such that sensation cannot be transmitted from the source of stimulation, such as a tooth or the periodontium, to the brain. Local anesthetics work by blocking the entry of sodium ions into their channels, thereby preventing the transient increase in permeability of the nerve membrane to sodium that is required for an action potential to occur (2).

The most commonly used Local anaesthetics in dentistry are lignocaine (lidocaine), followed by bupivacaine and mepivacaine. Research findings demonstrate that 2% lidocaine with 1:100,000 epinephrine and 0.5% bupivacaine with 1: 200,000 epinephrine showed no significant difference in terms of anaesthetic efficacy. However, the effect of bupivacaine with epinephrine was prolonged as compared to lidocaine with adrenaline (3). When used for an inferior alveolar nerve block (IANB), 3% mepivacaine plain and 4% prilocaine plain are as effective as 2% lidocaine with 1:100,000 epinephrine (4). For lignocaine, anaesthetic success of IANB has been shown to improve when supplementary buccal and lingual infiltrations are administered with 2% lignocaine with 1:100,000 adrenaline (5).

Hinkley and co-authors (6) have shown that 4% prilocaine with 1:200,000 epinephrine and 2% mepivacaine with 1:20,000 levonordefrin are also equivalent to 2% lidocaine with 1:100,000 epinephrine in an inferior alveolar nerve block in achieving pulpal anesthesia. Similarly, 3% mepivacaine and 2% lidocaine with 1:100,000 epinephrine were found to be equivalent for inferior alveolar nerve blocks in the case of symptomatic pulpitis (7). These studies should however be viewed with caution, as the technique of anaesthesia is an important factor determining success of injections.

Adding an infiltration injection of articaine after an inferior alveolar nerve block resulted in an 88% success rate for articaine in comparison with lidocaine, which showed a 71% success rate. Therefore, if the patient has pain after a clinically successful inferior alveolar nerve block (lip numbness), adding a cartridge of articaine could probably help in providing profound pulpal anaesthesia (8). However studies comparing the anaesthetic efficacy of articaine and lignocaine have yielded varying results. One study showed that 4% articaine with 1:100,000 epinephrine showed superior maxillary infiltration anaesthesia in the lateral incisor but not for molars (9).

Supplementary injections and pre-anaesthetic analgesics

From the aforementioned discussion, it appears evident that supplementary injections via infiltration enhances the anaesthetic success of nerve blocks. These supplementary injections are specifically required in cases where pulpal anaesthesia fails. Various mechanisms have been hypothesized to explain the failure of local anaesthetics, including anatomical variations, such as cross-innervations and accessory innervations from the lingual nerve, buccal nerve, mylohyoid nerve or cervical plexus, decreased local pH, tachyphylaxis of anaesthetic solutions and activation of nociceptors, including tetrodotoxin and capsaicin-sensitive transient receptor potential vanilloid type 1 (TRPV1) (10,11).

The two most common situations of relevance to endodontics are: lowered pH of the surrounding tissues, as in the case of abscess, wherein the amount of base form of anaesthetic to penetrate the nerve membrane is reduced. In these instances, there is less of the ionized form within the nerve to achieve anaesthesia. However, in the case of inflamed pulps, the condition termed "hot tooth" is clinically the most enigmatic in terms of pain relief. Hot tooth essentially implies a tooth whose pulp does not respond to LA. These inflamed pulps have altered resting potentials and decreased excitability thresholds (10,11).

These cases of hot pulp can be managed by two approaches: pre-anaesthetic analgesics and supplementary injections of local anaesthesia. The supplementary injections commonly employed are periodontal ligament injection (intra ligamentary injection), intra-osseous injection and intra pulpal injection. This review will discuss only on the use of pre-anaesthetic analgesics for enhancing success of LA.

Pre-anaesthetic medication with analgesics

NSAIDs reversibly inhibit cyclooxygenase (prostaglandin endoperoxide synthase), the enzyme-mediating production of prostaglandins (PGs) and thromboxane A2. Given the ability of NSAIDs in reducing nociceptor activation by decreasing the levels of inflammatory mediators, it has been hypothesized that pre-medication with NSAIDs will influence the success rate of local anaesthesia in patients with irreversible pulpitis (11).

Lornoxicam (8mg) and diclofenac potassium (50mg) were found to increase the success of IANB in teeth with irreversible pulpitis (11). Ibuprofen acts as an indirect analgesic blocking the production of prostaglandins. However, anaesthetic premedication with 800 mg ibuprofen, 45 minutes before the procedure, did not increase the success of IANB in patients with irreversible pulpitis (12). Preoperative administration of ibuprofen or ketorolac had no significant effect on success rate of inferior alveolar nerve block in patients with irreversible pulpitis (13). However another clinical study showed that premedication with ibuprofen and indomethacin significantly increased the success rates of inferior alveolar nerve block anaesthesia for teeth with irreversible pulpitis (14). Despite conflicting results, it has been observed in all clinical studies that premedication with NSAIDs increases success of IANB although this may not be statistically significant.

Inter-appointment pain management

The term flare up may be defined as an acute exacerbation of asymptomatic pulp or periradicular pathosis after the initiation or continuation of root canal treatment, manifested by excruciating pain and/or associated swelling, requiring active intervention by the dentist. Idiopathic flare ups have resulted in many treatments that have been empirically advocated for the prevention or alleviation of symptoms during root canal therapy. These include relief of occlusion, premedication of the pulp chamber or root canal, establishment of drainage through the root canal, or by the excision of the overlying tissues, and various medications applied to the root canal or administered systemically.

Antibiotics have been used, both locally and systemically, in anticipation of, or for the relief of pain during the course of endodontic therapy. The systemic use of antibiotics should be restrained generally but appears to have some value when the patient exhibits signs of systemic involvement, such as cellulitis, fever, malaise, and toxaemia. The overuse of antibiotics risks the induction of hypersensitivity or anaphylactic reactions, systemic side effects, and the development of resistant strains of microorganisms The use of the most popular antibiotic, penicillin, is based on the predominance of penicillin-sensitive microorganisms reportedly found in infected root canals. Increasing numbers of strains of pathogens, such as Streptococcus viridans and Staphylococcus aureus, originally susceptible to penicillin (15) are becoming increasingly resistant (16). There appears to be a trend toward an increase in the number of anaerobic dental infections. In such cases, some antibiotics such as clindamycin or tinidazole may be effective, but the organisms may be resistant to erythromycin, demeclocycline, or doxycycline (17).

There are no significant studies which show that any specific antibiotic is capable of reducing or eliminating painful exacerbations during endodontic therapy. An interesting finding is that, when ingested, tryptophan seems to have a positive effect in managing pain during flare up. A small amount is carried past the blood-brain barrier into the brain, utilized by certain brain neurons for conversion into serotonin (5-hydroxytryptamine). Centrally, serotonin plays a role in various behavioral responses, including elevation of pain threshold. It has been reported that 3 g of tryptophan given daily to patients, brought about a significant reduction in post endodontic treatment pain after 24 h, compared with a control group (18).

Non-narcotic analgesics

The nonnarcotic analgesics are a heterogeneous group of synthetic organic compounds. They may act at the receptor site, controlling the cause of the pain; at the cord, affecting the transmission of pain impulses, or, at a central level, altering the perception of pain. The analgesics that act at receptor sites presumably reduce the output of impulses from the receptors, but they may also counteract the chemical mediators produced as a result of the inflammatory response. One of the substances implicated as a pain mediatoris bradykinin. The thromboxanes and PG's E2 and F2 appear to exacerbate the pain induced by bradykinin (19,20). Among the analgesics that act primarily on the pain perception threshold are salicylates (aspirin); combinations of aspirin, phenacetin, and caffeine; acetophenetidin (Phenacetin); acetaminophen (Liquiprin, Tempra, Tylenol, and Valadol); and propoxyphene (Darvon).

NSAIDS

The anti-inflammatory and analgesic action of the NSAIDS is due to the inhibition of prostaglandin synthesis by inactivation of cyclooxygenase pathway and also inhibition of phosphodiesterase, leading to increase in cyclic AMP production (21). Recently, other non-steroidal anti-inflammatory agents have been reported to be more effective than aspirin, with less side effects (21).

Narcotic analgesics

Narcotic analgesics are most commonly prescribed for relief of severe pain. Most of the more potent analgesics (morphine, codeine, meperidine, pentazocine, and percodan) are primarily narcotics. They react with neurons in the brain stem, spinal cord, thalamus, and cerebral cortex (22), although the exact site of the action is unknown. The narcotic analgesics act primarily by controlling the reaction to pain. Sharp, localized pain is poorly relieved by the opiates, which effectively relieve duller, more chronic, and less severe pain. However, they are capable of raising the pain reaction threshold by causing relaxation, apathy, and freedom from anxiety. The commonly used narcotic analgesics consist of morphine, codeine, meperidine, and propoxyphene. Morphine is the drug of first choice for severe pain. Previously, morphine was not found to be effective when administered orally. Presently oral morphine is available and he most effective way of dealing with pain is the repeated administration of one agent at regular intervals to keep the threshold high (23). There is no specific analgesic that is preferentially effective for the pain induced during root canal therapy.

Post-operative pain management

Endodontic pain is often associated with chronic inflammation, the presence of bacterial by-products, influx of immune cells and activation of the cytokine network and other inflammatory mediators. The chronicity of pulpal and periapical inflammation permits sprouting of nociceptor terminals and thus change the peripheral anatomy of the pain system.

In humans, cortisol is the primary glucocorticoid that is continuously synthesized and secreted from the adrenal cortex. Glucocorticoids inhibit the inflammatory response by its effect on gene transcription that produces a decrease in the release of vasoactive and chemo attractive factors like bradykinin and certain cytokines that occur during periapical inflammation. Glucocorticoids when given over a short course is unlikely to be harmful although it is contraindicated with patients that have systemic fungal infection, patients that have hypersensitivity to the drug, patients with ulcerative colitis, pyogenic infection, diverticulitis, peptic ulcer, renal insufficiency, hypertension, osteoporosis, pregnancy, diabetes mellitus, ocular herpes, acute psychosis and history of TB. Steroids have been used as intracanal medicaments to control pain (24)

Oral dexamethasone, intraligamentary, intrasseous and intramuscular administration of steroids have shown decrease in endodontic post treatment pain. The studies show that they have the best efficacy and most appropriately used for those patients who present with moderate to severe pain and teeth with pulpal necrosis and associated radiolucencies (chronic inflammatory processes) than pain associated with irreversible pulpitis. Intraoral injection of 6-8mg of dexamethasone or 40mg of methylprednisolone or oral dose of 48mg methlprednisolone/day for 3 days and 10-12mg dexamethasone/day for 3 days is suggested by the literature reviewed (24). Antibiotics are not routinely recommended in conjuction with corticosteroids in the management of the otherwise healthy patient.

NSAIDs: COX-1 inhibitors

NSAIDs primarily through the inhibition of cyclooxygenase (COX) enzymes 1 and 2. COX-1 is expressed throughout the body and has a role in protection of stomach mucosa, kidney function and platelet action. COX-2 is induced by various endogenous compounds such as cytokines, mitogens and endotoxins in inflammatory cells and is responsible for the elevated production of prostaglandins during inflammation (25). Inhibiting COX-2 blocks prostaglandin formation and ultimately prevents inflammation and sensitization of the peripheral nociceptors. However, inhibiting COX-1 attenuates its protective actions (21). Nevertheless, numerous clinical studies have confirmed that moderate to severe pain of dental origin is best managed through the use of ibuprofen or other NSAIDs and its maximum analgesic effect is at least equal to that of standard doses of acetaminophen-opioid combinations. It is important to understand that NSAIDs generally require a higher dose to achieve maximum anti-inflammatory action than that to achieve analgesic action. Modaresi and colleagues showed that preoperative administration of ibuprofen, if not contraindicated, is a drug of choice 1 hour before local anesthesia injection as an effective method for achieving a deep anaesthesia during treatment of inflamed teeth (26). The same has been proven for lornoxicam and diclofenac potassium as well (11).

COX-2 inhibitors

Although NSAIDs are remarkably effective in the management of pain and inflammation, their use is limited by several adverse effects including gastrointestinal bleeding and ulceration, impaired renal function, and inhibition of platelet aggregation. Discovery of COX-2, led to the hypothesis that NSAIDs side effects could be decreased, as the inhibition of COX-2 is more directly implicated in ameliorating inflammation while the inhibition of COX-1 is related to adverse effects in the gastrointestinal tract. This stimulated the development of selective COX-2 inhibitors that are better tolerated than non-selective NSAIDs but comparable in analgesic efficacy (27).

A study comparing meloxicam with piroxicam and placebo in controlling postoperative endodontic pain was done in 51 patients who underwent root canal treatment. Results showed that there was no significant difference in the reduction of analgesic effect of meloxicam and piroxicam (28). The advantage of meloxicam over piroxicam was there were fewer gastro-intestinal side effects (28,29).

Comparative studies done with rofecoxib and ibuprofen on postendodontic pain management have shown prophylactic administration of 50 mg of rofecoxib before root canal therapy was more effective at reducing postendodontic pain at 12 and 24 h after initiation of treatment, when compared with 600 mg of ibuprofen or placebo (30). Prophylactic rofecoxib administration provides an effective reduction in postendodontic pain. Rofecoxib's analgesic efficacy, long duration of action, lower gastrointestinal toxicity, and apparent lack of inhibition of platelet function suggest that rofecoxib may be useful as a pre-emptive analgesic when postendodontic pain is anticipated (30).

Recent work suggests that the metabolite AM404 is responsible for all or part of the analgesic effects of acetaminophen. There has also been speculation that acetaminophen has some capacity as a COX-2 inhibitor, but this may be limited at the site of inflammation.

The FDA recommends the maximum single dose be limited to 1000 mg and the daily dose to 4000 mg. At these levels, adverse effects are rare but can include nausea and other stomach issues. At higher doses, APAP can cause acute hepatotoxicity. There has been more evidence supporting a combination of both ibuprofen and acetaminophen in the treatment of post-operative pain. The addition of acetaminophen to ibuprofen has an additive effect that can preclude the need for narcotic analgesics and thus avoid the undesired side effects.

Pre-emptive analgesia

The concept of preventing the development of central sensitization was first explored as a clinical strategy through a retrospective review of medical records (31). The preoperative administration of a local anesthetic delayed the postoperative request for a postoperative analgesic in patients immediately following a variety of surgical procedures performed under general anaesthesia.

The preoperative administration of a local anaesthetic and an opioid delayed the postoperative request for medication by approximately six and three hours respectively. The combination of a local anesthetic and an opioid resulted in an even greater delay suggestive of an additive effect.

It appears that optimal clinical benefits can be achieved by administering drugs such as local anaesthetics and NSAIDs before the onset of postoperative pain.

Administering these drugs before a surgical or an endodontic procedure may be of benefit for longer procedures or for minimizing peripheral sensitization, which is a result of the cascade of inflammatory mediators that are released by tissue injury and fuel the subsequent inflammatory process (11).

Antibiotics in endodontics

The effectiveness of an antibiotic is related to both the type and concentration of the antibiotic. However, it must be clearly understood that antibiotics per se do not play a role in pain control in endodontics. They serve purely as a means of infection control, if sufficient control cannot be achieved via intracanal disinfection, or in the presence of signs like abscess. Clearly, if antibiotics are to be effective in managing endodontic infections and reducing endodontic symptoms, they must reach the target tissues in therapeutic concentrations. This is especially a concern in pathological conditions, when the tissues may have reduced blood flow or may even become necrotic (32).

A placebo controlled-study was conducted to determine the effect of penicillin on pain in untreated teeth, diagnosed with moderate to severely painful irreversible pulpitis (33). The study revealed that there was no pain relief on administration of antibiotics. In view of odontogenic infections, different antibiotics were used that were effective against most odontogenic bacteria from culture and sensitivity testing, namely penicillin, amoxicillin, clindamycin, cephalosporin showed similar efficacy except that a study done with the co-amoxiclav combination (Augmentin) revealed faster pain reduction (34). The choices of penicillin (or amoxicillin) as the primary antibiotic prescribed, and clindamycin as the drug of second choice appear to be consistent with choices made by dentists or endodontists on recent surveys, although some dentists seem to favour erythromycin for patients with penicillin allergy (35, 36).

Ledermix

Ledermix is a paste that combines 1% triamcinolone acitonide (a corticosteroid) and dimethyl chlorotetracycline (demeclocycline, a tetracycline analog). It has been used as a pulp capping agent, and as a root canal medicament for both vital and necrotic cases because of its anti-inflammatory and antimicrobial properties (37) The concentration of demeclocycline in the root canal was shown to be much higher than is required to inhibit bacteria; however, this activity tends to decrease considerably by 7 days (37). Ledermix was shown to be effective against pulpal pain in some earlier studies, possibly because of its corticosteroid content. There is still no consensus on the use of this material in endodontics.

Macrolides

Macrolides are bacteriostatic antibiotics that exert their action by interfering with bacterial protein synthesis by binding to the 50S ribosomal subunit, it is thought by binding to the donor site during the translocation step (37) Among the more commonly prescribed macrolides are erythromycin, clarithromycin, azithromycin and roxithromycin. Erythromycin 950 mg qid) has been shown to be more effective than penicillin (500 mg qid) in patients with moderate to severe pain pre-operatively but there were no statistical reduction in pain post-obturation (38).

Clindamycin

There have been some trials evaluating clindamycin as an intracanal medicament. Clindamycin is a potent bactericidal antibiotic that binds to the 50S ribosomal subunit and interferes with protein synthesis. In a clinical study, clindamycin was shown to be comparable to calcium hydroxide in eliminating bacteria from root canals, and also in being not effective against enterococci (39). Recently, clindamycin-impregnated ethylene vinyl acetate fibers were investigated in vitro and found to be effective against other common endodontic pathogens (40) However, further investigations of this fiber in clinical situations have not been reported.

Tetracyclines

Tetracyclines are another group of bacteriostatic antibiotics that bind to the 30S ribosomal subunit of bacteria, and specifically inhibit the binding of aminoacyl-t-RNA synthetases to the ribosomal acceptor site. A number of beneficial non-antimicrobial properties have been described for tetracyclines and tetracycline analogs, even when used in subantimicrobial doses (41). The most important of these properties is the inhibition of expression and production of host matrix metalloproteinases (MMPs) (42). MMPs are a group of 11 or more endopeptidases that include collagenases, gelatinases and other enzymes that are up-regulated during inflammation, causing tissue destruction. It was shown that levels of MMP-9 (a gelatinase) were significantly higher in inflamed than in normal dental pulps (42). Tetracycline is also thought to inhibit osteoclasts, thereby reducing bone resorption, and can act synergistically with other agents that reduce bone resorption such as bisphosphonates (43) In this regard, doxycycline was recently shown to reduce crestal bone resorption following endodontic flap reflection (44).

Conclusion

Patients typically associate dental care with pain. For many patients, fear of dental pain and avoidance of dentistry are synonymous. Endodontic pre and post treatment pain continues to be a significant problem facing the dental profession. Therefore, it is evident that pre and post-treatment analgesic intervention is required in a variable percentage of endodontic cases. Further research from the pharmacology industry should focus on the possibility of locally delivering analgesics and antibiotics for effective pain relief in endodontics.

References

[1]   Sandkuhler J. Models and mechanisms of hyperalgesia and allodynia. Physiol Rev 2009; 89:707-58.

[2]   Haas DA. An update on local anesthetics in dentistry. J Can Dent Assoc 2002;68:546-51.

[3]   Parirokh M, Yosefi MH, Nakhaee N, Manochehrifar H, Abbott PV, Reza Forghani F. Effect of bupivacaine on postoperative pain for inferior alveolar nerve block anesthesia after single-visit root canal treatment in teeth with irreversible pulpitis. J Endod 2012; 38:1035-9.

[4]   McLean C, Reader A, Beck M, Meyers W. An evaluation of 4% prilocaine and 3% mepivacaine compared with 2% lidocaine (1:100,000 epinephrine) for inferior alveolar nerve block. J Endo 1993; 19:146-50.

[5]   Foster W, Drum M, Reader A, Beck M. Anesthetic efficacy of buccal and lingual infiltrations of lidocaine following an inferior alveolar nerve block in mandibular posterior teeth. Anesth Prog 2007; 54:163-9.

[6]   Hinkley S, Reader A, Beck M, Meyers W. An evaluation of 4% prilocaine with 1:200,000 epinephrine and 2% mepivacaine with 1:20,000 levonordefrin compared with 2% lidocaine with:100,000 epinephrine for inferior alveolar nerve block. Anesth Prog 1991; 38:84-9.

[7]   Cohen H, Cha B, Spangberg L. Endodontic anesthesia in mandibular molars: a clinical study. J Endod 1993; 19:370-3.

[8]   Haase A, Reader A, Nusstein J, Beck M, Drum M. Comparing anesthetic efficacy of articaine versus lidocaine as a supplemental buccal infiltration of the mandibular first molar after an inferior alveolar nerve block. J Am Dent Assoc 2008; 139:1228-35.

[9]   Evans G, Nusstein J, Drum M, Reader A, Beck M. A prospective, randomized, double-blind comparison of articaine and lidocaine for maxillary infiltrations. J Endod 2008; 34:389-93.

[10]   Wallace J, Michanowicz A, Mundell R, Wilson E. A pilot study of the clinical problem of regionally anesthetizing the pulp of an acutely inflamed mandibular molar. Oral Surg Oral Med Oral Pathol 1985; 59: 517-21.

[11]   Prasanna N, Subbarao CV, Gutmann JL. The efficacy of pre-operative oral medication of lornoxicam and diclofenac potassium on the success of inferior alveolar nerve block in patients with irreversible pulpitis: a double-blind, randomised controlled clinical trial. Int Endod J 2011; 44: 330-6.

[12]   Oleson M, Drum M, Reader A, Nusstein J, Beck M. Effect of preoperative ibuprofen on the success of the inferior alveolar nerve block in patients with irreversible pulpitis. J Endod 2010; 36:379-82.

[13]   Aggarwal V, Singla M, Kabi D. Comparative evaluation of effect of preoperative oral medication of ibuprofen and ketorolac on anesthetic efficacy of inferior alveolar nerve block with lidocaine in patients with irreversible pulpitis: A prospective, double-blind, randomized clinical trial. J Endod 2010; 36:375-8.

[14]   Parirokh M, Ashouri R, Rekabi AR, Nakhaee N, Pardakhti A, Askarifard S, Abbott PV. The effect of premedication with ibuprofen and indomethacin on the success of inferior alveolar nerve block for teeth with irreversible pulpitis. J Endod 2010; 36:1450-4.

[15]   Turner JE, Moore DW, Shaw BS. Prevalence and antibiotic susceptibility of organisms isolated from acute soft tissue abscesses secondary to dental caries. Oral Surg 1975; 39:848.

[16]   Hunt DE, Meyer RA. Continued evolution of the microbiology of oral infections. J Am Dent Assoc 1983; 107:53.

[17]   Heimdahl A, von Konow L, Nord CE. Isolation of lactamase producing bacteroides strains associated with clinical failures with penicillin treatment of human orofacial infections. Arch Oral Biol 1980; 25:689.

[18]   Shpeen SE, Morse DR, Furst ML. The effect of tryptophan on postoperative endodontic pain. Oral Surg 1984; 58:446.

[19]   Weissmann G. Pain mediators and pain receptors. Hospital practice special report: considerations in management of acute pain. New York: HP Publishing, 1977:28-30.

[20]   Flower RJ. Drugs which inhibit prostaglandin biosynthesis. Pharmacol Rev 1974; 26:33.

[21]   Crossley HL, Bergman SA, Wynn RL. Nonsteroidal anti-inflammatory agents in relieving dental pain: a review. J Am Dent Assoc 1983; 106:61.

[22]   Miller RR. Clinical effects of pentazocine in hospitalized and medical patients. J Clin Pharmacol 1975; 15:198.

[23]   Wiffen PJ, Wee B, Moore RA. Oral morphine for cancer pain. Cochrane Database Syst Rev 2013; 22(7):CD003868.

[24]   Marshall JG. Consideration of steroid for endodontic pain. Endod Topics 2002; 3:41-51.

[25]   Khan AA, Dionne RA. COX- 2 inhibitors for endodontic pain. Endod Topics 2002; 3:31-40.

[26]   Modaresi J, Dianat O, Mozayeni MA. The efficacy comparison of ibuprofen, acetaminophen-codeine, and placebo premedication therapy on the depth of anesthesia during treatment of inflamed teeth. Oral Surg Oral Med Oral Pathol Oral Radiol Endod 2006; 102:399-403.

[27]   Lee Y, Rodriguez C, Dionne RA. The role of COX-2 in acute pain and the use of selective COX-2 inhibitors for acute pain relief. Curr Pharm Des 2005; 11:1737-55.

[28]   Nekoofar MH, Sadeghipanah S, Dehpour AR. Evaluation of meloxicam (A Cox-2 Inhibitor) for management of postoperative endodontic pain: A double-blind placebo-controlled study. J Endod 2003; 29:634-7.

[29]   Dequeker J, Hawkey C, Kahan A, Steinbruck K, Alegre C, Baumelou E, et al. Improvement in gastrointestinal tolerability of the selective cyclooxygenase (COX)-2 inhibitor, meloxicam, compared with piroxicam: Results of the Safety and Efficacy Large-scale Evaluation of COX-inhibiting Therapies (SELECT) trial in osteoarthritis. Br J Rheumatol 1998; 37:946–51.

[30]   Gopikrishna V, Parameswaran A. Effectiveness of prophylactic use of rofecoxib in comparison with ibuprofen on postendodontic pain. J Endod 2003; 29:62-4.

[31]   Dionne R. To tame the pain. Compend Contin Educ Dent 1998; 19:421-6.

[32]   Fouad AF. Are antibiotics effective for endodontic pain? An evidence-based review. Endod Topics 2002; 3:52-66.

[33]   Nagle D, Reader A, Beck M, Weaver J. Effect of systemic penicillin on pain in untreated irreversible pulpitis. Oral Surg Oral Med Oral Pathol Oral Radiol Endod 2000; 90:636-40.

[34]   Lewis MA, Carmichael F, MacFarlane TW, Milligan SG. A randomised trial of co-amoxiclav (Augmentin) versus penicillin V in the treatment of acute dentoalveolar abscess. Br Dent J 1993; 175:169-74.

[35]   Yingling NM, Byrne BE, Hartwell GR. Antibiotic use by members of the American Association of Endodontists in the year: report of a national survey. J Endod 2000; 28:396-404.

[36]   Whitten BH, Gardiner DL, Jeansonne BG, Lemon RR.Current trends in endodontic treatment. report of a national survey. J Am Dent Assoc 1996; 127:1333-41.

[37]   Abbott PV, Hume WR, Pearman JW. Antibiotics and endodontics. Aust Dent J 1990; 35:50-60.

[38]   Torabinejad M, Cymerman JJ, Frankson M, Lemon RR, Maggio JD, Schilder H. Effectiveness of various medications on postoperative pain following complete instrumentation. J Endod 1994; 20: 345-54.

[39]   Molander A, Reit C, Dahlen G. Microbiological evaluation of clindamycin as a root canal dressing in teeth with apical periodontitis. Int Endod J 1990; 23:113-8.

[40]   Gilad JZ, Teles R, Goodson M, White RR, Stashenko P. Development of a clindamycin-impregnated fiber as an intracanal medication in endodontic therapy. J Endod 1999; 25:722-7.

[41]   Golub LM, Lee HM, Ryan ME, Giannobile WV, Payne J, Sorsa T. Tetracyclines inhibit connective tissue breakdown by multiple non-antimicrobial mechanisms. Adv Dent Res 1998; 12:12-26.

[42]   Gusman H, Santana RB, Zehnder M. Matrix metalloproteinase levels and gelatinolytic activity in clinically healthy and inflamed human dental pulps. Eur J Oral Sci 2002; 110:353-7.

[43]   Llavaneras ANS et al. A combination of a chemically modified doxycycline and a bisphosphonate synergistically inhibits endotoxin-induced periodontal breakdown in rats. J Periodontol 2001; 72: 1069-77.

[44]   Cummings GR, Torabinejad M. Effect of systemic doxycycline on alveolar bone loss after periradicular surgery. J Endod 2000; 26:325-7.

In: Pain Management Yearbook 2013
Editor: Joav Merrick

ISBN: 978-1-63117-944-0
© 2014 Nova Science Publishers, Inc.

Chapter 37

Occlusal splint treatment in temporomandibular disorder

Vinitha Elizabeth Stephen[1]*and V. Kamakshi[2]

[1]Saveetha Dental College, Saveetha University
[2]Department of Prosthodontics, Saveetha Dental College, Saveetha University

Abstract

The term temporomandibular disorder (TMD) describes the collection of symptoms that are associated with the temporomandibular joint (TMJ), Splints are widely used in the management of temperomandibular disorders. This article focuses on different splints used for different types of disorders. This article is an overview on splints, their mode of action and different types used in the management of temperomandibular disorders. If splint therapy is unsuccessful then the splint should be discarded and a more effective treatment modality to be carried out. If splint therapy is successful, then the patient can retain the splint to use on an 'as needed' basis, reassured that they will never do themselves any harm by wearing the splint, even on a temporary basis.

Keywords: Temporomandibular disorder, temporomandibular joint, occlusal splint

Introduction

Temperomandibular disorders (TMJ) is a collective term which refers to large number of clinical problems that involve the masticatory muscles, temperomandibular joint (TMJ) or both the associated structures (1-2). It may be related to an imbalance among occlusal, anatomical, psychological and neuromuscular factors, providing neck and head structural dysfunction (1-3). Occlusal spints are the most widely employed treatment of

---

* Corresponding author: Vinitha Elizabeth Stephen, Saveetha Dental College, Saveetha University, Chennai, India.
  E-mail: vinithaelizabeth91@gmail.com.

temperomandibular disorders (TMD). Splint therapy is considered effective to recapture the displaced disc (4).

Occlusal splint

Occlusal splint or occlusal device is a removable artificial occlusal surface used for diagnosis or therapy, affecting the relationship of maxilla to the mandible. It may be used for occlusal stabilization, for treatment of temporomandibular disorders or prevent wear of the dentition.

Occlusal splints can perform one basic function. They can prevent the existing occlusion from controlling the jaw to jaw relationship at maximum intercuspation. When the occlusal surfaces are covered, either partially or completely, the splint material becomes the occluding surface and the way the occluding surface is contoured determines how the mandible must be positioned to occlude the teeth with the splint. What occlusal splints cannot do? It cannot violate the mechanical laws and does not unload the condyles.

It has been shown that the nature of patients occlusion is a valuable predictor of success of splint therapy in pain dysfunction syndrome (5,6). A pretreatment record should be made of the patient's occlusion before any splint therapy (5). Whether or not a reorganized approach is being undertaken, pretreatment analysis of occlusion is mandatory (5,7). All splints will have the common mode of action:

1) All splints will decrease occlusal forces.
2) All splints will have a placebo effect (cognitive awareness effect).
3) All splints will alter occlusal contacts.

Several splint designs are in frequent use in management of TMD namely (5):

- Soft vacuum formed splint, usually made on lower arch
- Localized occlusal interference splint.
- Stabilization splint.
- Anterior repositioning splint.
- NTI-tss splint

Soft bite guard is the commonly prescribed splint. It is quick to fabricate and can be provided as an emergency treatment for patients with acute TMD. The splint is tolerated in the lower arch than the upper arch as there is no satisfactory way of thinning the margins of splint while keeping good retention. It is less expensive and easy to fabricate. These appliances are usually worn only at night. The appliance is made out of 2mm polyvinyl (5).

Indications for treatment are patients exhibiting high levels of clenching and bruxism, they help dissipate some heavy loading forces encountered during parafunctional activity.

Localized occlusal interference splint are also called interceptor appliance and their indications: Patients with or without TMD who show active signs of bruxism, may be regarded as a 'habit breaker' and they can be used at night and also on occasions when patient is aware of parafunctioning.(5)

The appliance is constructed after making impression following which the patient's centric occlusion is recorded. The splint has a palatal plate, which can be retained by Adams clasp or ball end clasp around the first molar or second premolar and bears ball end wires anteriorly. The ball end of these wires is usually fitted against the mesial marginal ridge of the first premolar or against the cingulum of the maxillary canine such that the tips of the cusp of either the mandibular canines or mandibular first premolar occlude against it. Thus the teeth do not touch during closure in centric occlusion and deliberately increases the load on the proprioceptive fibres of the periodontal membrane of four teeth. The hypothesis is that in this way, parafunctioning is prevented.

These splints do not result in wearing of teeth occluding against splint, primarily because their use stops parafunctional habit.

Stabilization splint aim to stabilize the mandible against the maxilla. There are different names for this type like: Michigan splints-upper splints, Tanner splints-lower splints, Fox appliance or centric relation appliance. They are indicated for myofacial pain and TMJ pain, bruxism associated toothwear or tooth mobility from occlusal disharmony.

The stabilization splint is ideally constructed from heat activated polymethyl-methacrylate. Full time wearing is normally recommended for patients with (8): Increase in vertical dimension and patients with increased tooth mobility (periodontal disease should be treated before splint therapy). Night time wear is suggested for nocturnal parafunction.

The appliance is constructed after impressions are made and centric relation recorded with posterior teeth apart by 1.5-2mm, thickness of the intended splint. If the jaw is stiff, a Lucia jig can help in providing relaxation and at the same time establishes the intended interocclusal clearance. The jig should be adjusted to have a flat biting surface to allow a single lower incisor to trace out a gull wing appearance when marked with occlusal indicating foil. Beauty hard wax is preferred to register the occlusion. "Horseshoe" wax base is fabricated to cover the occlusal surface, incisal edges and into the palate. Buccal overlap by 1.0 to 1.5 mm is provided. Occlusal plane is built up into even contact with opposing teeth without indentations. Build incisal ramp into contact with opposing incisors and develop protrusive guidance and canine guidance ramps for lateral excursions.(8)

Fitting

Stability, retention and tightness of the splint is checked, before examining the occlusion (8). After adjusting the patient should be able to put the splint in and take it out comfortably and fitting problems are corrected by relining.

Adjusting centric relation contact aim is to eliminate any premature or deflective contacts. With the patient in supine position and the splint in place ask the patient to close gently guiding them into centric relation. The patient is then asked to point to the contact and observe whether the jaw is forced to shift forward or laterally as he/she continues to close. To mark this contact, the articulating foil (blue or black) is placed and patient is asked to close slowly until teeth first hit the splint. Take the splint out and grind this point and check again and repeat the grinding to spread single points of contact equally against all opposing teeth with slightly lighter contacts anteriorly.

Having established a stable platform on the splint in centric relation, interferences are eliminated during lateral and protrusive movements and smooth guidance for all excursions provided (8). Red articulating paper may be used to show excursive contacts. Interference may be removed in the following order: non-working side, working side and finally protrusive interference. Always check that the markings are smooth and unbroken. A smooth well finished splint is better than one with a rough surface and sharp edges.

It is a full coverage splint constructed on upper arch and guides the mandible downwards and forwards into a protruded position. It is the splint of choice for treatment of patients suffering from disc displacement with reduction (9,10).

A click usually arises because of anterior, more usually anteromedial-intra-articular displacement of disc. It is suggested that this splint can be used when the opening and closing clicks are eliminated, if patient opens from a protrusive mandibular position.

A diagnostic test need to be done before using this splint to determine whether the click disappears when the patient is asked to open from and close into a protrusive mandibular position. In a patient with class I skeletal relationship this position is usually incisal edge to edge.

In case of an increased overjet (class II div 1) there may be no need to advance the mandible this far for the disc displacement to be reduced). By such anterior repositioning the click should be eliminated because while the mandible is anteriorly positioned, the head of condyle moves downwards and forwards and when in this position, normal relationship is restored.

The aim of providing this splint is to maintain the mandible in a temporary therapeutic positioning in which click is eliminated and thereby allowing the disc to reposition. During fitting of the appliance the upper teeth should fit into the indentations prepared, else tooth movement could occur. To achieve a success, 24 hours a day for three months is suggested followed by gradual wearing off period when time without using the splint is increased slowly.

NTI tss splint- Nociceptive Trigeminal Inhibition tension suppression system is indicated for the prevention and treatment of bruxism, temporomandibular disorders (TMDs), occlusal trauma, tension-type headaches and/or migraine (11,12). The NTI-tss device is a small pre-fabricated anterior bite stop which covers the two maxillary (or mandibular) central incisors. The fit along the teeth is accomplished at the chair side by filling either an autopolymerizing acrylic or a thermoplastic material into the base of the device, which is subsequently adapted along the central incisors, thereby increasing the vertical dimension between the upper and lower jaw.

Adjustments along the outer surface of the bite stop are made by the dentist to ensure that at jaw closure and during excursive movements tooth contacts are present only between the intraoral device and the incisal embrasures of the antagonistic teeth.

Complications

Patients who wears splint for 24 hours a day will have anterior open bite (11-12), sensitivity in the lower front teeth (11-13), dryness of the mouth because of forced upper jaw in these patients (11-13), tongue thrusting, increased salivation (11-14), tenderness in teeth while wearing the device (11-14) and mobility and local bone loss (11-15).

General considerations

The objectives of providing splint to the patient should be defined to the patient. Splints are used for facial pain, muscle pain, joint sounds and to stabilize the mandibular position. Splint appropriate to the diagnosis should be designed.

Full coverage splints should be used, especially if designed for wear on 24 hour basis and treatment should be coordinated with the diagnosis. The occlusion must be examined and recorded before any splint therapy and it is not necessary to perform a "second phase of treatment." While considering treatment of stabilization splint, improvement in the patient's symptoms may not be linear.

Clear advice on oral hygiene should be given and patients with splint advocated for headache, should be referred to a neurologist for examination.

Conclusion

This article is an overview on splints, their mode of action and different types used in the management of temperomandibular disorders. If splint therapy is unsuccessful then the splint should be discarded and a more effective treatment modality to be carried out. If splint therapy is successful, then the patient can retain the splint to use on an 'as needed' basis, reassured that they will never do themselves any harm by wearing the splint, even on a temporary basis.

References

[1]   Strini PJ, Machado NA, Gorreri MC, Ferreira Ade F, Sousa Gda C, Fernandes Neto AJ. Postural evaluation of patients with temporomandibular disorders under use of occlusal splints. J Appl Oral Sci 2009; 17(5):539-43.

[2]   Parker MW. A dynamic model of etiology in temporomandibular disorders. J Am Dent Assoc 1990; 120(3):283-90.

[3]   Clark GT, Green EM, Dornan MR, Flack VF. Craniocervical dysfunction levels in a patient sample from a temporomandibular joint clinic. J Am Dent Assoc 1987; 11(2):251-6.

[4]   Huanga I, Wub J, Kaoa Y, Chena C, Chena C, Yangd Y.Splint therapy for disc displacement with reduction of the temperomandibular joint. Part1: Modified mandibular splint. Kaohsiung J Med Sci 2011; 27(8):323-9.

[5]   Gray RJM, Davies SJ. Occlusal splints and TMD: "Why, when, how?" Dent Update 2001; 28:194-9.

[6]   Gray RJM, Davies SJ, Quale AA. A comparison of two splints in the treatment of TMJ pain dysfunction. Can occlusal analysis be used to predict the success rate of splint therapy. Br Dent J 1991; 17:55-8.

[7]   Wise MD. Introduction to occlusal adjustment and posterior restoration. In: Wise MD, ed. Occlusion and restorative dentistry for the general dental practitioner. London: BDJ Publications, 1986:111-2.

[8]   Moufti MA, Lillco JT, Wassell RW. How to make a well fitting stabilization splint? Dent Update 2007; 34:398-408.

[9]   Gray RJM, Davies SJ. The pattern of splint usage in the management of two common TMD. Part I: The anterior repositioning splint in the treatment of disc displacement with reduction. Br Dent J 1997; 183(6): 199-203.

[10]   Clark GT. Treatment of jaw clicking with temperomandibular repositioning:analysis of 25 cases. J Craniomandibular Pract 1984; 2:263-70.

[11]   Stapelmann H, Türp JC. The NTI-tss device for the therapy of bruxism, temporomandibular disorders, and headache. Where do we stand? A qualitative systematic review of the literature. BMC Oral Health 2008;8:22 doi:10.1186/1472-6831-8-22

[12]   Clark GT, Minakuchi H. Oral appliances. In: Laskin DM, Greene CS, Hylander WL, eds. Temporomandibular disorders. An evidence-based approach to diagnosis and treatment. Chicago, IL: Quintessence, 2006:377-90.

[13]   Jokstad A, Mo A, Krogstad BS. Clinical comparison between two different splint designs for temporomandibular disorder therapy. Acta Odontol Scand 2005; 63:218-26.

[14]   Magnusson T, Adiels AM, Nilsson HL, Helkimo M. Treatment effect on signs and symptoms of temporomandibular disorders. Comparison between stabilisation splint and a new type of splint (NTI). A pilot study. Swed Dent J 2004; 28:11-20.

[15]   Fitins D: Överbelastade incisiver – en effekt av NTI-skenan. Ajour Odont 2002; 3:5. [Swedish]

In: Pain Management Yearbook 2013
Editor: Joav Merrick

ISBN: 978-1-63117-944-0
© 2014 Nova Science Publishers, Inc.

Chapter 38

Symptom clusters analysis in bone metastases patients using the European Organization for Research and Treatment of Cancer Quality of Life Questionnaire Bone Metastases Module (EORTC QLQ-BM22)

Leonard Chiu[1], Edward Chow, MBBS [1]*, Nicholas Chiu[1],
Liying Zhang[1], Gillian Bedard, BSc(C)[1], Alysa Fairchild[2],
Vassilios Vassiliou[3], Mohamed A Alm El-Din [4],
Reynaldo Jesus-Garcia[5], Fabien Forges[6], Ling-Ming Tseng[7],
Ming-Feng Hou[8], Wei-Chu Chie[9], Takefumi Satoh[10],
Brigette BY Ma[11], Henry Lam[1] and Andrew Bottomley[12]

[1]Department of Radiation Oncology, Odette Cancer Centre,
University of Toronto, Toronto, Ontario, Canada
[2]Department of Radiation Oncology, Cross Cancer Institute, Edmonton, Alberta, Canada
[3]Department of Radiation Oncology, Bank of Cyprus Oncology Centre, Nicosia, Cyprus
[4]Department of Clinical Oncology, Tanta University Hospital, Tanta Faculty of
Medicine, Tanta, Egypt
[5]Department of Orthopedic Oncology,
Federal University of Sa~o Paulo, Sa~o Paulo, Brazil
[6]Department of Pharmacy, Lucien Neuwirth Cancer Institute,
Saint-Priest en Jarez, France

---

* Corresponding author: Professor Edward Chow MBBS, MSc, PhD, FRCPC Department of Radiation Oncology, Odette Cancer Centre, Sunnybrook Health Sciences Centre, 2075 Bayview Avenue, Toronto, ON Canada. Email: Edward.Chow@sunnybrook.ca.

[7]Department of Surgery, Taipei Veterans General Hospital,
National Yang-Ming University, Taipei, Taiwan
[8]Department of Gastroenterologic Surgery,
Kaohsiung Medical University Hospital, Kaohsiung, Taiwan
[9]Department of Public Health and Institute of Epidemiology and Preventative Medicine,
National Taiwan University, Taipei, Taiwan
[10]Department of Urology, Kitasato University School of Medicine, Kanagawa, Japan
[11]Department of Clinical Oncology, Prince of Wales Hospital,
Shatin, New Territories, Hong Kong, SAR
[12]European Organisation for Research and Treatment of Cancer,
EORTC Headquarters, Brussels, Belgium

Abstract

The objectives were to compare the symptom cluster compositions of radiotherapy and bisphosphonates patients at baseline and to examine whether symptom cluster composition in the bone metastases patient cohort changed over time. We employed principal component analysis (PCA) to extract symptom clusters in data collected from patients with bone metastases using the European Organization for Research and Treatment of Cancer (EORTC) Bone Metastases Module (QLQ-BM22). A total of 626 patients across 8 countries participated in this study with questionnaires administered to the patients at baseline and follow-up a month later. Radiotherapy and bisphosphonates patients were isolated from the total patient sample and PCA was used to identify clusters in these groups. At baseline, general bone metastases patients had different symptom clusters than those of radiotherapy and bisphosphonates patients. General bone metastases patients rarely had symptom clusters that included both psychosocial and pain symptoms concurrently while radiotherapy and bisphosphonates patients did. At follow-up, with the exception of bisphosphonates patients, all patients had similar symptom cluster composition with all psychosocial items separated from pain symptoms. Psychosocial items and symptom items of the QLQ-BM22 are more likely to coexist in symptom clusters of radiotherapy and bisphosphonates patients than those of general bone metastases patients. Moreover, treatment from baseline till follow-up seemed to influence most patients to reduce the association of painful symptoms with thoughts or worries about how their illnesses would affect their life; bisphosphonates patients did not experience this effect from treatment however.

Keywords: Symptom cluster, bone metastases, Principal Component Analysis (PCA), radiotherapy, bisphosphonates, QLQ-BM22, palliative care

Introduction

Bone metastases are common in advanced cancer patients (1). Patients with primary cancer of the prostate, breast, and lung are especially susceptible to bone metastases, with approximately 65-75% of prostate and breast cancer patients and 30-40% of lung cancer patients developing bone metastases (2,3). Due to the advanced nature of bone metastases, the disease is commonly associated with many complications. In addition, patients with bone metastases often experience multiple symptoms concurrently, which can act in concert to significantly affect the quality of life (QoL) of patients.

When two or more interrelated symptoms occur concurrently, the group of related symptoms is defined as a symptom cluster (4). Symptoms in the group must share more characteristics with each other than with symptoms outside of the cluster. Of course, it is important to differentiate between symptoms that actually induce the existence of one another and symptoms which merely occur simultaneously (5). It is the strong correlation of a related group of symptoms—not simply the most prevalent symptoms in patients—that is of interest. Moreover, it is also important to distinguish between symptom clusters and symptom burdens. While the latter measures the impact and severity of multiple symptoms on a patient, the former is concerned with identifying a group of symptoms that strongly influence the presence of one another.

Symptom cluster research is very useful in oncology settings. Examining the patterns of association and synergy between concurrent symptoms can lead to increased understanding of symptom management for health care professionals (6). As such, it will aid in the development of ideal treatments and interventions to manage multiple concurrent symptoms and aid in attempting to improve the quality of life (QoL) of patients suffering from many symptoms simultaneously.

In this study, we employed principal component analysis (PCA) to extract symptom clusters in data collected from patients with bone metastases using the European Organization for Research and Treatment of Cancer (EORTC) Bone Metastases Module (QLQ-BM22). The QLQ-BM22 is a 22-item bone metastases module used to supplement the 30-item QLQ-C30, a core questionnaire used to measure QoL in general cancer patients (7).

The primary objective of this study was to compare the symptom clusters of different patient cohorts at baseline. More specifically, this study examined whether symptom clusters change when patients are due to undergo radiotherapy as opposed to bisphosphonate treatment. The secondary objective was to examine whether symptom cluster composition in a particular patient cohort changed over time.

Methods

A total of 626 patients across 8 countries participated in this study. Over half of the patients were from Canada, with another 36 percent from Taiwan. Of the 626 patients, 180 of the patients underwent radiotherapy and 122 went through bisphosphonate treatments. As expected, the three most common primary cancer sites originated from the breast (34%), prostate (29%), and lung (12%) (Table 1).

QLQ-BM22 questionnaires were administered during routine clinical assessment at baseline and a month later at follow-up. The QLQ-BM22 is a 22 item module that specifically addresses the QoL of patients with bone metastases (7). The QLQ-BM22 four subscales address painful sites, pain characteristics, functional characteristics, and psychosocial aspects. The questionnaire is scored on a scale from 1 to 4, with 1 indicating "not at all", 2 indicating "at little", 3 indicating "quite a bit", and 4 indicating "very much" (Table 2).

Statistical analysis

To examine whether any interrelationships existed between symptoms, a principal component analysis with varimax rotation *(PCA)* was performed on the 22 items at baseline and at follow-up (Q21 and Q22 used inversed scores in order to keep the same direction as other items).

The PCA is an appropriate procedure that transforms a number of observed variables into a smaller number of variables (called principal components). The first principal component accounts for as much of the variability in the data as possible. The number of significant principal components was selected with an eigenvalue higher than 1.0 and each component explained more than 5% of the variance. The highest factor loading score predicted the assignment of individual symptoms to an independent factor. The internal consistency and reliability of the derived clusters was assessed with Cronbach's alpha. Robust relationship and correlation among symptoms were displayed with the biplot graphic.

Table 1. Patients at baseline (n = 626)

Patient characteristics (n = 626)

Age (years)		
n	625	
Mean ± SD	59.5 ± 12.8	
Median (range)	59 (26 – 95)	
Karnofsky Performance Status		
n	615	
Mean ± SD	80.6 ± 16.1	
Median (range)	80 (30 – 100)	
KPS > 80		
No	373	(60.65%)
Yes	242	(39.35%)
Sex		
Female	416	(66.45%)
Male	210	(33.55%)
Country		
Canada	315	(50.32%)
Taiwan	226	(36.10%)
Cyprus	47	(7.51%)
Brazil	12	(1.92%)
Egypt	11	(1.76%)
France	6	(0.96%)
Japan	5	(0.80%)
Hong Kong	4	(0.64%)
Language		
English	315	(50.32%)
Mandarin	230	(36.74%)
Greek	47	(7.51%)

Portuguese	12	(1.92%)
Arabic	11	(1.76%)
French	6	(0.96%)
Japanese	5	(0.80%)
Education		
High School	160	(40.82%)
University	118	(30.10%)
Elementary School	41	(10.46%)
Masters Or PhD	22	(5.61%)
Others	51	(13.01%)
Employment status		
Retired	207	(53.08%)
Employed	124	(31.79%)
Unemployed	58	(14.87%)
Cohabitant		
Spouse	187	(46.63%)
Spouse and child(ren)	86	(21.45%)
Alone	66	(16.46%)
Child(ren)	34	(8.48%)
Others	28	(6.98%)
Age (years)		
Married Status		
Married	263	(67.44%)
Single	38	(9.74%)
Widowed	37	(9.49%)
Partner	11	(2.82%)
Others	41	(10.51%)
Primary Cancer Site		
Breast	356	(56.87%)
Prostate	111	(17.73%)
Lung	67	(10.70%)
Renal Cell/Kidney	20	(3.19%)
Colorectal	16	(2.56%)
Multiple Myeloma	11	(1.76%)
Liver	5	(0.80%)
Oesophagus	4	(0.64%)
Ovarian	3	(0.48%)
Bladder	2	(0.32%)
Pancreas	2	(0.32%)
Stomach	2	(0.32%)
Others	25	(3.99%)
Unknown	2	(0.32%)
Out/In-patients status		
Outpatient	574	(91.84%)
Inpatient	51	(8.16%)

Table 1. (Continued)

Accrual location		
Medical Oncology Clinic	324	(51.76%)
Radiation Oncology Clinic	219	(34.98%)
Hospital Ward	13	(2.08%)
Others	70	(11.18%)
No. of Bone Metastases		
1	112	(19.21%)
2 to 3	147	(25.21%)
>3	324	(55.57%)
Previous SRT		
No	186	(46.38%)
Yes	215	(53.62%)
Previous Systemic Treatment		
No	90	(22.44%)
Yes	311	(77.56%)
Radiotherapy		
No	446	(71.25%)
Yes	180	(28.75%)
Bisphosphonates Treatment		
No	504	(80.51%)
Yes	122	(19.49%)
Spinal Cord Compression		
No	201	(92.20%)
Yes	17	(7.80%)
Pathological Fracture		
No	162	(74.31%)
Yes	56	(25.69%)
Hypercalcemia		
No	208	(95.41%)
Yes	10	(4.59%)
Orthopaedic Surgery		
No	180	(82.57%)
Yes	38	(17.43%)

The longer the length and the closer together the arrows were, the higher the correlation between symptoms. The PCA statistical approach was performed with varimax rotation on the 22 items of the QLQ-BM22 at baseline and at one-month follow-up. Results are separated into analysis of symptom clusters for all patients, for radiotherapy patients, and for bisphosphonate patients.

Table 2. QLQ-BM22 Questionnaire

	During the *past week* have you had *pain* in any of the following parts of your body?
1. Painful sites	1. in your back?
	2. in your leg(s) or hip(s)?
	3. in your arm(s) or shoulder(s)?
	4. in your chest or rib(s)?
	5. in your buttock(s)?
2. Pain characteristics	**During the *past week*:**
	6. Have you had constant pain?
	7. Have you had intermittent pain?
	During the *past week* have you had *pain* in any of the following parts of your body?
	8. Have you had pain not relieved by pain medications?
3. Functional interference	9. Have you had pain while sitting or lying down?
	10. Have you had pain when trying to stand up?
	11. Have you had pain while walking?
	12. Have you had pain with activities such as bending or climbing stairs?
	13. Have you had pain with strenuous activity (e.g., exercise, lifting)?
	14. Has pain interfered with your sleeping at night?
	15. Have you had to modify your daily activities because of your illness?
3. Functional interference	16. Have you felt isolated from those close to you (e.g., family, friends)?
	17. Have you been thinking about your illness?
	18. Have you worried about loss of mobility because of your illness?
	19. Have you worried about becoming dependent on others because of your illness?
	20. Have you worried about your health in the future?
	21. Have you felt hopeful your pain will get better?
	22. Have you felt positive about your health?

For QLQ-BM22, 1 indicates "not at all", 2 indicates "at little", 3 indicates "quite a bit", and 4 indicates "very much".

Results

A total of 626 patients participated in the QLQ-BM22 questionnaire for symptom cluster analysis. At baseline, there were four symptom clusters identified by the PCA, which extracted four clusters with eigenvalues greater than 1.0. Cluster 1 contained the items "Q2, Q5, Q6, Q8, Q10-Q14, and Q16"; Cluster 2 contained the items "Q1, Q3, Q4, Q7, Q9, Q15"; Cluster 3 included "Q17-Q20"; and Cluster 4 included "Q21-Q22". Table 2 lists the specific questions that the question numbers refer to in the QLQ-BM22. The first cluster accounts for 41% of total variance, the second accounts for 8%, the third accounts for 7%, and the fourth accounts for 6%. These 4 clusters account for 61.5% of the total variance, and each component explained more than 5% of the variance. As well, the final communality estimates ranged from 0.30 for Q17 to 0.84 for Q19, showing that all variables are well accounted for by the 4 components. Moreover, the internal reliabilities of the first and third clusters were 0.92 and 0.82, which have good internal consistency (Table 3). Figure 1 shows the biplot among the first 4 principal components.

Table 3. Factor loadings and final communality from the PCA of QLQ BM-22 items for all patients at baseline (score 1-4)

Item	Component 1	Component 2	Component 3	Component 4	Final communality
Q2	**0.76**	-0.03	0.17	-0.02	0.603
Q5	**0.62**	0.03	0.17	-0.09	0.418
Q6	**0.57**	0.56	0.15	-0.08	0.663
Q8	**0.49**	0.45	0.14	-0.08	0.468
Q10	**0.56**	0.56	0.18	-0.07	0.662
Q11	**0.73**	0.36	0.22	0.02	0.713
Q12	**0.83**	0.18	0.22	0.05	0.767
Q13	**0.76**	0.30	0.26	0.02	0.740
Q14	**0.71**	0.37	0.26	0.02	0.709
Q16	**0.51**	0.41	0.40	0.02	0.582
Q1	0.33	**0.57**	0.21	-0.02	0.482
Q3	-0.09	**0.62**	0.05	0.07	0.401
Q4	0.06	**0.67**	0.09	0.01	0.459
Q7	0.43	**0.45**	0.18	0.13	0.437
Q9	0.39	**0.70**	0.16	-0.05	0.672
Q15	0.41	**0.61**	0.21	0.04	0.588
Q17	0.32	0.08	**0.50**	-0.03	0.366
Q18	0.35	0.17	**0.80**	0.03	0.792
Q19	0.23	0.21	**0.86**	0.07	0.842
Q20	0.11	0.18	**0.82**	0.05	0.715
Q21	-0.05	0.03	0.04	**0.85**	0.727
Q22	0.01	-0.01	0.03	**0.85**	0.722
% of variance	41%	8%	7%	6%	
Cronbach's alpha	0.92	0.78	0.82	0.61	

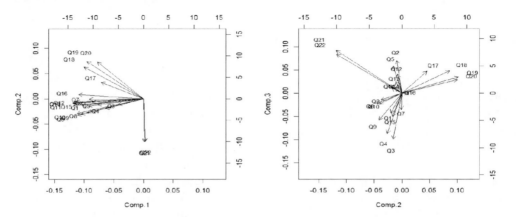

Figure 1. (Continued).

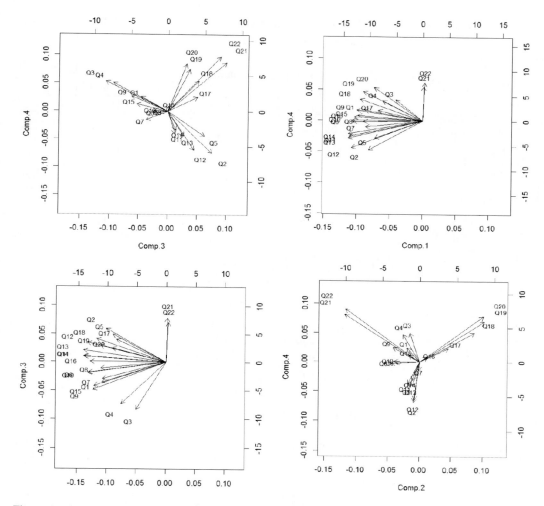

Figure 1. Biplot among four principal clusters *of all patient responses at baseline*, depicting the planes of a three-dimensional model. The arrows of longer length and closer proximity suggest a higher correlation between symptoms.

At follow-up

At follow-up, there were still four symptom clusters identified by PCA. However, the clusters had slightly different compositions. More items from the QLQ-BM22 were added to Cluster 1 and other items were moved to different clusters. The only cluster that still consisted of the same items at follow-up was Cluster 4, which still consisted of the items "Have you felt hopeful your pain will get better?" and "Have you felt positive about your health?" At follow-up, Cluster 1 contained the items "Q1, Q2, Q5, Q6, Q7, Q8, Q9-Q15," Cluster 2 contained the items "Q16-Q20," Cluster 3 included "Q3 and Q4," and Cluster 4 included "Q21-Q22." The four clusters account for 41%, 8%, 7%, and 6% of the total variance. These 4 clusters account for 61.7% of the total variance, and each component explained more than 5% of the variance (Table 4) (Figure 2). The first two clusters have good internal consistency compared to the last two clusters (Cronbach's alpha: 0.93, 0.83, 0.58, and 0.61).

Table 4. Factor loadings and final communality from the PCA of QLQ BM-22 items for all patients at follow-up (score 1-4)

Item	Component 1	Component 2	Component 3	Component 4	Final communality
Q1	**0.46**	0.22	0.44	0.07	0.456
Q2	**0.63**	0.09	0.22	-0.07	0.453
Q5	**0.58**	0.04	0.22	-0.08	0.545
Q6	**0.69**	0.14	0.28	0.06	0.581
Q7	**0.54**	0.30	0.33	0.01	0.395
Q8	**0.66**	0.16	0.10	0.01	0.580
Q9	**0.63**	0.12	0.40	0.04	0.489
Q10	**0.74**	0.20	0.17	0.01	0.474
Q11	**0.83**	0.19	0.08	0.12	0.574
Q12	**0.84**	0.21	-0.02	0.05	0.624
Q13	**0.80**	0.25	0.08	0.03	0.748
Q14	**0.76**	0.31	0.12	0.01	0.758
Q15	**0.59**	0.24	0.42	0.02	0.714
Q16	0.53	**0.54**	0.08	-0.04	0.683
Q17	0.31	**0.48**	-0.31	0.15	0.582
Q18	0.25	**0.86**	0.16	0.03	0.584
Q19	0.25	**0.82**	0.22	0.03	0.453
Q20	0.10	**0.81**	0.26	0.02	0.826
Q3	0.20	0.11	**0.69**	0.11	0.784
Q4	0.29	0.21	**0.67**	0.02	0.741
Q21	0.01	0.01	0.21	**0.84**	0.751
Q22	0.02	0.07	-0.07	**0.88**	0.784
% of variance	41%	8%	7%	6%	
Cronbach's alpha	0.93	0.83	0.58	0.61	

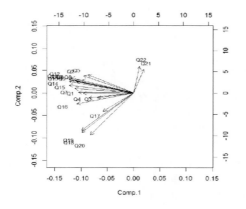 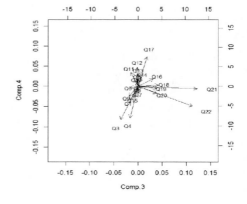

Figure 2. (Continued).

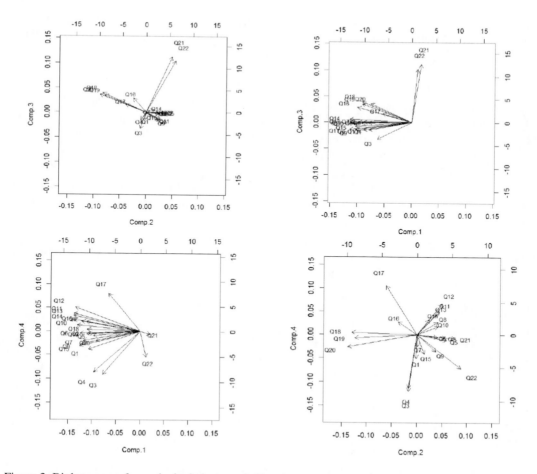

Figure 2. Biplot among four principal clusters of all patient responses at follow-up, depicting the planes of a three-dimensional model. The arrows of longer length and closer proximity suggest a higher correlation between symptoms.

Symptom clusters for patients with radiotherapy

At baseline

One hundred and seventy-seven radiotherapy patients participated in the QLQ-BM22 questionnaire for symptom cluster analysis. Similar to the symptom clusters derived from the responses from all patients who participated in the study, four symptom clusters were identified at baseline from the radiotherapy patient responses. The two sets of symptom clusters (all patient responses versus radiotherapy patient responses) consisted of a slightly different composition of items. Differences between the two sets of clusters can be attributed to the shuffling of certain items between the first three clusters. In the end, the symptom cluster composition for patients with radiotherapy consisted of Cluster 1 containing the items "Q1, Q4, Q6, Q8, Q9, Q10, and Q15-Q17", Cluster 2 containing the items "Q2, Q5, Q11-Q14", and Cluster 3 containing the items "Q3, Q7, Q18-Q20". Cluster 4 remained the same with the items "Q21 and Q22".

Leonard Chiu, Edward Chow, Nicholas Chiu et al.

The first cluster accounts for most of the total variance (42%). These 4 clusters account for 63.2% of the total variance, and each component explained more than 5% of the variance with good internal consistency (Table 5) (Figure 3).

At follow-up

The symptom clusters for patients with radiotherapy at follow-up had a different symptom cluster composition. At follow-up, Cluster 1 contained the items "Q2, Q5, Q7, Q8, Q10-Q15." Cluster 2 contained the items "Q4, Q16-Q20," Cluster 3 included "Q1, Q3, Q6, and Q9", and Cluster 4 included "Q21-Q22".

The first cluster accounts for 41% of total variance, the second accounts for 10%, the third accounts for 8%, and the fourth accounts for 5%. These 4 clusters account for 64.2% of the total variance, and each component explained more than 5% of the variance (Table 6) (Figure 4).

Table 5. Factor loadings and final communality from the PCA of QLQ BM-22 items for radiotherapy patients at baseline (score 1-4)

Item	Component 1	Component 2	Component 3	Component 4	Final communality
Q1	**0.64**	0.16	0.30	-0.07	0.535
Q4	**0.45**	0.05	0.41	-0.11	0.391
Q6	**0.72**	0.40	0.11	-0.25	0.746
Q8	**0.70**	0.32	0.06	0.03	0.604
Q9	**0.82**	0.17	0.19	-0.17	0.760
Q10	**0.76**	0.31	0.25	-0.22	0.788
Q15	**0.68**	0.33	0.18	0.05	0.605
Q16	**0.51**	0.43	0.38	0.06	0.590
Q17	**0.55**	-0.09	0.33	0.16	0.446
Q2	0.07	**0.82**	0.01	-0.05	0.680
Q5	0.17	**0.73**	0.11	-0.05	0.578
Q11	0.55	**0.56**	0.28	-0.03	0.699
Q12	0.29	**0.72**	0.32	-0.05	0.704
Q13	0.36	**0.69**	0.38	-0.04	0.755
Q14	0.43	**0.58**	0.40	0.02	0.688
Q3	0.22	-0.02	**0.33**	-0.08	0.165
Q7	0.36	0.18	**0.39**	0.15	0.332
Q18	0.14	0.48	**0.73**	0.01	0.781
Q19	0.23	0.27	**0.83**	0.03	0.815
Q20	0.18	0.22	**0.81**	-0.12	0.750
Q21	-0.07	-0.07	-0.16	**0.85**	0.765
Q22	-0.07	-0.02	0.08	**0.84**	0.722
% of variance	42%	8%	7%	6%	
Cronbach's alpha	0.88	0.90	0.74	0.67	

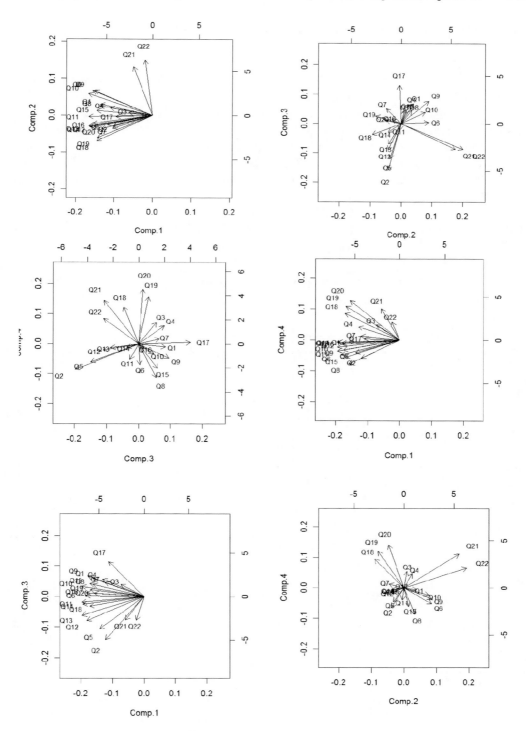

Figure 3. Biplot among four principal clusters of *radiotherapy patient responses at baseline*, depicting the planes of a three-dimensional model. The arrows of longer length and closer proximity suggest a higher correlation between symptoms.

Symptom clusters for patients with bisphosphonates

At baseline

One hundred and twenty-one bisphosphonates patients participated in the QLQ-BM22 questionnaire for symptom cluster analysis, indicating that symptom profiles of general cancer patients and those that have undergone bisphosphonates are generally similar. At baseline, there were four symptom clusters that were identical to the four symptom clusters created from the responses of all patients who participated in the study. Cluster 1 contained the items "Q4, Q7, Q16-Q20".Cluster 2 contained the items "Q1, Q3, Q6, Q8, Q9, Q10, Q15". Cluster 3 included the items "Q2, Q5, Q11-Q14", and Cluster 4 included items "Q21 and Q22".

Table 6. Factor loadings and final communality from the PCA of QLQ BM-22 items for radiotherapy patients at follow-up (score 1-4)

Item	Component 1	Component 2	Component 3	Component 4	Final communality
Q2	**0.76**	-0.14	0.20	-0.16	0.662
Q5	**0.72**	0.09	0.28	-0.20	0.639
Q7	**0.58**	0.43	-0.06	-0.09	0.534
Q8	**0.48**	0.30	0.32	-0.15	0.441
Q10	**0.64**	0.22	0.46	-0.10	0.684
Q11	**0.80**	0.19	0.35	0.09	0.809
Q12	**0.87**	0.14	0.19	0.02	0.815
Q13	**0.79**	0.23	0.26	0.08	0.750
Q14	**0.75**	0.25	0.18	-0.06	0.666
Q15	**0.61**	0.31	0.32	-0.02	0.571
Q4	0.14	**0.50**	0.49	-0.13	0.526
Q16	0.13	**0.60**	0.36	-0.09	0.508
Q17	-0.06	**0.53**	0.20	0.15	0.342
Q18	0.37	**0.79**	0.11	0.08	0.782
Q19	0.44	**0.73**	0.08	0.06	0.739
Q20	0.14	**0.83**	0.09	-0.13	0.737
Q1	0.35	0.26	**0.65**	0.14	0.634
Q3	0.24	0.11	**0.55**	0.10	0.376
Q6	0.26	0.10	**0.75**	-0.12	0.653
Q9	0.49	0.21	**0.56**	0.06	0.604
Q21	-0.06	-0.07	0.02	**0.90**	0.827
Q22	-0.08	0.06	0.01	**0.90**	0.826
% of variance	41%	10%	8%	5%	
Cronbach's alpha	0.93	0.81	0.74	0.65	

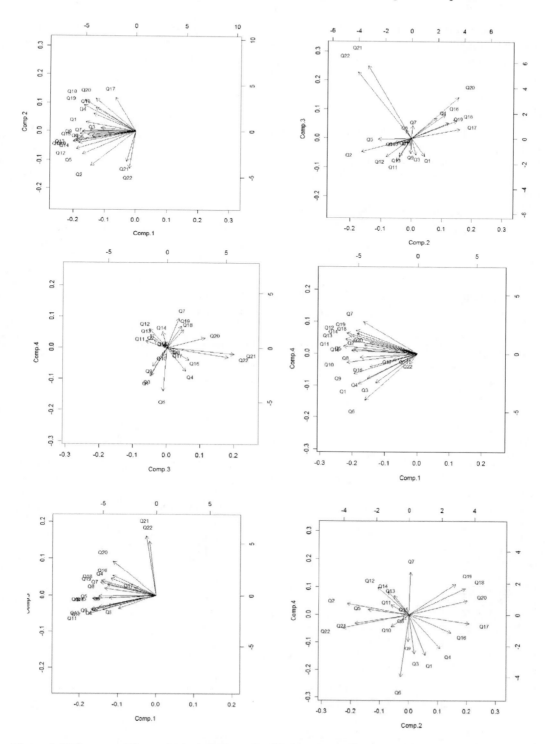

Figure 4. Biplot among four principal clusters of ***radiotherapy patient responses at follow-up***, depicting the planes of a three-dimensional model. The arrows of longer length and closer proximity suggest a higher correlation between symptoms.

The first cluster accounts for 39% of total variance, the second accounts for 9%, the third accounts for 7%, and the fourth accounts for 6%. These 4 clusters account for 61% of the total variance, and each component explained more than 5% of the variance (Table 7) (Figure 5).

At follow-up

Symptom clusters at follow-up for bisphosphonate patients were different than the clusters constructed at baseline. The symptom cluster for bisphosphonates patients at follow had Cluster 1 containing the items "Q1, Q2, Q3, Q5, Q7-Q15" Cluster 2 containing the items "Q4, Q16, Q18-Q20," Cluster 3 containing "Q6 and Q17", and Cluster 4 included "Q21-Q22".

The first cluster accounts for 37% of total variance, the second accounts for 10%, the third accounts for 9%, and the fourth accounts for 7%. These 4 clusters account for 63.4% of the total variance, and each component explained more than 5% of the variance (Table 8) (Figure 6).

Table 7. Factor loadings and final communality from the PCA of QLQ BM-22 items for bisphosphonates patients at baseline (score 1-4)

Item	Component 1	Component 2	Component 3	Component 4	Final communality
Q4	**0.42**	0.39	-0.34	0.1	0.455
Q7	**0.47**	0.14	0.13	0.13	0.276
Q16	**0.72**	0.35	0.06	0.24	0.699
Q17	**0.73**	0.03	0.14	0.13	0.569
Q18	**0.73**	0.28	0.27	0.11	0.704
Q19	**0.79**	0.24	0.27	0.05	0.748
Q20	**0.81**	0	0.09	-0.13	0.689
Q1	0.36	**0.48**	0.27	0.26	0.503
Q3	-0.11	**0.55**	-0.06	0.01	0.315
Q6	0.2	**0.65**	0.32	-0.28	0.641
Q8	0.33	**0.65**	0.18	-0.06	0.568
Q9	0.29	**0.73**	0.23	-0.03	0.674
Q10	0.48	**0.59**	0.19	-0.09	0.623
Q15	0.15	**0.69**	0.23	0.19	0.588
Q2	0.02	0.05	**0.78**	-0.04	0.617
Q5	0.09	0.27	**0.37**	0.32	0.324
Q11	0.49	0.3	**0.66**	0.04	0.764
Q12	0.49	0.22	**0.66**	0.01	0.732
Q13	0.53	0.33	**0.58**	0.18	0.759
Q14	0.45	0.32	**0.59**	0.16	0.680
Q21	-0.05	-0.06	0.1	**0.88**	0.786
Q22	0.35	-0.02	-0.05	**0.76**	0.696
% of variance	39%	9%	7%	6%	
Cronbach's alpha	0.84	0.86	0.89	0.65	

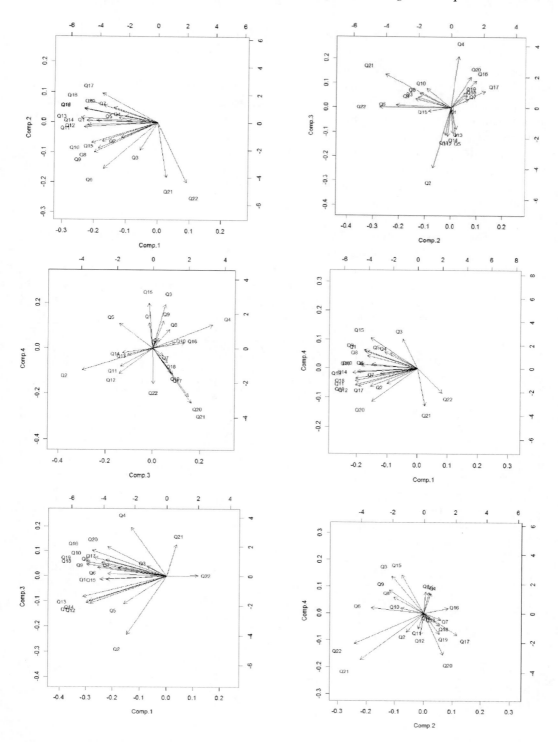

Figure 5. Biplot among four principal clusters of *bisphosphonates patient responses at baseline*, depicting the planes of a three-dimensional model. The arrows of longer length and closer proximity suggest a higher correlation between symptoms.

Discussion

When multiple symptoms occur simultaneously, the group of symptoms is termed a symptom cluster (4). Health care professionals use symptom cluster research to better understand the patterns of symptoms that arise in different types of patients. In gaining more knowledge on these symptoms, health care professionals can develop more appropriate treatments for patients and improve QoL (6).

In our study, we derived our symptom clusters from the QLQ-BM22, a questionnaire used to assess the QoL of patients suffering from bone metastases. Using the PCA Method, we found that at baseline the symptom clusters of general bone metastases patients differ slightly from those of radiotherapy patients and bisphosphonates patients.

Table 8. Factor loadings and final communality from the PCA of QLQ BM-22 items for bisphosphonates patients at follow-up (score 1-4)

Item	Component 1	Component 2	Component 3	Component 4	Final communality
Q1	**0.66**	0.25	0.19	-0.14	0.558
Q2	**0.71**	-0.11	-0.17	0.08	0.549
Q3	**0.29**	0.14	-0.21	-0.17	0.176
Q5	**0.57**	-0.18	0.28	0.08	0.440
Q7	**0.62**	0.30	0.18	0.06	0.512
Q8	**0.52**	0.25	0.32	-0.21	0.478
Q9	**0.61**	0.01	0.53	0.14	0.677
Q10	**0.62**	0.08	0.48	-0.10	0.629
Q11	**0.82**	0.34	-0.03	0.11	0.794
Q12	**0.80**	0.25	-0.03	0.18	0.730
Q13	**0.73**	0.50	-0.08	0.14	0.812
Q14	**0.81**	0.38	-0.08	-0.01	0.810
Q15	**0.46**	0.38	0.29	0.24	0.499
Q4	0.16	**0.69**	-0.21	-0.39	0.699
Q16	0.24	**0.64**	0.36	-0.07	0.607
Q18	0.36	**0.75**	0.22	0.34	0.849
Q19	0.32	**0.69**	0.20	0.32	0.729
Q20	0.08	**0.84**	0.12	-0.07	0.728
Q6	0.04	0.11	**0.74**	-0.04	0.557
Q17	-0.12	0.45	**0.66**	0.10	0.660
Q21	0.01	-0.11	-0.10	**0.85**	0.738
Q22	0.16	0.19	0.10	**0.81**	0.727
% of variance	37%	10%	9%	7%	
Cronbach's alpha	0.91	0.80	0.36	0.49	

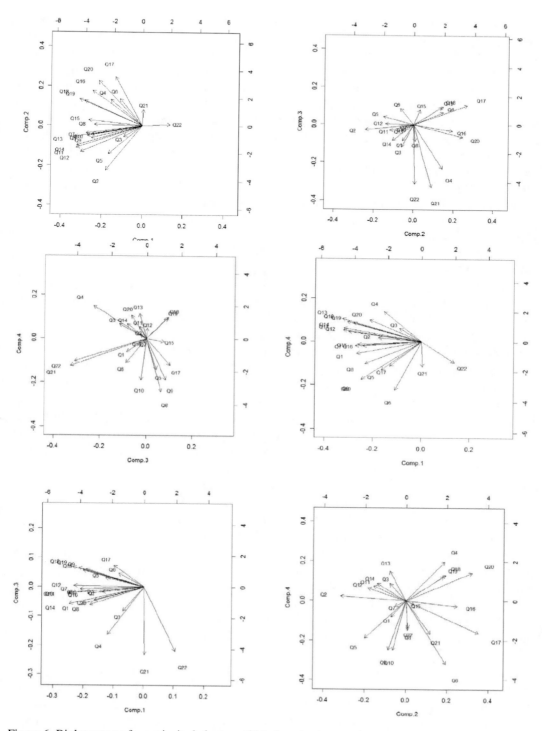

Figure 6. Biplot among four principal clusters of *bisphosphonates patient responses at follow-up*, depicting the planes of a three-dimensional model. The arrows of longer length and closer proximity suggest a higher correlation between symptoms.

The symptom clusters of general bone metastases rarely exhibited pain symptoms in the same symptom cluster as psychosocial items. Apart from the psychosocial item "Have you felt isolated from those close to you?",Cluster 1 and Cluster 2 were only comprised of items from the QLQ-BM22 that measured the severity, frequency, or location of the pain experienced by the patient. Cluster 3 and Cluster 4 on the other hand, were only comprised of items that addressed the psychosocial aspects of bone metastases, such as "Have you been thinking about your illness?" or "Have you felt positive about your health?"

In contrast, the symptom clusters of bisphosphonates and radiotherapy patients included a mixture of pain symptoms and psychosocial items. In the case of bisphosphonates patients, two questions from the QLQ-BM22 that addressed the pain aspects of bone metastases ("Have you had pain in your chest or rib(s)?" and "Have you had intermittent pain?") were included in a cluster made predominantly of psychosocial items.

In the case of radiotherapy patients, there was an even greater overlap of pain symptoms and psychosocial items. Questions from the QLQ-BM22 that addressed the pain aspects of bone metastases were included in the same cluster as questions that focused more on the psychosocial aspects of the disease, and vice versa.

For example, pain items such as "Have you had pain in your arm(s)?" were included in clusters that addressed psychosocial items like "Have you worried about your health in the future?" and psychosocial items such as "Have you felt isolated from those close to you?" were included in clusters made of questions addressing pain symptoms.

This overlap in psychosocial items and pain symptoms seems to indicate that radiotherapy patients who had answered highly (the QLQ-BM22 is scored on a 1-4 scale with 1 indicating "not at all", 2 indicating "at little", 3 indicating "quite a bit", and 4 indicating "very much") to "Have you had pain in your arm(s) and shoulder(s)", were also answering highly to questions like "Have you worried about your health in the future?" In addition to comparing the symptom cluster composition of general bone metastases, bisphosphonates and radiotherapy patients, the symptom clusters were also examined at follow-up to examine whether symptom cluster composition changed over time, particularly from baseline till the first follow-up session. The results of this study found that at follow-up, with the exception of bisphosphonates patients, all patients had similar symptom cluster composition, with most psychosocial items separated from pain symptoms. In the radiotherapy patient cluster at follow-up, only the pain item "Have you had pain in your chest or rib(s)?" was placed in a cluster among psychosocial items. Even the one psychosocial item that was previously present in a symptom cluster with only pain symptom ("Have you felt isolated from those close to you?") was placed in a new cluster with only psychosocial items. If radiotherapy at baseline had influenced patients to answer psychosocial items and pain symptoms of the QLQ-BM22 in the same way, treatment of any type—with the exception of bisphosphonates—influenced them to answer those two different aspects of the questionnaire differently.

Speculation on the implications behind these results should be done cautiously, as causation in symptom clusters is very different from correlation. The clear separation of psychosocial items and pain items in symptom clusters after radiotherapy treatment may or may not indicate a decrease in the severity or frequency of pains experienced by these patients. When interpreting these findings, limitations to this study should be taken into consideration. Firstly, the symptom clusters constructed in this study were created solely from using one accepted statistical method, the PCA. Indeed, there is no consensus on which symptom analysis technique is the most accurate in creating symptom clusters. Other symptom analysis techniques should be used to validate the results found in this study. Secondly, comparisons between all patients, radiotherapy patients, and bisphosphonates patients may be confounded because the radiotherapy patients and bisphosphonates patients used in this study were also included in the "all patients" cohort that was compared with the before mentioned cohorts. As such, if the symptom clusters of a certain cohort were very similar to that of the "all patients" cohort, this may actually be due to the fact that a large proportion of the all patients group of 626 patients consisted of bisphosphonates patients. A final limitation to this study is due to the heterogeneity in the patient cohort included in this study. Although all patients in this study had bone metastases, they experienced a wide array of primary cancers (Table 1). As such, the impact of the original cancer, as well as the stage of development of the primary cancer may have influenced the scores of the QLQ-BM22. Future studies should divide patients into cohorts with homogenous primary cancer sites and validate the findings from this study with more of the independent variables controlled.

Conclusion

Our findings indicated that at baseline, general bone metastases patients had different symptom clusters than those of radiotherapy patients and bisphosphonates patients. General bone metastases patients rarely had symptom clusters that included both psychosocial and pain symptoms concurrently, while bisphosphonates and especially radiotherapy patients did. Moreover, our study found that at follow-up, with the exception of bisphosphonates patients, all patients had similar symptom cluster composition, with all psychosocial items separated from pain symptoms. Finally, although there are limitations to this study—including results based on solely one symptom analysis technique, confounders from comparing a total patient cohort with its substituent, and the heterogeneity in site of the primary cancer in patients included in this study—it should be noted that this study is based on a large sample size of 626 patients spanning 8 countries, and has major implications. Future studies should aim to transcend the limitations presented in this study and confirm our findings.

Acknowledgments

We thank the generous support of the Bratty Family Fund, Michael and Karyn Goldstein Cancer Research Fund, Joseph and Silvana Melara Cancer Research Fund, and the Ofelia Cancer Research Fund.

References

[1]   Xiao C. The state of science in the study of cancer symptom clusters. Eur J Oncol Nurs 2010; 14(5): 417–34.

[2]   Kang Y, Siegel P, Shu W, Drobnjak M, Kakonen S, Cardon-Cardo C, Guise T, Massague J. A multigenic program mediating breast cancer metastasis to bone. Cancer Cell Press 2003; 3: 537-49.

[3]   Coleman RE. Skeletal complications of malignancy. Cancer 1997; 80(8 Suppl): 1588-94.

[4]   Kim, HJ, McGuire DB, Tulman L, Barsevick AM. Symptom clusters: Concept analysis and clinical implications for cancer nursing. Cancer Nurs 2005; 28: 270.

[5]   Chen E, Khan L, Zhang L, Nguyen J, Zeng L, et al. Symptom clusters in patients with brain metastases—a reanalysis comparing different statistical methods. J Radiat Oncol 2013; 2(1): 95-102.

[6]   Barsevick AM, Whitmer K, Nail LM, Beck SL, Dudley WN. Symptom cluster research: conceptual, design, measurement, and analysis issues. J Pain Symptom Manage 2006; 31(1): 85-95.

[7]   Chow E, Bottomley A. Understanding the EORTC QLQ-BM22, the module for patients with bone metastases. Expert Rev Pharmaecon Outcomes Res 2009; 9(5): 461-5.

In: Pain Management Yearbook 2013
Editor: Joav Merrick

ISBN: 978-1-63117-944-0
© 2014 Nova Science Publishers, Inc.

Chapter 39

Spinal cord compression as a first presentation of cancer: A case report

Nicholas Lao, Michael Poon, BSc(C), Marko Popovic, BHSc(C), Cheryl Yip and Edward Chow, MBBS*

Rapid Response Radiotherapy Program, Department of Radiation Oncology,
Odette Cancer Centre, Sunnybrook Health Sciences Centre, University of Toronto,
Toronto, Ontario, Canada

Abstract

Bone metastases occur in up to 90% of patients with advanced breast or prostate cancer. Spinal cord compression (SCC) is an oncologic emergency and is considered a complication of bone metastases. If SCC is left untreated, it can result in a loss of feeling, motor control, and eventually paralysis. In most cases, cancer will be first diagnosed in early stages. We present the case of a 71 year-old male who, upon initial presentation, had a spinal cord compression and associated lower extremity weakness and gait difficulty. At this time, he had no prior history of cancer or confirmed tissue diagnosis of cancer.

Keywords: Cancer, palliative radiotherapy, spinal cord compression

Introduction

In 2011, there were 240,890 new diagnoses of prostate cancer with 33,720 deaths from the disease in the United States (1). Men with well-differentiated prostate cancer have an

* Corresponding author: Professor Edward Chow MBBS, MSc, PhD, FRCPC Department of Radiation Oncology, Odette Cancer Centre, Sunnybrook Health Sciences Centre, 2075 Bayview Avenue, Toronto ON, Canada. E-mail: Edward.Chow@sunnybrook.ca.

excellent prognosis, often surviving 10-20 years without intervention (1). Prostate cancer often presents with localized symptoms such as bladder outlet obstruction, but terminal stages can be associated with bone pain and weight loss (1).

One of the most common sites of prostate cancer metastasis is the bone. Bone metastases can cause extreme pain and skeletal-related events (SRE) such as fracture and spinal cord compression (SCC) (2). Spinal cord compression is an unfortunate complication that results from extradural tumor growth along the spinal cord or vertebral collapse from tumour growth within the vertebrae (3). Metastatic epidural SCC occurs in 5-14% of cancer patients (4).

In the case of prostate cancer, men who are at risk are screened regularly using a prostate-specific antigen (PSA) test. If cancer is suspected, an ultrasound in addition to a biopsy may help confirm the diagnosis. The use of both of these tools increases the chance of detecting prostate cancer early. As a result of appropriate screening regimens, SCC is infrequently the first presentation of prostate cancer. However, even if not shown by a PSA test, patients may detect local symptoms of prostate cancer, including bladder outlet obstruction. In the rare case of an undetected cancer metastasizing to bone, bone pain is often the first symptom that triggers diagnosis of the underlying malignancy.

In this report we present the case of a 71 year-old male with spinal cord compression as his first presentation of cancer.

Case Report

A 71 year-old male was referred to the Rapid Response Radiotherapy Program (RRRP), Odette Cancer Centre at Sunnybrook Hospital. He presented on June 18, 2013 with lower extremity weakness and increased gait difficulty beginning roughly 24 hours prior to his visit. A MRI scan performed showed probable diffuse metastatic bone disease and cord compression at T3 (figures 1 and 2). However, the patient neither had a prior tissue diagnosis nor a prior history of cancer, which created a challenge in determining whether to radiate or not. However, given the impending risk of paralysis, an operative opinion was needed. As a result, the neurosurgeon was consulted and agreed to perform a surgical decompression of the spinal cord as well as retrieve a tissue diagnosis.

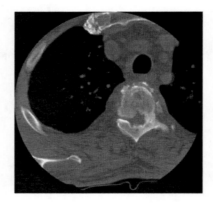

Figure 1. Axial MRI of the spine showing mildly compressive right lateral pedicle epidural soft tissue at T3.

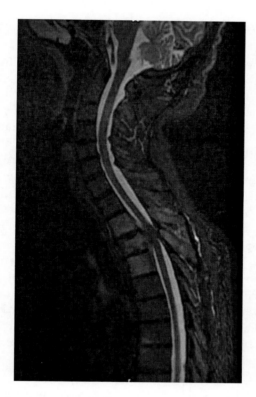

Figure 2. MRI of the spine showing metastatic disease present from T3-T5 and mildly compressive right lateral pedicle epidural soft tissue at T3.

The surgical decompression was performed the same day. The spinous processes were removed from T2, T3 and T4, and a laminectomy was performed at T3 and T4. Soft tissue specimens of the spinal cord compression were sent out for tissue analysis.

The surgical pathology returned indicating that the tissue was positive for cancerous malignancy from a likely prostatic origin. The patient returned to the RRRP on July 15 for post-operative radiation therapy and received 20 Gy in five fractions to the T1-T5 thoracic area for palliative consolidation. Subsequently, the patient started hormonal therapy for his prostate cancer.

Discussion

This case report was unique in that no symptoms of primary prostate cancer or bone metastases were experienced before the onset of SCC. In the case of prostate cancer, symptoms such as bladder outlet obstruction are common (1). When the cancer metastasizes to bone, bone pain is a common symptom that is usually treated using palliative radiotherapy.

In the literature, there are few articles discussing patients who present with SCC as their first indication of cancer. In patients with prostate cancer, only one article outlined an approximate incidence of SCC as the first presentation of cancer (5). Iacovou et al. reported that, of 37 men who underwent laminectomy for SCC, 11 (29%) were previously undiagnosed with cancer (5).

Patients with SCC often present with local or radicular pain, numbness and motor weakness in the lower extremities. Treatment of spinal cord compression in patients with prostate cancer has a relatively favourable clinical course compared to other types of tumours (3). Over 50% of patients see improvements in neurological symptoms with the median survival above 1 year (3). The keys to obtaining these results are rapid diagnosis and treatment.

Treatment options include laminectomy to decompress the spinal cord followed by post-operative radiation therapy. However, radiation therapy alone can be administered directly to the site of SCC. Patchell et al. performed a randomised trial exploring the effectiveness of each treatment regimen. Surgery followed by radiotherapy in selected patients was found to be significantly superior in survival time, continence, muscle strength, and functional ability. In some patients however, surgical decompression may not be an option. Patients with poor performance status may also not be suitable candidates for surgery. To provide tumour shrinkage and promote bone healing, multiple fraction treatment regimens may be given. Common schedules include 2000cGy in five fractions or 3000cGy in ten fractions. In a phase III randomized trial, Marazano et al. compared 16Gy in 2 weeks (short course) with 30Gy in 2 weeks (split course) radiotherapy regimens. They were both found to be effective and carry acceptable toxicity, however, it was concluded that the short course regimen would provide more convenience to patients and allow for greater machine-time for other patients because of the fewer fractions needed in patients with poor prognosis (6).

In the case of this 71 year-old gentleman, no tissue diagnosis had been performed previous to his initial presentation of SCC and he had no prior history of cancer. This created a challenge when deciding whether to proceed with radiotherapy. However, surgical decompression and tissue diagnosis were performed because of the impending risk of paralysis. Only later was it revealed that the patient did in fact have bone metastases from a prostate origin. In patients with SCC that have no confirmed malignancy, there is always the possibility of a benign tumour as a differential diagnosis. Performing radiotherapy to a benign tumour may increase the risk of malignancy at that site.

Conclusion

It is not common for a patient to experience SCC as their first presentation of cancer. More often, patients with cancer experience local symptoms at the primary site of cancer or bone pain at the site of bone metastases before symptoms of SCC are experienced. When treating SCC, two main treatment modalities exist: surgical decompression followed by post-operative radiotherapy, or radiotherapy alone in an attempt to shrink the lesion. In patients with SCC and who are good surgical candidates, the former is favoured. In patients with impending SCC, the latter is common. Patients with SCC and without tissue diagnosis benefit from the option of surgical decompression and tissue diagnosis to prevent the possible radiation of a benign tumour.

Acknowledgments

We thank the generous support of the Bratty Family Fund, Michael and Karyn Goldstein Cancer Research Fund, Joseph and Silvana Melara Cancer Research Fund, and the Ofelia Cancer Research Fund.

References

[1]   Albertsen PC. What is the risk posed by prostate cancer? J Natl Cancer Inst Monogr 2012; 2012(45): 169-74.

[2]   Sun L, Yu S. Efficacy and safety of denosumab versus zoledronic acid in patients with bone metastases. Am J Clin Oncol 2013; 36(4): 399-403.

[3]   Smith JA Jr, Soloway MS, Young MJ. Complications of advanced prostate cancer. Urology 1999; 54(6A Suppl): 8-14.

[4]   Patchell RA, Tibbs PA, Regine WF, et al. Direct decompressive surgical resection in the treatment of spinal cord compression caused by metastatic cancer: a randomised trial. Lancet 2005; 366(9486): 643-8.

[5]   Iacovou JW, Marks JC, Abrams PH et al. Cord compression and carcinoma of the prostate: is laminectomy justified? BJU Int 1985; 57(6): 733-6.

[6]   Maranzano E, Bellavita R, Rossi R et al. Short-course versus split-course radiotherapy in metastatic spinal cord compression: results of a phase III, randomized, multicenter trial. J Clin Oncol 2005; 23(15): 3358-64.

In: Pain Management Yearbook 2013
Editor: Joav Merrick

ISBN: 978-1-63117-944-0
© 2014 Nova Science Publishers, Inc.

Chapter 40

Particle disease versus bone metastases

Nicholas Lao, Michael Poon, BSc(C), Marko Popovic, BHSc(C), Cheryl Yip and Edward Chow, MBBS*

Rapid Response Radiotherapy Program, Department of Radiation Oncology,
Odette Cancer Centre, Sunnybrook Health Sciences Centre, University of Toronto,
Toronto, Ontario, Canada

Abstract

Following arthroplasty, complications resulting from wear of the prosthesis, namely particle disease, can arise. Due to the rarity of the disease, its similar appearance to a lytic lesion in diagnostic imaging, and similar clinic presentation to bone metastases, it can be misdiagnosed (1). We present the case of a 47 year-old woman who presented with what was believed to be a lytic lesion, but was later found to be consistent with particle disease.

Keywords: Particle disease, bone metastases

Introduction

Often when a patient's joint deteriorates due to necrosis or arthritis, if a conservative option is not suitable, an arthroplasty is performed. This procedure involves the surgical replacement of the affected joint with prosthesis. However, long term complications can arise from the procedure including particle disease. Particle disease usually occurs 5 years after initial

---
* Corresponding author: Professor Edward Chow MBBS, MSc, PhD, FRCPC Department of Radiation Oncology, Odette Cancer Centre, Sunnybrook Health Sciences Centre, 2075 Bayview Avenue, Toronto ON, Canada. E-mail: Edward.Chow@sunnybrook.ca.

surgical arthroplasty (2). It occurs as a result of abrasive wear of the prosthesis from normal gait. Foreign particles from the prosthesis, such as polyethylene or methylmethacrylate cement are shed and cause a granulomatous response which presents as osteolysis. Particle disease is generally asymptomatic until substantial bone loss. However, when particle disease becomes symptomatic, pain, shortening of limb, and reduced range of motion are common symptoms.

Particle disease can be mistaken for a lytic lesion resulting from metastases because of its rarity and similar appearance on x-ray imaging within the oncologic setting (1). In addition, both particle disease and lytic lesions from cancer can cause significant bone pain. In this report, we present the case of a 47 year-old woman who presented with what was believed to be a lytic lesion secondary to cancer, but was found to be consistent with particle disease.

Case Report

A 47 year-old female was referred to the Rapid Response Radiotherapy Program, Odette Cancer Centre at Sunnybrook Hospital. She presented on June 20, 2013 with increasing hip pain. In 1996, she suffered a trauma which resulted in a hip dislocation and a fracture of the acetabulum. She was treated with a reduction of the hip and an open reduction with internal fixation of the acetabular fracture. In 2002 the patient developed severe pain in her hip. She was diagnosed with avascular necrosis and underwent a total hip athroplasty in Sri Lanka.

Since her initial minor trauma, the patient stated that she did not have much pain. However, she did describe start-up pain after prolonged inactivity. She localized this to the lateral/posterolateral aspect of her hip/proximal femur. She denied significant changes in her weight recently. On examination, the patient walked with a normal gait. Trendelenburg sign was negative. Range of motion of her right hip was 0 to 120 degrees of flexion, 45 degrees of external, and 30 degrees of internal rotation. Leg lengths were equal. Neurovascular examination revealed normal sensation in the deep and superficial peroneal, tibial, sural, saphenous nerve distributions. She was able to flex and extend her ankle and toes and evert the foot normally on the right side. However, there was a global decrease in power on the left side. An x-ray of her hip and right femur was taken and showed what was believed to be a lytic lesion. An x-ray of bi-lateral femurs and hip was taken at Sunnybrook Hospital. The prosthetic showed wear of the polyethylene as well as two areas of osteolysis, consistent with small particle disease. In the pertrochanteric region there were two areas of osteolysis particularly involving the posterolateral cortex just distal to the greater trochanter that appear to be an uncemented implant. The implant itself appears to be ingrown with no signs of loosening, subsidence or mal-alignment (Figure 1). Therefore, the patient was referred to orthopaedic care. Following workup, the patient has been informed that she will require a revision of her total hip arthroplasty.

Discussion

Particle disease occurs as a result of abrasive wear of the prosthesis from normal gait. The resulting foreign polyethylene particles can cause a granulomatous response at the join, leading to osteolysis. This can cause pain, shortening of limbs, and decreased range of motion in patients.

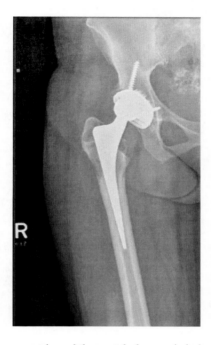

Figure 1. The femoral head is asymmetric and the acetabular cup is in keeping with extensive polyethylene wear. Focal osteolysis in the proximal femur in the greater and lesser trochanters as well as a large cortical osteolytic lesion in the posterolateral cortex measuring 5 cm in dimension. The appearance is in keeping with small particle disease and not tumor.

In this case of a 47 year-old woman, the particle disease was mistaken for a lytic lesion forming in the bone. She was subsequently referred to Radiation Oncology at Odette Cancer Centre. Because of the rarity and similar appearance to a lytic lesion, particle disease can be incorrectly diagnosed (1). Kuo et al. suggests the use of a 3-phase bone scan and 18F-Fluoride PET/CT to differentiate metastases and particle infection (2). However, in many cases such as this one, x-ray imaging can be sufficient in providing a proper diagnosis. Oncologists should take extra care when assessing patients with prosthesis and to explore the possible diagnosis of particle disease. Management of particle disease usually consists of surgical revision. In a case study by Taylor et al., biocompatible cement was used to fill the affected area followed by a tibial allograft to stabilize the area (3). Rehabilitation of the joint is an important step in post-operative management. Although, compared to primary replacements, revisions are usually rehabilitated more conservatively (3).

Conclusion

Particle disease can be mistaken for a lytic lesion because of its rarity, similar appearance on some imaging, and its similar symptoms to bone metastases. Employing the use of a 3-phase bone scan and 18F-Fluoride PET/CT can be an effective method to differentiate metastases and particle disease (2). Oncologists should take extra care when assessing patients with prosthesis and to explore the possible diagnosis of particle disease.

Acknowledgments

We thank the generous support of the Bratty Family Fund, Michael and Karyn Goldstein Cancer Research Fund, Joseph and Silvana Melara Cancer Research Fund, and the Ofelia Cancer Research Fund.

References

[1]   Parwani AV, Yang B, Clark DP, et al. Particle disease: Cytopathologic findings of an unusual case. Diagnostic Cytopathology 2004; 31(4): 259-62.
[2]   Kuo J, Foster C, Shelton D. Particle disease on flouride-18 (NaF) PET/CT imaging. J Radiol Case Rep 2011; 5(5): 24-30.
[3]   Taylor DW, Taylor JE, Raizman I et al. Total revision of the hip using allograft to correct particle disease induced osteolysis: A case study. McGill J Med 2009; 12(1): 21-4.

In: Pain Management Yearbook 2013
Editor: Joav Merrick

ISBN: 978-1-63117-944-0
© 2014 Nova Science Publishers, Inc.

Chapter 41

Radiotherapy for a cervix cancer Patient with Ehlers-Danlos syndrome: A case report

Leonard Chiu, Nicholas Chiu, Michael Poon, BSc(C),
Gillian Bedard, BSc(C), Marko Popovic, BHSc(C),
Erin Wong, BSc(C), Henry Lam, Edward Chow, MBBS
*and Elizabeth A Barnes**

Rapid Response Radiotherapy Program, Department of Radiation Oncology,
Odette Cancer Centre, Sunnybrook Health Sciences Centre, University of Toronto,
Toronto, Ontario, Canada

Abstract

Early stage cervix cancer can be treated successfully with radiotherapy or surgery, with advantages and disadvantages for each modality. Ehlers-Danlos syndrome Type IV is a rare connective tissue disorder associated with vascular tear due to mutation in the gene for type III procollagen. This care report outlines the management of a patient with stage IB2 cervical cancer and Ehlers-Danlos Type IV Syndrome.

Keywords: Ehlers-Danlos Syndrome, cervical cancer, radiation, chemotherapy, surgery

Introduction

---

* Corresponding author: Elizabeth A Barnes MD, FRCPC, Affiliate Scientist, Department of Radiation Oncology, Odette Cancer Centre, Sunnybrook Health Sciences Centre, 2075 Bayview Avenue, Toronto, ON Canada. E-mail: toni.barnes@sunnybrook.ca.

Ehlers-Danlos Syndrome is a group of congenital connective tissue disorders characterized by skin hypersensitivity, easy bruising, skin fragility and joint hypermobility (1). The internal manifestations of this disease are associated with significant morbidity and mortality (2). In particular, the type IV strain is characterized by possible vascular and major organ rupture (3) and has been found to result in premature death (4). Due to the nature of the disease, life-threatening complications can arise during surgery, and modification of anesthetic and surgical techniques is necessary (2).

Treatment options for stage IB cervix cancer are either radical hysterectomy and pelvic node dissection, or concurrent chemoradiotherapy with both external beam radiation and brachytherapy (5). For young patients with tumors ≤3 cm, we often recommend primary surgery in order to allow for ovarian preservation and to avoid the late morbidity associated with radiotherapy. Larger IB primary tumors are typically treated with definitive chemoradiotherapy. In this report, we present the case of a 36-year-old woman with Ehlers-Danlos Type IV Syndrome, who presented with a FIGO stage IB2 5 cm squamous cell carcinoma of the cervix. The competing morbidities of surgery versus radiotherapy were discussed at length in a multi-disciplinary tumor board. Consultation with rheumatology and vascular surgery was sought, and a literature review conducted. No case reports of radiotherapy for patients with cervix cancer and Ehlers-Danlos syndrome were found, and only two case reports regarding radiotherapy for any malignancy were found (6,7). Likewise, no reports in the literature were found on radical hysterectomy in patients with Ehlers-Danlos syndrome.

Case Report

A 36-year-old female presented with a 2-month history of post-coital bleeding. Previous annual PAP smears had been normal. A cervical biopsy showed an invasive squamous cell carcinoma. She was referred to our center and seen by gynecologic oncology and radiation oncology in a multidisciplinary gynecology cancer clinic. Pelvic examination showed an abnormally enlarged, hard 5 cm cervix cancer involving full thickness of the cervical stroma with no obvious parametrial invasion. Staging investigations included a pelvic MRI which reported a cervical mass that measured 4.4 cm x 3.5 cm x 3.5 cm in size, completely replacing the cervical stroma with early left parametrial invasion. A CT scan of the abdomen and pelvis confirmed no adenopathy and CXR was normal.

This patient had a known diagnosis of Ehlers-Danlos Type IV syndrome. Previous surgeries included one diaphragmatic hernia repair, four inguinal hernia repairs, as well as two cesarean sections. No complications had arisen from these procedures. She had seen rheumatology in the past, and was followed with annual ECG and blood work through her family physician. On exam, classic facial characteristics of Ehler-Danlos Syndrome were seen along with skin hyperelasticity.

The treatment recommendation for a stage IB2 5 cm cervical cancer at our center would be concurrent chemoradiotherapy, with an expected 5-year local control rate of 80-85%. However, radical hysterectomy with postoperative pelvic radiotherapy was also considered, as this would avoid the morbidity of brachytherapy, which would deliver a high dose of radiation to the rectum. After consultation with vascular surgery and rheumatology, it was believed that there could be considerable risk related to vascular injury during surgery. This could lead to spontaneous vessel rupture and aneurysm formation or dissection, which may not be clinically manifested until several years later. The potential late side effects of radiotherapy due to vessel injury were a concern, particularly as a result of the brachytherapy. A literature review was conducted for further information, however, only a few case reports on the use of radiotherapy for patients with Ehlers-Danlos syndrome were found (6,7). Given that both treatments would be equally efficacious in controlling the patient's disease, and balancing the risks of each treatment modality, it was believed that primary radiotherapy would be the less morbid procedure.

The patient received 45Gy in 25 fractions to the pelvis using a 4 field box technique followed by a 2 field parametrial boost of 5.4Gy in 3 fractions with a 4 cm midline shield. Five cycles of concurrent weekly cisplatin (40 mg/m^2) were given. The patient tolerated the weekly cisplatin chemotherapy well. Acute toxicity related to the radiotherapy included grade 2 gastrointestinal side effects, with loss of appetite, diarrhea, and 20 lb of weight (10% of her body weight). The patient also developed a brisk erythematous skin reaction over her buttocks. In addition, while positioning the patient on the procedure table during her first HDR brachytherapy procedure, a superficial perineal tear occurred that required suturing. Three fractions of HDR delivering 700 cGy at Point A were administered.

The patient was seen in follow-up 6 weeks after treatment and was subsequently seen every 3-4 months after that. She is now 24 months from treatment completion. She has had a complete local response to treatment with eradication of her cervical disease, and remains free from local and distant disease based on clinical examination and radiological investigations. Symptoms of hot flashes and sweats from the radiation-induced menopause were ameliorated with estrogen and progesterone. Depression occurred secondary to her ongoing gastrointestinal difficulty, and an SSRI was initiated. Grade 2 (Common Terminology Criteria Adverse Events 3.0 criteria) late gastrointestinal side effects from her radiotherapy treatment occurred with pain on defecation, fecal incontinence and urgency, diarrhea, and intermittent pelvic pain. Consultation was sought with gastroenterology. She was started on low dose loperamide which was effective in reducing her episodes of diarrhea.

Discussion

This care report outlines the management of a patient with stage IB2 cervical cancer and Ehlers-Danlos Type IV Syndrome. We found only two case reports on the use of radiotherapy in patients with Ehlers-Danlos syndrome in the literature. One describes a fatal outcome after radiotherapy to the brain with a rupture of the Circle of Willis (7). The authors of this report hypothesized that this may have been the result of incomplete repair of the arterial wall after radiotherapy. Another case report showed no increase in late toxicity after radiotherapy to the mediastinum in a patient with epitheliod hemangioendothelioma (6).

Definitive chemoradiotherapy for cervix cancer is associated with up to a 11% risk of grade 3/4 (Common Terminology Criteria Adverse Events 3.0 criteria) late gastrointestinal and genitourinary toxicity in patients with no known predisposing comorbidities (8). The use of radiotherapy in patients with other connective tissue disorders has been reported in the literature with conflicting results. It is thought there may be a moderate increase in acute and late toxicity seen in patients with systemic lupus erythematous, but the authors concluded that this should not prohibit the use of radiotherapy (9). In addition, a case report on the use of radiotherapy to the breast and axilla in a patient with mixed connective tissue disease reported marked early and late toxicity to skin and subcutaneous tissue toxicity (10). Another case report showed fatal pelvic necrosis after pelvic radiotherapy for cervix cancer (11). It is thought that patients with connective tissue diseases have an increased risk of fibrosis after radiotherapy due to abnormal vasculature. Furthermore, there is the distinct possibility of rectal bleeding and fistula formation (12).

As even mild agitation of the patient's skin during her first brachytherapy insertion resulted in skin tear, it is reasonable in hindsight to believe that surgical removal of the cancer may have resulted in excessive bleeding. Indeed, consultation with a vascular surgeon during the deliberation process confirmed this possibility. The surgeon recommended that the patient not be brought to the operating room if at all possible as tying off the uterine artery at its origin at the internal iliac artery may result in massive hemorrhage and the possibility of major morbidity and mortality.

This case demonstrates the constant dilemmas faced by physicians in deciding between various treatments. Specifically, it highlights the necessity of a multidisciplinary team to be involved in the diagnosis of difficult cases involving issues in various medical fields; in this case, for instance, the referral to a rheumatologist in assessing the severity of the Ehlers-Danlos Type IV Syndrome, as well as further deliberation with surgeons and radiation oncologists, were necessary in reaching a final decision for treatment.

Conclusion

This case report demonstrates that radical chemoradiotherapy was an effective treatment option for our patient with cervix cancer and Ehlers-Danlos Type IV Syndrome. She has had a complete response to treatment, with no evidence of local or distant disease. While she did experience grade 2 late gastrointestinal toxicity, which may have been a result of her connective tissue disorder, this is now improving with conservative measures. We believe that definitive radiotherapy was the appropriate treatment option, given the surgical risk of excessive hemorrhage. For such patients, referral to a rheumatologist and further consultation with surgeons and oncologists should aid in the deliberation process in choosing the appropriate treatment. Regular follow-ups after chemoradiotherapy treatment are necessary to manage the potential late toxicity of treatment.

References

[1]   Hamel BCJ. Ehlers-Danlos syndrome. Neth J Med 2004;62(5):140-2.
[2]   Wesley JR, Mahour H, Woolley MM. Multiple surgical problems in two patients with Ehlers-Danlos syndrome. Surgery 1980; 87(3): 319-24.
[3]   Penin M, Schwarze U, Superti-Furga A, Byers PH. Clinical and genetic features of Ehlers-Danlos syndrome type IV, the vascular type. N Engl J Med 2000; 342(10): 673-80.
[4]   Sykes EM. Colon perforation in Ehlers-Danlos syndrome report of two cases and review of the literature. Am J Surg 1984; 147: 410-3.

[5]   Landoni F, Maneo A, Colombo A, Placa F, Milani R, Perego P, Favini G, Ferri L, Mangioni C. Randomised study of radical surgery versus radiotherapy for stage Ib-IIa cervical cancer. Lancet 1997; 350(9077): 535-40.

[6]   Begbie SD, Bell DR, Nevell DF. Mediastinal epithelioid hemangioendothelioma in a patient with type IV Ehlers-Danlos syndrome: A case report and review of the literature. Am J Clin Oncol 1997; 20(4): 412-5.

[7]   Holodny AI, Deck M, Petito CK. Induction and subsequent rupture of aneurysms of the circle of Willis after radiation therapy in Ehlers-Danlos syndrome: A plausible hypothesis. Am J Neuroradiol 1996; 17(2): 226-32.

[8]   Forrest JL, Ackerman I, Barbera L, Barnes EA, Davidson M, Kiss A, Thomas G. Patient outcome study of concurrent chemoradiation, external beam radiotherapy, and high-dose rate brachytherapy in locally advanced carcinoma of the cervix. Int J Gynecol Cancer 2010; 20(6): 1074-8.

[9]   Pinn ME, Gold DG, Petersen IA, Osborn TG, Brown PD, Miller RC. Systemic lupus erythematosus, radiotherapy, and the risk of acute and chronic toxicity: The Mayo Clinic experience. Int J Radiat Oncol Biol Phys 2008; 71(2): 498-506.

[10]   Mayr NA, Riggs Jr. CE, Saag KG, Wen BC, Pennington EC, Hussey DH. Mixed connective tissue disease and radiation toxicity. Cancer 1997; 79(3): 612-8.

[11]   Olivotto A, Fairey, RN, Gillies JH, Stein H. Fatal outcome of pelvic radiotherapy for carcinoma of the cervix in a patient with systemic lupus erythematosis. Clin Radiol 1989; 40: 83-4.

[12]   McKusick VA. Heritable disorders of connective tissue. St. Louis: CV Mosby, 1972.

In: Pain Management Yearbook 2013
Editor: Joav Merrick

ISBN: 978-1-63117-944-0
© 2014 Nova Science Publishers, Inc.

Chapter 42

Pathological fracture from metastatic bone disease of an unknown primary cancer

Cheryl Yip, Marko Popovic, BHSc(C), Nicholas Lao,
Natalie Pulenzas, BSc(C) and Edward Chow, MBBS *

Rapid Response Radiotherapy Program, Department of Radiation Oncology,
Odette Cancer Centre, Sunnybrook Health Sciences Centre, University of Toronto,
Toronto, Ontario, Canada

Abstract

Cancer of unknown primary (CUP) is a common malignancy that accounts for approximately 3 to 5% of all cancer diagnosis. When patients suffer from pathological fractures secondary to bone metastases, specifically those with poor performance status, surgery is usually not indicated due to poor prognosis. Instead, pain management may become the primary concern. In this report, we present the case of a 65 year old male with widespread bone metastases from a CUP. The patient suffered from severe bone pain and pathological fractures in the right acetabulum as well his right humerus. Consequently, he was unable to walk and felt extremely weak. The patient originally was scheduled to receive palliative radiotherapy of 30 Gy in 10 fractions, but the dose was later reduced to 20 Gy in 5 fractions.

Keywords: Cancer of unknown primary, palliative radiotherapy, bone metastases

---

* Corresponding author: Professor Edward Chow MBBS, MSc, PhD, FRCPC Department of Radiation Oncology, Odette Cancer Centre, Sunnybrook Health Sciences Centre, 2075 Bayview Avenue, Toronto, ON Canada. Email: Edward.Chow@sunnybrook.ca.

Introduction

Cancer of unknown primary (CUP) accounts for approximately 3 to 5% of all cancer diagnosis (1). A patient is diagnosed with a CUP when it is histologically confirmed that a cancer has metastasized, but the primary site is unidentifiable (2). In order to manage the treatment of patients with CUP, these patients are often placed into specific risk categories, which help with predicting prognosis (3). Classification criteria include determining which organs are involved and how favourable the prognosis is (3). For example, patients categorized with the most differentiated and chemo-sensitive tumors carry a more favourable prognosis (3). On the other hand, a diagnosis of systemic bone disease is considered an unfavourable predictor (3). Hence, CUP patients with a diagnosis of widespread bone metastases would generally have a poor prognosis.

In this report, we present the case of a 65 year old man with rapidly progressing and widespread bone metastases from a CUP. As a result, the patient had sustained a fracture of the lesser trochanter in the left hip. This fracture worsened his performance status, caused him to experience severe pain and, consequently, he was unable to walk. Palliative radiotherapy was originally planned. However, on the day of radiation planning, the patient sustained a second pathological fracture of the right humerus. As the patient was too weak for surgery, the provision of pain relief as immediately as possible became the primary concern.

Case Report

A 65 year old male was referred to the Rapid Response Radiotherapy Program at the Odette Cancer Centre, Sunnybrook Health Sciences Centre on July 29, 2013. He was diagnosed with metastatic disease from a CUP. A CAT scan of the thorax, abdomen, and pelvis was performed on July 30 and revealed lesions in the rib, liver, right adrenal gland, and thoracic spine at T6. A lytic lesion found in the posterior of the right acetabulum was in keeping with bone metastases. A bone scan was also conducted, revealing a lytic bony reaction in the femur, which was also in keeping with bony metastatic disease. An X-ray of the pelvis showed destruction in both the right acetabulum and the left hip lesser trochanter (see figure 1). A biopsy of the skin showed invasive poorly-differentiated squamous cell carcinoma; pathology concluded it was high-grade adeno-squamous carcinoma, with an uncertain primary site. The patient had a low performance status and was unable to walk because of the severe pain in both hips.

On the same day the scans were performed, orthopaedics felt the patient was not a suitable candidate for surgery due to his weak condition; therefore, radiotherapy was recommended. As the cancer was widespread and rapidly progressing, the intention was to control pain in his bones as well as for potential prophylaxis of future fractures. Bilateral hips and upper femurs would be treated with 30 Gy in 10 fractions and lesions in the rib cage and the T-spine would receive 20 Gy in 5 fractions. After simulation and radiotherapy planning was completed on the same day, the patient went home and fractured his right humerus. The fracture was through a lytic lesion with a butterfly fragment displaced laterally by one quarter shaft width (Figure 2).

Due to the patient's weak condition, the orthopedic surgeon again did not recommend surgery. Palliative radiotherapy to the right humerus was added. The patient, who was admitted as an in-patient at a local hospital, travelled to the Odette Cancer Centre daily by ambulance for radiation treatment. Transportation of the patient became an issue because at least 10 scheduled trips to Sunnybrook Health Sciences Centre would have to be made to complete treatment. As such, treatment of both hips and upper femurs were modified to 20 Gy in 5 fractions instead of 30 Gy in 10 fractions in order to minimize the pain and suffering associated with trips by ambulance. As surgery was not an option, pain management and decrease in symptomatic suffering from palliative radiotherapy became the primary concern in the management of this patient. The patient tolerated the radiotherapy and received pain relief from the radiation.

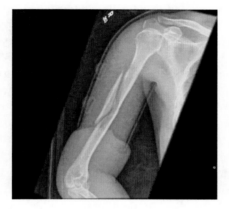

Figure 1. Pathologic fracture mid humeral shaft through a lytic lesion with a butterfly fragment displaced laterally by one quarter shaft width.

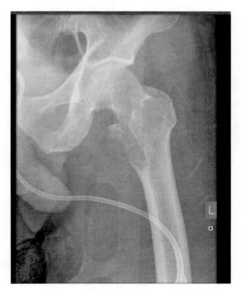

Figure 2. Destructive lytic lesion with a pathologic fracture through the lesser trochanter, along with destructive lytic lesion lateral right acetabulum with a small avulsion of the lateral acetabular margin.

Discussion

When deciding the best therapeutic method for a patient, a physician takes factors such as performance status, disease-specific variables, and survival estimates into account (4). It is important to be able to accurately predict survival and judge a patient's performance status, since an invasive treatment method like surgery would not be optimal for a patient in a fragile condition. The most common treatment options available for CUP patients include chemotherapy or radiotherapy, while combinative options, such as that of chemotherapy and radiotherapy, chemotherapy and surgery, radiotherapy and surgery, radiotherapy and endocrine therapy, or endocrine treatment alone are used to treat a smaller proportion of patients (3).

Given that the prognosis of CUP patients with widespread bone metastases and multiple sites of pathological fracture are poor (3), palliative radiotherapy is a recommended non-invasive option. In fact, most CUP patients carry a poor prognosis as only a minority (15-20%) of patients belong to a subgroup associated with a more favourable prognosis (3).

After the patient sustained the fracture to his right humerus, the dose of radiotherapy that the patient was to receive to the bilateral hips and upper femurs was changed from 30 Gy in ten fractions to 20 Gy in five fractions. The intent of radiotherapy for this patient was not only to control pain, but also for potential prophylaxis of further fractures in other sites. Radiation would allow for recalcification of the bones, which could prevent further fractures. In a study done by Koswig et al., it was found that there is a greater extent of recalcification in patients that are treated with multiple fractions of radiation versus only a single fraction (5). No such information exists between treatment of 30 Gy in 10 fractions and 20 Gy in 5 fractions. Nonetheless, this reduction in dose was done in order to allow for fewer radiotherapy-related trips on the ambulance, as well as for providing recalcification of the affected areas and an equal amount of pain relief.

Conclusion

In general, it is important to accurately predict the prognosis of CUP patients. The poor prognosis of CUP patients in certain risk categories makes surgery an unfavorable option, especially in the treatment of patients with poor performance status. Management of pathological fractures secondary to bone metastases patients through radiotherapy requires a balance in assessing what the treatment hopes to achieve, as well as the needs and conditions of the patient in question.

Acknowledgments

We thank the generous support of the Bratty Family Fund, Michael and Karyn Goldstein Cancer Research Fund, Joseph and Silvana Melara Cancer Research Fund, and the Ofelia Cancer Research Fund.

References

[1] Pavlidis N, Pentheroudakis G. Cancer of unknown primary site: 20 questions to be answered. Ann Oncol 2010; 21(7): 303-7.

[2] Pavlidis N, Briascoulis E, Hainsworth J et al. Diagnostic and therapeutic management of cancer of an unknown primary. Eyr J Cancer 2003; 39(14): 1990-2005.

[3] Stella GM, Senetta R, Cassenti A et al. Cancers of unknown primary origin: current prospectives and future therapeutic strategies. J Transl Med 2012; 10: 12.

[4] Forsberg JA, Sjoberg D, Chen QR et al. Treating metastatic disease: Which survival mode is best suited for the clinic? Clin Orthop Relat Res 2013; 471(3): 843-50.

[5] Koswig S, Budach V. Recalcification and pain relief following radiotherapy for bone metastases. A randomized trial of 2 different fractionation schedules (10 x 3 Gy vs 1 x 8 Gy). Strahlenther Onkol 1999; 175(10):500-8.

In: Pain Management Yearbook 2013
Editor: Joav Merrick

ISBN: 978-1-63117-944-0
© 2014 Nova Science Publishers, Inc.

Chapter 43

Palliative radiotherapy for brain and Bone metastases from a papillary Thyroid carcinoma

Cheryl Yip, Nicholas Lao, Marko Popovic, BHSc(C),
Natalie Pulenzas, BSc(C) and Edward Chow, MBBS *

Rapid Response Radiotherapy Program, Department of Radiation Oncology,
Odette Cancer Centre, Sunnybrook Health Sciences Centre, University of Toronto,
Toronto, Ontario, Canada

Abstract

Metastases from papillary thyroid cancers (PTC) are an uncommon occurrence. When metastases do occur, the most common sites are to the lung and bone; conversely, metastases to the brain from a thyroid primary are extremely rare. Complications can arise from bone metastases, including pathological fractures. Treatment of fractures consists of surgical intervention and/or radiation treatment. The decision of whether or not to operate on a patient is affected by the patient's condition and survival expectancy; for the latter, brain metastases are a known marker of poor prognosis. In this case report, we present the case of a 78 year-old male with PTC who was diagnosed with both brain and bone metastases and suffered from a pathological fracture to the right humerus. The patient was treated with radiation treatment of 20 Gy in five fractions to the whole brain and to the right humerus. Current treatment strategies for patients in this population are reviewed and discussed.

Keywords: Papillary thyroid carcinoma, bone metastases, brain metastases, palliative radiotherapy, pain management

* Corresponding author: Dr Edward Chow MBBS, MSc, PhD, FRCPC Department of Radiation Oncology, Odette Cancer Centre, Sunnybrook Health Sciences Centre, 2075 Bayview Avenue, Toronto, ON Canada. Email: Edward.Chow@sunnybrook.ca.

Introduction

Papillary thyroid carcinoma (PTC) is the most common thyroid malignancy and accounts for 65 to 80% cases of thyroid carcinomas (1). The clinical course of PTC is usually associated with little or no pain and generally a good prognosis (2). Distant haematogenous metastases from papillary thyroid carcinoma are relatively uncommon and usually involve the lung and bone in 1 to 7% of papillary thyroid carcinoma patients (1). Brain metastases from the thyroid are especially uncommon and, in reported series, occur in 0.1 to 5% of cases (2). A patient with a diagnosis of distant metastases has a significantly worse prognosis and these patients face a higher mortality rate (1).

PTC patients with bone metastases can experience complications, such as pathological fractures. When a fracture does occur, the physician's objective is to relieve pain in the area as well as to promote healing of the bone. In these cases, the question of whether or not to achieve these objectives with surgery or radiation alone is raised. An important factor used in this decision process is the expected survival rate of the patient. In the case of PTC patients, a diagnosis associated with metastases significantly worsens prognosis, which is unfavourable for undergoing surgery.

In this report, we present the case of a 78 year old male with papillary thyroid carcinoma and with accompanying brain, liver, and bone metastases. The patient suffered from headaches as well as a pathological fracture of the right humerus secondary to the bone metastasis. The patient was treated with palliative radiation treatment of 20 Gy in five fractions to the whole brain as well as 20 Gy in five fractions to the right humerus. The patient was reported to have tolerated the radiation treatment and felt relief from the pain.

Case report

A 78 year-old male was referred to the Rapid Response Radiation treatment Program (RRRP), Odette Cancer Centre at Sunnybrook Health Sciences Centre on July 10, 2013. He was referred for palliative radiation treatment of his brain metastases, as well as for pain in his right upper arm. The source of the pain was from a fracture of the metaphyseal region of his right humerus, just distal to his metastasis (Figure 1). The fracture occurred about 3 weeks before the referral and the patient was placed in a splint in which he experienced minimal pain. The patient had previously been diagnosed with papillary thyroid carcinoma with brain, liver, and bone metastases on June 26, 2013.

On the same day as the referral, the patient began whole brain radiation treatment of 20 Gy in five fractions. The purpose of the palliative treatment was to relieve the headaches the patient was experiencing. Potential side effects included fatigue, alopecia, raised intracranial pressure, nausea, and vomiting. The patient was to continue with dexamethasone in order to help reduce the swelling in the brain. The patient tolerated the treatment and received pain relief.

Planning for radiation treatment of the right humerus fracture was also considered but not immediately arranged because the fracture was found to be misaligned. The patient was to be assessed by an orthopaedic surgeon with the intent of scheduling a surgical fixation, after which the need for postoperative radiation treatment to the humerus would be assessed.

However, on July 15, the orthopaedic surgeon advised the patient to proceed with only radiation treatment to the right humerus without any surgical intervention to align the fracture. It was noted that surgical management would require preoperative embolization of the arm, which would put the patient at high risk for bleeding. Additionally, recovery from the surgery would not be indolent, since he was wheelchair dependent and his unsteadiness required almost 24-hour care. The patient consequently started the radiation treatment of 20 Gy in five fractions to the right humerus fracture on July 18.

Discussion

Metastases are uncommon when the primary cancer is located in the thyroid, and brain metastases are an especially rare occurrence. Metastases can create complications in prognosis, as these patients tend to have more aggressive carcinomas (3). Consequently, the treatment of patients with brain metastases from PTC is generally for palliative purposes and to control symptoms. In this case report, the patient presented with papillary thyroid carcinoma and brain, liver, and bone metastases.

There have not been enough cases of brain metastases from PTC reported in the literature for a consensus regarding the optimal therapeutic approach to have been reached (2). In a case series by Tahmasebi et al., patients with both brain metastasis and metastases were presented. It was found that common treatment options included resection, radiation treatment, and radioactive iodine (1).

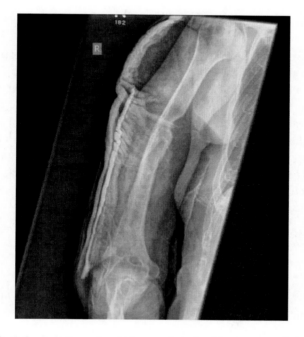

Figure 1. Spiral pathologicfracture through mid-humeral shaft with varus angulation measuring twelve degrees and posterior displacement by one shaft width. Lytic destructive lesion involving the medial humeral shaft immediately above the fracture that measures approximately 1 by 4 cm.

Upon the patient's completion of palliative radiation treatment for his brain metastases, the question of whether or not to surgically fixate his right humerus was raised. Two options were presented: surgical intervention followed by radiation treatment for pain control or palliative radiation treatment alone. Depending on the conditions of patients with fractures secondary to bone metastases, surgical intervention may not always be available as an option.

The decision of whether to operate is a vital step, as there should not be the risk of under- or over-treating patients with bone metastases (4). Often times, estimations of factors like survival rates, demographic and disease-specific variables, patient- or physician-derived performance status, and laboratory analysis are used to guide the decision of whether or not surgical treatment is appropriate. (4) For example, a revised scoring system developed by Tokuhashi et al. for pre-treatment evaluation of metastatic spinal tumor prognosis emphasizes the importance of predicting a patient's chances of survival before selecting a treatment method (5). Overtreatment of a patient could result in a difficult recovery period and decrease in quality of life of a fragile patient. On the other hand, under-treatment could result in a less invasive method being chosen and leading to potential complications in the future.

The patient presented in this case continued with radiation treatment of the fractured right humerus without first having the operation to align the fracture. Given that the patient had complications from liver, bone, and brain metastases, as well as his dependency on 24-hour care, surgical intervention was not an appropriate option. Therefore, along with the patient's age of 78 years old, the less invasive option, palliative radiation treatment to control the pain without surgical intervention, became the best option.

Conclusion

Brain metastases from papillary thyroid carcinoma are a rare diagnosis. This case demonstrates the potential difficulty of deciding a treatment option for a patient with a poor prognosis due to risk of complications. Further documentation of patients with brain metastases from the thyroid in case reports and reviews would help clarify and improve treatment options available to such patients. This could improve treatment options available to patients with metastases from PTC and could also aid in surgical decision-making. It is important to be able to make an accurate statement about a patient's diagnosis which can help determine their prognosis. This will allow pain and symptoms of metastases to be treated without risking the chance of either an overly-invasive treatment option for fragile patients or an under-effective treatment for stable patients.

Acknowledgments

We thank the generous support of the Bratty Family Fund, Michael and Karyn Goldstein Cancer Research Fund, Joseph and Silvana Melara Cancer Research Fund, and the Ofelia Cancer Research Fund.

References

[1] Tahmasebi FC, Farmer P, Powell SZ et al. Brain metastases from papillary thyroid carcinomas. Virchows Arch 2013; 462(4): 437-80.

[2] Aguiar PH, Agner C, Tavares FR et al. Unusuaul brain metastases from papillary thyroid carcinoma: case report. Neurosurgery 2001; 49(4): 1008-13.

[3] Chiu AC, Delpassand ES, Sherman SI. Prognosis and treatment of brain metastases in thyroid carcinoma. J Clin Endocrinol Metab 1997; 82(11): 3637-42.

[4] Forsberg JA, Sjoberg D, Chen QR et al. Treating metastatic disease: Which survival mode is best suited for the clinic? Clin Orthop Relat Res 2013; 471(3):843-50.

[5] Tokuhashi Y, Matsuzaki H, Oda H et al. A revised scoring system for preoperative evaluation of metastatic spine tumor prognosis. Spine 2005; 30(10):2186-91.

SECTION FIVE: ACKNOWLEDGMENTS

In: Pain Management Yearbook 2013
Editor: Joav Merrick

ISBN: 978-1-63117-944-0
© 2014 Nova Science Publishers, Inc.

Chapter 44

About the editor

Joav Merrick, MD, MMedSci, DMSc, is professor of pediatrics, child health and human development affiliated with Kentucky Children's Hospital, University of Kentucky, Lexington, Kentucky, United States and the Division of Pediatrics, Hadassah Hebrew University Medical Center, Mount Scopus Campus, Jerusalem, Israel, the medical director of the Division for Intellectaul and Developmental Disabilities, Ministry of Social Affairs and Social Services, Jerusalem, the founder and director of the National Institute of Child Health and Human Development. Numerous publications in the field of pediatrics, child health and human development, rehabilitation, intellectual disability, disability, health, welfare, abuse, advocacy, quality of life and prevention. Received the Peter Sabroe Child Award for outstanding work on behalf of Danish Children in 1985 and the International LEGO-Prize ("The Children's Nobel Prize") for an extraordinary contribution towards improvement in child welfare and well-being in 1987.

Contact

Office of the Medical Director,
Health Services,
Division for Intellectual and Developmental Disabilities,
Ministry of Social Affairs and Social Services,
POBox 1260, IL-91012 Jerusalem, Israel.
E-mail: jmerrick@zahav.net.il

In: Pain Management Yearbook 2013
Editor: Joav Merrick

ISBN: 978-1-63117-944-0
© 2014 Nova Science Publishers, Inc.

Chapter 45

About the National Institute of Child Health and Human Development in Israel

The National Institute of Child Health and Human Development (NICHD) in Israel was established in 1998 as a virtual institute under the auspicies of the Medical Director, Ministry of Social Affairs and Social Services in order to function as the research arm for the Office of the Medical Director. In 1998 the National Council for Child Health and Pediatrics, Ministry of Health and in 1999 the Director General and Deputy Director General of the Ministry of Health endorsed the establishment of the NICHD. In 2011 the NICHD became affiliated with the Division of Pediatrics, Hadassah Hebrew University Medical Center, Mt Scopus Campus in Jerusalem.

Mission

The mission of a National Institute for Child Health and Human Development in Israel is to provide an academic focal point for the scholarly interdisciplinary study of child life, health, public health, welfare, disability, rehabilitation, intellectual disability and related aspects of human development. This mission includes research, teaching, clinical work, information and public service activities in the field of child health and human development.

Service and academic activities

Over the years many activities became focused in the south of Israel due to collaboration with various professionals at the Faculty of Health Sciences (FOHS) at the Ben Gurion University of the Negev (BGU). Since 2000 an affiliation with the Zusman Child Development Center at the Pediatric Division of Soroka University Medical Center has resulted in collaboration around the establishment of the Down Syndrome Clinic at that center. In 2002 a full course on "Disability" was established at the Recanati School for Allied Professions in the Community, FOHS, BGU and in 2005 collaboration was started with the Primary Care Unit of the faculty and disability became part of the master of public health course on "Children and society". In the academic year 2005-2006 a one semester course on "Aging with disability" was started as part of the master of science program in gerontology in our collaboration with the Center for Multidisciplinary Research in Aging. In 2010 collaborations with the Division of Pediatrics, Hadassah Hebrew University Medical Center, Mt Scopus Campus, Jerusalem, Israel.

Research activities

The affiliated staff have over the years published work from projects and research activities in this national and international collaboration. In the year 2000 the International Journal of Adolescent Medicine and Health and in 2005 the International Journal on Disability and Human development of De Gruyter Publishing House (Berlin and New York), in the year 2003 the TSW-Child Health and Human Development and in 2006 the TSW-Holistic Health and Medicine of the Scientific World Journal (New York and Kirkkonummi, Finland), all peer-reviewed international journals were affiliated with the National Institute of Child Health and Human Development. From 2008 also the International Journal of Child Health and Human Development (Nova Science, New York), the International Journal of Child and Adolescent Health (Nova Science) and the Journal of Pain Management (Nova Science) affiliated and from 2009 the International Public Health Journal (Nova Science) and Journal of Alternative Medicine Research (Nova Science).

National collaborations

Nationally the NICHD works in collaboration with the Faculty of Health Sciences, Ben Gurion University of the Negev; Department of Physical Therapy, Sackler School of Medicine, Tel Aviv University; Autism Center, Assaf HaRofeh Medical Center; National Rett and PKU Centers at Chaim Sheba Medical Center, Tel HaShomer; Department of Physiotherapy, Haifa University; Department of Education, Bar Ilan University, Ramat Gan, Faculty of Social Sciences and Health Sciences; College of Judea and Samaria in Ariel and in 2011 affiliation with Center for Pediatric Chronic Diseases and Center for Down Syndrome, Department of Pediatrics, Hadassah Hebrew University Medical Center, Mount Scopus Campus, Jerusalem.

International collaborations

Internationally with the Department of Disability and Human Development, College of Applied Health Sciences, University of Illinois at Chicago; Strong Center for Developmental Disabilities, Golisano Children's Hospital at Strong, University of Rochester School of Medicine and Dentistry, New York; Centre on Intellectual Disabilities, University of Albany, New York; Centre for Chronic Disease Prevention and Control, Health Canada, Ottawa;

Chandler Medical Center and Children's Hospital, Kentucky Children's Hospital, Section of Adolescent Medicine, University of Kentucky, Lexington; Chronic Disease Prevention and Control Research Center, Baylor College of Medicine, Houston, Texas; Division of Neuroscience, Department of Psychiatry, Columbia University, New York; Institute for the Study of Disadvantage and Disability, Atlanta; Center for Autism and Related Disorders, Department Psychiatry, Children's Hospital Boston, Boston; Department of Paediatrics, Child Health and Adolescent Medicine, Children's Hospital at Westmead, Westmead, Australia; International Centre for the Study of Occupational and Mental Health, Düsseldorf, Germany; Centre for Advanced Studies in Nursing, Department of General Practice and Primary Care, University of Aberdeen, Aberdeen, United Kingdom; Quality of Life Research Center, Copenhagen, Denmark; Nordic School of Public Health, Gottenburg, Sweden; Scandinavian Institute of Quality of Working Life, Oslo, Norway; Centre for Quality of Life of the Hong Kong Institute of Asia-Pacific Studies and School of Social Work, Chinese University, Hong Kong.

Targets

Our focus is on research, international collaborations, clinical work, teaching and policy in health, disability and human development over the life span and to establish the NICHD as a permanent institute in Israel in order to conduct model research and together with other partners establish at least four university affiliated centers of excellence for people with intellectaul and developmental disability and also together with academic partners establish a national master and doctoral program in disability and human development at the institute to secure the next generation of professionals working in this often non-prestigious/low-status field of work.

Contact

Joav Merrick, MD, DMSc
Professor of Pediatrics, Child Health and Human Development
Medical Director, Health Services,
Division for Intellectual and Developmental Disabilities,
Ministry of Social Affairs and Social Services, POB 1260,
IL-91012 Jerusalem, Israel.
E-mail: jmerrick@inter.net.il

Index

B

C

D

E

F

G

J

K

L

M

Index

N

O

S

T

U

V

X

W

Y